Baillière's
CLINICAL
OBSTETRICS
AND
GYNAECOLOGY
INTERNATIONAL PRACTICE AND RESEARCH

Baillière's

CLINICAL OBSTETRICS AND GYNAECOLOGY

INTERNATIONAL PRACTICE AND RESEARCH

Volume 1/Number 4
December 1987

Renal Disease in Pregnancy

MARSHALL D. LINDHEIMER
JOHN M. DAVISON
Guest Editors

Baillière Tindall
London Philadelphia Toronto Sydney Tokyo

Baillière Tindall 24–28 Oval Road
W. B. Saunders London NW1 7DX, UK

West Washington Square
Philadelphia, PA 19105, USA

1 Goldthorne Avenue
Toronto, Ontario M8Z 5T9, Canada

Harcourt Brace Jovanovich Group (Australia) Pty Ltd
Post Office Box 300,
North Ryde, NSW 2113, Australia

Exclusive Agent in Japan:
Maruzen Co. Ltd. (Journals Division)
3–10 Nihonbashi 2-chome, Chuo-ku, Tokyo 103, Japan

ISSN 0950–3552

ISBN 0–7020–1224–6 (single copy)

Baillière's Clinical Obstetrics and Gynaecology is published four times each year by
Baillière Tindall. Annual subscription prices are:

TERRITORY	ANNUAL SUBSCRIPTION	SINGLE ISSUE
1. UK & Republic of Ireland	£35.00 post free	£15.00 post free
2. USA & Canada	US$68.00 post free	US$25.00 post free
3. All other countries	£45.00 post free	£18.50 post free

The editor of this publication is Seán Duggan, Baillière Tindall, 24–28 Oval Road,
London NW1 7DX, UK.

Baillière's Clinical Obstetrics and Gynaecology was published from 1974 to 1986 as
Clinics in Obstetrics and Gynaecology.

Printed in Great Britain at the Alden Press, Oxford

Contributors to this issue

JOHN C. ATHERTON BSc, PhD, Senior Lecturer, Department of Physiological Sciences, Stopford Building, University of Manchester, Manchester M13 9PT, UK.

WILLIAM M. BARRON MD, FACP, Assistant Professor, Departments of Medicine and Obstetrics and Gynecology, University of Chicago, Pritzker School of Medicine, 5841 S. Maryland Avenue, Chicago, IL 60637, USA.

CHRISTINE BAYLIS BSc, PhD, Associate Professor, Department of Physiology, West Virginia University, Morgantown WV 26505, USA.

MARK A. BROWN MB BS, FRACP, Staff Nephrologist St George Hospital, Belgrave Street, Kogarah, NSW 2217, Australia.

FREDRIC L. COE MD, FACP, Professor of Medicine and Physiology, University of Chicago, Chief Nephrology Program, University of Chicago, Box 28–5841 S Maryland, Chicago, IL 60637, USA.

F. GARY CUNNINGHAM MD, FACOG, Professor and Chairman, Department of Obstetrics and Gynecology, University of Texas Health Science Center, Dallas; Chief of Obstetrics and Gynecology, Parkland Memorial Hospital, Dallas, Texas 75235, USA.

JOHN M. DAVISON BSc, MD, MSc, FRCOG, Consultant Obstetrician and Gynaecologist, MRC Human Reproduction Group, Princess Mary Maternity Hospital, Great North Road, Newcastle upon Tyne NE2 3BD, UK.

WILLIAM DUNLOP PhD, MB ChB, FRCOG, FRCS Ed, Professor of Obstetrics and Gynaecology, University of Newcastle upon Tyne, Princess Mary Maternity Hospital, Great North Road, Newcastle upon Tyne NE2 3BD, UK.

DOMINIQUE FORGET MD, Research Fellow, Département de Néphrologie, Hôpital Necker, 161 Rue de Sèvres, 75743 Paris Cedex 15, France.

LILLIAN W. GABER MD, Formerly Research Fellow, Department of Pathology, University of Chicago, Chicago; presently Assistant Professor, Department of Pathology, Gailor Clinic, Tennessee, TN, USA.

E. D. M. GALLERY MD, FRACP, Staff Specialist in Renal Medicine, Royal North Shore Hospital, St Leonards, NSW 2065, Australia.

ROGER GREEN MB, ChB, MSc, Professor of Physiology, Department of Physiological Sciences, Stopford Building, University of Manchester, Manchester M13 9PT, UK.

JEAN-PIERRE GRUNFELD MD, Professor of Nephrology, Université René Descartes, Hôpital Necker, 161 Rue de Sèvres, 75743 Paris Cedex 15, France.

JOHN P. HAYSLETT MD, Professor of Medicine, Yale School of Medicine, 333 Cedar Street, New Haven, CT 04510, USA.

SUSAN HOU MD, Assistant Professor of Medicine; University of Chicago; Director, Renal Failure Program, Michael Reese Hospital, 2929 S Ellis Avenue, Chicago, IL 60616, USA.

PASCAL HOULLIER MD, Département de Néphrologie, Hôpital Necker, 161 Rue de Sèvres, 75743 Paris Cedex 15, France.

PAUL JUNGERS MD, Département de Néphrologie, Hôpital Necker, 161 Rue de Sèvres 75743 Paris Cedex 15, France.

ADRIAN I. KATZ MD, FACP, Professor of Medicine, University of Chicago Medical Center, Chicago, IL 60637, USA.

VICTORIA S. LIM MD, Associate Professor, Department of Medicine, University of Iowa Hospitals and Clinics, Iowa City, Iowa 52242, USA.

MARSHALL D. LINDHEIMER MD, FACP, Professor of Medicine and Obstetrics and Gynecology, University of Chicago; Director Medical High Risk Clinic, Chicago Lying-in Hospital, 5841 Maryland Avenue, Chicago, IL 60637, USA.

PATSY MAIKRANZ MD, Fellow, Nephrology Program, University of Chicago. Currently at Dallas Nephrology Associates, 3604 Live Oak, Dallas, TX 75204, USA.

JOAN H. PARKS MBA, Research Associate, (Assistant Professor) Nephrology Program, University of Chicago, 5841 S Maryland Avenue, Chicago IL 60637, USA.

NATHALIE PERTUISET MD, Ancien Chef de Clinique de Clinique-assistant, Service de Néphrologie du Professeur Crosnier, Hôpital Necker, 161 Rue de Sèvres, 75743 Paris Cedex 15, France.

E. ALBERT REECE MD, Associate Professor of Obstetrics and Gynaecology, Attending Perinatologist, Director of the Diabetes-in-Pregnancy Study Unit, Yale University School of Medicine; Department of Obstetrics and Gynecology, 333 Cedar Street, New Haven CT 06510, USA.

BENJAMIN SPARGO MD, Professor, Department of Pathology, University of Chicago, 5841 South Maryland, Hospital Box 327, University of Chicago Medical Center, Chicago IL 60637, USA.

Table of contents

RECENT ISSUES

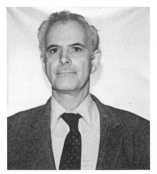 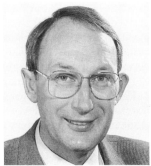

Foreword

'Children of women with renal disease used to be born dangerously – or not at all – not at all, if their doctors had their way, (Editorial: *Lancet* ii: 801, 1975).

This quotation summarized the opinions of many obstetricians and nephrologists during the early 1970s. The author of the Editorial concluded that the literature did not support such a drastic view, and in fact many closely supervised pregnancies would indeed succeed. To do this he (or she) had cited retrospective data much of which were incomplete and limited in scope. In essence, less than 15 years ago, the kidney in pregnancy was a grossly understudied area of reproductive physiology, pathology and medicine, and considerably more research was required if physicians were to be properly informed on how to counsel patients with renal disease wishing to conceive, or how to manage those already pregnant.

Fortunately, both the late 1970s and this decade have witnessed a great deal of progress due to work performed by investigators with a diversity of interests (e.g. physiologists, pathologists, clinicians). Animal models have been utilized to gain insight into questions such as why glomerular filtration (GFR) increases in normal pregnancy or the fate of single nephron dynamics in the kidneys of rodents with experimentally produced renal disease. Advances have been made concerning the kidney in volume and water homeostasis during both normal and abnormal pregnancies, and there are now several large and carefully conducted studies, in which morphological diagnoses from renal biopsies have been correlated with pregnancy outcome and the natural history of the specific disease. Similar studies have been performed in transplant populations. Finally, we have gained insight into the endocrine disturbances which accompany renal insufficiency and their effects on fertility; on how to manage gravidas undergoing dialytic therapy and to treat pregnancies complicated by acute renal failure.

The exciting progress alluded to above, forms the basis of this issue. Your editors, who reside in two different continents, have invited contributions from an international faculty, chosen because of their many contributions to the areas they review. The initial articles, devoted primarily to changes in renal function and volume homeostasis during normal pregnancy, include data derived from animal models, underscoring our belief that insight into the mechanisms of the striking humoral and functional alterations of normal gestation is a prerequisite to a complete understanding of the interactions between kidney disease and pregnancy. Such an approach will eventually lead to improvements in management too.

Renal disease and pregnancy constitutes the second part of this issue. Several articles are devoted to acute problems such as sudden renal failure, stone passage and urinary tract infections. There is an overview of the natural history and management to chronic renal disease in general, while specific chapters are devoted to diabetes (given the frequency of this disorder in gestational populations), and to reflux nephropathy. Since many texts and symposia have already been devoted to hypertension and pregnancy, pre-eclampsia is discussed only in the context of its characteristic renal lesion, and the recent claims that it can cause residual glomerular sclerosis in the kidney. The final chapters include general discussions on reproductive endocrinology in women with renal insufficiency, presenting guidelines for managing women who have conceived while undergoing dialytic therapy, or who are recipients of a kidney transplant.

Finally, we note that current knowledge, though far greater than the 1975 Editorial quoted above, is still incomplete with several controversies remaining unresolved. For instance there is still uncertainty on the effects of pregnancy in women with moderate renal insufficiency (creatinine levels between 1.4 and 3 mg dl^{-1}) at conception major disagreements remain concerning the effects of gestation on patients with a specific disease (e.g. IgA nephropathy, focal glomerular sclerosis, or reflux nephropathy). Another area requiring further study, includes the safety of protein restriction, considered of use in non-pregnant populations with renal dysfunction and/or nephrotic syndrome, on fetal development. Hopefully, the above and other problems will be resolved when future editions of this series are devoted to the kidney in pregnancy.

MARSHALL D. LINDHEIMER

JOHN M. DAVISON

1

Renal haemodynamics and tubular function in human pregnancy

WILLIAM DUNLOP
JOHN M. DAVISON

Understanding of abnormality must be based upon a realistic appreciation of normality. Without this, the significance of changes observed in disease may be overlooked. This is especially true of the interpretation of early studies of renal function during human pregnancy. Inappropriate control data were obtained from women haphazardly selected during the last few weeks of pregnancy or the first few days of the puerperium or even from men; results were indiscriminately 'corrected' to a standard body surface area and the numbers investigated during any single study were small. As a result, it was incorrectly assumed that renal function changed little during pregnancy and the significance of the changes detected by some workers in women with renal complications was considerably underestimated.

This chapter surveys current information about the substantial alterations that are now known to occur in renal haemodynamics and in renal tubular function during normal human pregnancy. Accurate information is difficult to acquire because of the limitations imposed upon research workers by the use of experimental subjects who are not only human but pregnant. Many of the techniques used have been indirect and experimental design has thus on occasions lacked the rigour that can be achieved using animal subjects. However there are important inter-species differences in the renal adaptation to pregnancy. Furthermore, there is no single acceptable animal model for many of the important renal complications of pregnancy, including pre-eclampsia. Such evidence as we have, despite its lack of precision, is therefore of considerable clinical importance.

MAJOR HAEMODYNAMIC CHANGES OF PREGNANCY

The substantial changes which occur in renal haemodynamics during human pregnancy are best appreciated in the context of the overwhelming physiological readjustment which occurs in general cardiovascular physiology. As early as the eighth week of pregnancy, cardiac output can be shown to have increased significantly, the result of a combination of increases in heart rate and stroke volume (Robson et al, 1987a); by the second trimester, increments of at least 30% in cardiac output can be demonstrated (Walters et al, 1966). Changes occurring during the third trimester are still in dispute. Early workers noted a decrease towards term (Hamilton, 1949) but this finding was subsequently alleged to be artefactual. It was noted that investigations had been performed predominantly in the supine position, which could be shown to be associated with a reduction in cardiac output (Vorys et al, 1961), attributable to reduction in venous return resulting from compression of the inferior vena cava by the large gravid uterus (Kerr et al, 1964). Serial studies performed in the left lateral position appeared to show that cardiac output remained elevated throughout the third trimester (Lees et al, 1967). However, not all subsequent studies have confirmed this finding and disagreement persists (Ueland et al, 1969; Atkins et al, 1981a, 1981b; Blake et al, 1983; Newman et al, 1983; McLennan et al, 1987; Rawles et al, 1987). While discrepant results of this sort may engender considerable interest in academic circles, it can be argued that the controversy is of little practical consequence. Whatever effect maternal position may have upon measurements made in the physiology laboratory, there seems little doubt that the normal ambulant pregnant woman experiences a decrease in cardiac output during the final weeks of pregnancy (Blake et al, 1982).

After childbirth, there is an immediate rise in cardiac output (Kjeldsen, 1979; Robson et al, 1987b) as the result of an increase in stroke volume and despite a concomitant decrease in heart rate (Robson et al, 1987c). Cardiac output remains elevated for at least 48 hours (Robson et al, 1987c) but thereafter decreases rapidly, reaching values near to non-pregnant levels within two weeks of delivery (Robson et al, 1987d). These findings are compatible with recent reports of increments in blood pressure in the early puerperium, in women who have previously been normotensive (Walters et al, 1986) as well as in those who have been hypertensive (Walters and Walters, 1987; Crawford et al, 1987). Interestingly, the early puerperal increment in cardiac output appears to be associated with an increase in left atrial dimension (Robson et al, 1987e) at a time when an increase has been reported in circulating atrial natriuretic peptide (Steegers et al, 1987) and when there appears to be an associated natriuresis (Rutherford et al, 1987).

The exact distribution of the increased output from the heart during pregnancy remains largely conjectural (Table 1). Although blood flow to the liver and brain has not been shown to alter significantly during pregnancy, there is evidence of substantial increases in other parts of the maternal circulation. The most marked changes occur in the uterine and mammary circulations, which together appear to take up almost half of the increased cardiac output at term. However, it seems that the blood flow to these organs increases progressively throughout pregnancy (Assali et al, 1960; Hytten, 1954). Increase in cardiac output during early pregnancy must therefore result in enhancement of blood flow elsewhere in the body. By the second trimester, part of this increment will be diverted through the dilated resistance vessels responsible for the decrease in systemic arterial pressure (MacGillivray et al, 1969); part is also diverted through the renal circulation.

Table 1. Cardiovascular alterations during human pregnancy.

Function	Units	Non-pregnant	12th week	28th week	40th week
Cardiac output	l min^{-1}	4.5	6.0	6.0	6.0
stroke volume	ml	64	71	71	71
heart rate	beats min^{-1}	70	85	85	85
Plasma volume	ml	2600	2700	3600	3800
Blood flow	ml min^{-1}				
uterus		< 50	50	200	500
kidneys		480	840	890	775
skin		450			800
liver		1500	1500	1500	1500
brain		750	750	750	750
breasts		< 100			250
Arterial pressure	mmHg				
systolic		115	115	115	115
diastolic		70	55	60	70
Total peripheral arterial resistance	dyn s cm^{-5}	1700	980	1010	1250
Venous pressure	cmH$_2$O				
right atrium		4.5	4.5	4.5	4.5
femoral vein		4.5	10.0	20.0	25.0

RENAL HAEMODYNAMIC CHANGES

Renal blood flow has not been measured directly in human subjects. An estimate of blood flow can be obtained by determining the renal clearance of a substance which is freely filtered at the glomerulus and is then so actively secreted by the renal tubules that it is almost entirely removed from the glomerular plasma during a single passage through the nephron. A suitable substance is *p*-amino hippurate (PAH), which has a renal extraction of 92% when plasma concentrations are low (Warren et al, 1944; Smith, 1951). Since the determination of renal extraction involves renal vein catheterization which cannot be performed routinely in human subjects, PAH clearance is conventionally said to represent 'effective renal plasma flow' (ERPF).

In 1950, at the International Physiological Congress in Copenhagen, Bucht presented data, later published in full (Bucht, 1951), suggesting for the first time that substantial increases in renal blood flow could be demonstrated during human pregnancy. He also confirmed that assumptions about PAH extraction were likely to be valid during human pregnancy by performing renal vein catheterization during the first trimester in two women, an exploit that has not since been repeated. His major conclusion was rapidly endorsed by several other groups of workers (Lanz and Hochuli, 1955; Brandstetter and Schüller, 1956; Buttermann, 1958; Gylling, 1961), all of whom performed single investigations in women at different gestations. The magnitude of the increases and the pattern of change demonstrated during pregnancy differed considerably from study to study, in part as the result of substantial intersubject variability. It was clear that serial studies, whereby each woman

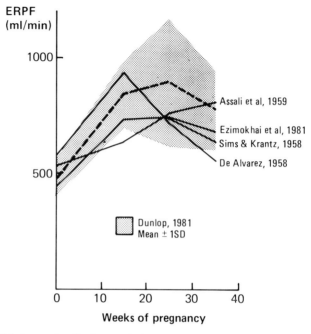

Figure 1. Serial changes in effective renal plasma flow (ERPF). Changes reported by several workers, superimposed upon the mean (dashed line) ± one standard deviation (shaded area). From the study of Dunlop (1981).

could act as her own control, were necessary to overcome this problem. Within a very short space of time, the results of several such studies were reported (Sohar et al, 1956; Sims and Krantz, 1956; 1958; De Alvarez, 1958; Dignam et al, 1958; Assali et al, 1959). Unfortunately, there were numerous discrepancies in study design (Chesley, 1960) and a uniform pattern of change was not apparent from these investigations. More recent analysis of the problem (Dunlop, 1982a) suggests that the results of these studies have been widely misinterpreted. It now appears probable that ERPF increases by some 80% between conception and the second trimester of pregnancy and then decreases significantly during the third trimester to a value which is still some 60% greater than the non-pregnant norm (Dunlop, 1981). Such a pattern of change is compatible with those of previous workers when allowance is made for inappropriate corrections to a standard body surface area (Chesley and Williams, 1945; Davison and Dunlop, 1980) (Figure 1).

It had been suggested that the decrease in renal blood flow during the third trimester reported by previous workers might have been a postural artefact similar to that reported for cardiac output (Vorys et al, 1961) and 'corrections' for this alleged discrepancy were frequently made in reviews of the subject (Pippig, 1969; Hytten and Leitch, 1971; Lindheimer and Katz, 1975). It was known that when women in the third trimester of normal pregnancy were investigated lying alternately on their backs and on their sides, the supine position was associated with decreased excretion of water (Walker et al, 1934) and of Na$^+$ (Hendricks and Barnes, 1955; Pritchard et al, 1955; Klopper, 1964). However, a similar effect of posture upon ERPF (Buttermann, 1958) could not be confirmed by all workers (Hendricks and Barnes, 1955; Pritchard et al, 1955; Sims and Krantz, 1958). In view of the confusion, a formal study of the problem was undertaken by Chesley and Sloan (1964). They demonstrated that the supine position was associated with decreases in urinary output and Na$^+$ excretion of about 60% together with reductions of ERPF and glomerular filtration rate (GFR) of about 20%. Almost half of the women initially recruited for study were eliminated from the final analysis, the majority for technical reasons, and there was evidence among these subjects of increases in clearance values and flow rates with time (similar to those reported by Hendricks and Barnes (1955)), perhaps suggesting a physiological readjustment to overcome the effect of posture. The authors stated that they had 'insufficient grounds for a strong argument' and their conclusions were not corroborated by a later larger study (Dunlop, 1976). However, this study also was bedevilled by technical problems resulting from inadequate equilibration during the initial clearance period. Furthermore the very substantial inter-subject variability could have prevented the detection of small postural differences in haemodynamics. A further serial study was therefore undertaken in which 17 women were investigated in the lateral position alone on two occasions eight weeks apart during the third trimester of pregnancy (Ezimokhai et al, 1981). ERPF decreased in 15 (Figure 2). There were also substantial changes in the renal handling of sodium and water under these circumstances (Dunlop, 1982b), suggesting that a more profound alteration in renal physiology might be occurring independently of posture.

It is of interest to compare these postulated changes in renal blood flow with other haemodynamic events occurring during pregnancy. The modified version of Poiseuille's equation conventionally used to describe flow in biological systems is as follows:

$$F = (P_A - P_B) \times \pi/8 \times 1/\eta \times r^4/L$$

where F = flow
$(P_A - P_B)$ = pressure difference between ends of vessel
η = viscosity of fluid
r = radius of vessel
L = length of vessel

This equation implies that, under otherwise constant physiological conditions, flow will be influenced greatly by relatively small changes in vessel radius. Now, under these circumstances, the radius of a blood vessel is inversely related to the intravascular hydrostatic pressure. Thus it will be apparent that there may be an inverse relationship between flow and pressure of the blood in a given system. It is therefore interesting to note that the pattern of change of arterial blood pressure during normal pregnancy (Schwarz, 1964; MacGillivray et al, 1969; Walters and Lim, 1975) forms virtually a mirror image of the pattern of change of ERPF described above. While it would be unwise to speculate from such data as are available about

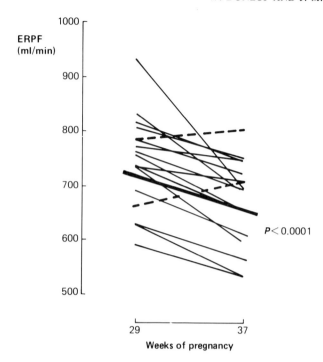

Figure 2. Serial changes in effective renal plasma flow (ERPF) during the third trimesters of the normal pregnancies of 17 healthy women investigated in the left lateral position. Only two subjects did not follow a downward trend.

complex intrarenal circulatory adjustments, it does seem possible that, at least in early pregnancy, peripheral vasodilatation may be responsible simultaneously for increases in renal blood flow and decreases in systemic blood pressure.

Intraglomerular changes during pregnancy

Inulin, a metabolically inert mixture of fructose polymers with a mean molecular weight of 5200 Da, is freely filtered at the glomerulus and is thereafter neither reabsorbed nor secreted by the renal tubules. The renal clearance of inulin therefore provides an index of the glomerular filtration rate (GFR) and the substance has been used for this purpose for more than fifty years (Shannon and Smith, 1935). The first studies of inulin clearance in pregnancy (Dill et al, 1942; Welsh et al, 1942; Kariher and George, 1943) compared results obtained from women investigated during late pregnancy with those obtained during the early puerperium. Little difference was found. Once again, it was not until women were investigated at earlier gestations that evidence of a substantial increase in GFR was obtained (Bosnes and Lange, 1950). It is now generally accepted that inulin clearance increases by about

Table 2. Diurnal variation in creatinine clearance during pregnancy.

Subject	Creatinine clearance (ml min^{-1})				CV* (%)
	08.00–12.00	12.00–16.00	16.00–20.00	20.00–08.00	
1	109	157	155	88	26.9
2	154	229	99	43	60.5
3	66	144	142	104	32.4
4	95	100	68	122	23.1
5	77	108	106	104	14.8
6	240	142	187	184	21.3
7	175	171	54	166	41.3
8	159	131	129	121	12.3
9	121	97	139	58	33.8
CV (%)	41.3	29.1	35.3	41.4	

* CV = coefficient of variation.

50% during pregnancy, probably from the first trimester (Sims and Krantz, 1958; Buttermann, 1958; Gylling, 1961), and is maintained at this augmented level at least until the 36th week of pregnancy (Davison and Hytten, 1974; Dunlop, 1981; Ezimokhai et al, 1981).

Since GFR increases less than ERPF during early pregnancy, the ratio of GRF to ERPF, known as the filtration fraction, falls. Late pregnancy is associated with an increase in filtration fraction to values similar to the non-pregnant norm (Dunlop, 1981). This pattern of change, although previously unsuspected, can be detected in the reports of previous workers (Davison and Dunlop, 1980; Dunlop, 1982a). Thus it seems possible that the mechanism controlling glomerular filtration may be altered to some extent during normal human pregnancy.

The factors that govern glomerular filtration have been extensively investigated by Brenner and his colleagues (Brenner et al, 1971). Their studies involved micropuncture of superficial nephrons in anaesthetized non-pregnant Munich–Wistar rats. Considerable caution must be observed in translating their conclusions to the very different circumstances of the normal pregnant woman. Nevertheless it is interesting to consider the implications of their findings in this context. A mathematical model of glomerular ultrafiltration has been devised (Deen et al, 1972) and tested under varying physiological circumstances. Among the factors regulating the rate of glomerular filtration are plasma flow (Brenner et al, 1972), hydrostatic and oncotic pressure differences between fluids in the glomerular capillary and in Bowman's space and the permeability of the capillary wall (Brenner et al, 1976). Under physiological circumstances in the rat, a point is reached within the glomerulus at which the opposing forces of hydrostatic and oncotic pressures are equalized and net filtration ceases (Brenner et al, 1971). This is the concept of filtration pressure equilibrium. When renal plasma flow (RPF) is increased experimentally, this equilibrium is progressively delayed and GFR increases in parallel with RPF, filtration fraction remaining constant.

Ultimately, at very high rates of RPF, filtration pressure equilibrium can no longer be achieved within a glomerulus of finite dimensions. GFR is no longer elevated to the same extent as RPF and filtration fraction decreases (Robertson et al, 1972). Furthermore, alterations in oncotic pressure influence this process. At a constant rate of RPF, a sufficient decrease in plasma oncotic pressure will prevent the attainment of filtration pressure equilibrium (Deen et al, 1973). Under these circumstances of disequilibrium, the net ultrafiltration pressure (balance of hydrostatic and oncotic forces) almost exclusively mediates flow-induced changes in GFR.

Micropuncture studies in pregnant Munich–Wistar rats have produced interesting data (see Chapter 2). In 6-day pregnant animals, no alteration of renal haemodynamics was detected (Baylis, 1980a) but approximately equal increments in GFR and RPF were present at days 9 (Baylis, 1982) and 12 (Baylis, 1980b) of pregnancy, which normally lasts for 22 days in all. It should be noted that at these early gestations there were no differences in hydrostatic and oncotic pressures. Baylis therefore attributed these renal haemodynamic changes in part to plasma volume expansion. It is important to be cautious about extrapolating from conclusions derived from work in this animal model to the human, however interesting the results. Not only do pregnant women show significant alterations in hydrostatic and oncotic pressures during early pregnancy (Robertson and Cheyne, 1972) but the maximum increase in plasma volume does not occur until the third trimester of pregnancy (Hytten and Paintin, 1963), by which time, it appears, human renal blood flow is already waning. Alterations in glomerular function under these circumstances must remain highly speculative.

Creatinine clearance

Rehberg (1926) was the first to suggest that the renal handling of creatinine could be used to estimate GFR. He acknowledged, however that his work was based upon the assumption that no tubular secretion of creatinine occurred. The validity of this assumption was soon questioned. Studies on various vertebrate species (Marshall and Grafflin, 1932; Clarke and Smith, 1932; Shannon et al, 1932; Shannon, 1934) and in humans (Joliffe and Chasis, 1933; Shannon, 1935) suggested that under certain circumstances tubular secretion of creatinine could make a significant contribution to clearance results. It seems probable that, for human subjects at least, this tubular contribution was overestimated by these early workers (Brod and Sirota, 1948) so that creatinine clearance still has a place in clinical practice today. Nevertheless it must be remembered that under conditions of substantial nephron loss the technique may result in considerable inaccuracy in the estimation of GFR (Shemesh et al, 1985).

Endogenous 24-hour creatinine clearance is a convenient, non-invasive technique which may be used to assess probable changes in GFR when infusion studies are impracticable. The method has proved particularly valuable for serial studies at frequent intervals during pregnancy and may be used with complete safety over the period of fetal organogenesis. Thus studies performed at weekly intervals over conception have shown that 24-hour creatinine clearance increases by 25% four weeks after the last menstrual period and by 45% at nine weeks (Davison and Noble, 1981). Weekly investigations during the third trimester have demonstrated a consistent and significant decrease to non-pregnant values preceding delivery (Davison et al, 1980); and daily investigations have suggested a small increase during the first few days of the puerperium (Davison and Dunlop, 1984). However, it is important to stress once again that these changes provide only indirect evidence of alterations in GFR and these are not all corroborated by the scanty evidence available from infusion studies. Thus, in the study of Sims and Krantz (1958) two women had inulin clearances performed between 6 and 9 weeks after the last menstrual period: increases of only 13% and 8% (as compared with non-pregnant data) were noted. Furthermore, no third-trimester reduction of inulin clearance has been convincingly demonstrated in serial studies up to the 37th week of pregnancy (Davison and Hytten, 1974; Dunlop, 1981; Ezimokhai et al, 1981) although one of the first reports of the technique in pregnancy suggested that a decrease might occur thereafter (Bonsnes and Lange, 1950).

Values for GFR estimated from 24-hour creatinine clearances are consistently less than those obtained from the clearances under infusion conditions of endogenous creatinine or inulin (Davison and Hytten, 1974). In part, this is due to diurnal variation in GFR and in part to specific fluctuations in creatinine clearance (Edwards et al, 1969). Table 2 illustrates the considerable magnitude of variations which were recorded when creatinine clearance was estimated over varying time intervals in well-motivated, carefully supervised, normally pregnant, ambulant women whose intake of food and fluid was unrestricted (W. Dunlop and L. M. Hill, unpublished data). It is obvious that considerable caution must be observed in interpreting renal function from such information.

Glomerular hyperfiltration

Eating a meat meal results in increases in the clearances not only of creatinine, but also of inulin (Bosch et al, 1983) and PAH (Hostetter, 1986). Other stimuli that have been shown to enhance GFR in humans include prolonged glycosuria (Brøchner-Mortensen, 1971; 1973) and increased renal arterial osmolality (Young and Rostorfer, 1973). It is considered that these changes are a reflection of increased glomerular perfusion and that this phenomenon may itself ultimately result in glomerular damage and relative renal impairment (Brenner et al, 1982). Could the glomerular hyperperfusion of human pregnancy lead to similar progressive nephropathy?

Early glomerular damage may result in increased permeability to albumin and microalbuminuria may develop early in the nephropathy of diabetes mellitus (Mogensen, 1971) or after unilateral nephrectomy (Hakim et al, 1984), both conditions that may be associated with glomerular hyperperfusion (Brenner et al, 1982). During normal human pregnancy there is an increase in total protein excretion (Davison, 1985) and a small increase in albumin excretion in particular has been reported during the third trimester and early puerperium (Lopez-Espinoza et al, 1986) but these changes are probably due to altered tubular function. In a recent report, Wright et al (1987b), although unable to detect an overall increase in albumin excretion during normal pregnancy, reported that ratios between clearances and urinary concentrations of albumin and creatinine increased progressively throughout pregnancy. The same group of workers has also suggested that these changes are more marked in women of high than of low parity, approximately matched for age (Wright et al, 1987a). It should be noted, however, that these results were based upon collection of urine during a 2-hour period during the afternoon, a protocol that must give rise to reservations about the validity of creatinine clearance estimations.

Preliminary data from long-term studies in groups of women with normal renal function, with single healthy kidneys, with renal allografts and with chronic renal diseases, some of whom achieved pregnancies and some of whom did not, have failed to demonstrate convincing evidence of an independent effect of pregnancy upon deterioration of renal function, whether assessed by 24-hour creatinine clearance, by inulin clearance or by total protein excretion (Davison, 1985; 1987). Clearly this important area needs further investigation and is discussed in detail in Chapter 2.

TUBULAR CONSEQUENCES OF GLOMERULAR CHANGES

Even allowing for small decrements in many plasma constituents during pregnancy, their filtered load will still increase. These changes must be accompanied by parallel increments in tubular reabsorption unless massive depletion would ensue.

Renal handling of Na^+

Renal Na^+ is the prime determinant of volume homeostasis, a topic discussed in detail in Chapters 4 and 5. Suffice it to say that the filtered load of sodium increases from nonpregnant levels of about 20 000 mmol per day to about 30 000 mmol per day. The adaptive increment in renal tubular reabsorption not only equals the increase in filtered load, but in addition 2–6 mmol of Na^+ are reabsorbed daily for fetal and maternal stores. This change represents the largest renal adjustment of pregnancy; nevertheless, the pregnant woman is probably not prone to excessive Na^+ retention. Furthermore, she handles ingested salt as she would when non-pregnant or may even be a subtle sodium waster (Lindheimer and Katz, 1986).

While existing clinical methods have been ideal for defining whole kidney function it has been impossible to quantify reabsorption at individual nephron segments. This has arisen in part because of difficulties in finding a suitable marker for the delivery of sodium (and water) from the proximal tubule to distal nephron segments. There is now evidence that lithium clearance (with simultaneous measurement of GFR and urinary volume) can be used for this purpose (Thomsen and Olesen, 1984). Preliminary data in the human suggest that Na^+ reabsorption is enhanced not only in the proximal tubule but also in distant nephron segments (Atherton et al, 1987).

Renal handling of urate

Only about 10% of the original filtered urate load appears in the urine. The renal handling of urate is, however, more complex than a simple tubular reabsorption, so that while a large proportion is reabsorbed proximally, any final excretion depends on the subsequent balance between active secretion and further reabsorption. It has been suggested that the hypouricaemia of normal pregnancy reflects a decrement in net tubular reabsorption. As pregnancy advances, however, the kidney appears to excrete a smaller proportion of filtered urate, and this increment in net reabsorption is associated with a rising plasma urate concentration (Dunlop and Davison, 1977), which approach or reach nonpregnant levels in the late third trimester.

Renal handling of glucose

In theory, the increased excretion of glucose in pregnancy could be due to the inability of renal tubules to accept the increased filtered glucose load resulting from increased GFR, a change in tubular reabsorptive capacity or a combination of both of these factors (Welsh and Sims, 1960). From serial studies of renal glucose handling under infusion conditions in women with varying degrees of glycosuria, it was demonstrated that glucose reabsorption was less complete during pregnancy than postpartum. Reabsorption was even less complete in pregnant women with obvious glycosuria. These women, although no longer clinically glycosuric following pregnancy, still showed less complete reabsorption under infusion conditions postpartum (Davison and Hytten, 1975).

The physiology of renal glucose reabsorption is complex and the concept of a tubular maximal reabsorptive capacity for glucose (Tm_G) is no longer tenable (Kurtzman and Pillay, 1973; Ullrich et al, 1976). In fact, glucose is always present in the urine, probably as a result of defective reabsorption from the 5% of filtered glucose that normally escapes proximal tubule reabsorption. Why the renal handling of glucose is altered in pregnancy is not known. Two major physiological adaptations of pregnancy have the potential to affect glucose reabsorption in opposite ways: volume expansion inhibits glucose reabsorption by inhibiting the reabsorption of sodium; whereas increased GFR stimulates glucose reabsorption. The hormones of pregnancy, particularly the sex steroids, might modify tubular function, and their concentrations do decline rapidly after delivery in much the same way as glucose excretion. Whatever the explanation, there must also be subtle, moment-by-moment intrarenal changes to account for the intermittency of glucose excretion.

Renal handling of protein

Much of the protein that normally appears in urine is thought to be the result of selective glomerular filtration and of non-selective tubular reabsorption, chiefly in the proximal tubule (Pesce and First, 1979). Proteins of a molecular weight of about 50 000 Da (like albumin) are just barely filtered through the filtration barrier and fixed negative charge of normal glomerular capillaries. It has been estimated that 10 g of protein is filtered every 24 hours, and only 150 mg (25% of which is albumin, the rest globulin) appears in the urine. Actually, 20% of normal urinary protein is Tamm-Horsfall protein, a mucoprotein of molecular weight of 7 000 000 Da, which is not present in plasma but is thought to be delivered from cells lining the distal nephron.

Total protein excretion increases during normal pregnancy and may reach 300 mg in 24 hours (Young et al, 1984; Davison, 1985). Albumin excretion, however, shows only a minimal increment, limited to the third trimester (range 10–36 mg) and persisting during the first postnatal week (Lopez-Espinoza et al, 1986). It is likely that the changes in renal handling of protein in normal pregnancy are due to altered tubular function.

CLINICAL RELEVANCE OF RENAL ALTERATIONS

Assessment of renal function

Changes in plasma creatinine and urea. Plasma creatinine levels decrease from a non-pregnant value of 73 μmol l^{-1} to 65, 51, and 47 μmol l^{-1}, respectively, in successive trimesters; plasma urea levels fall from non-pregnancy values of 4.3 mmol l^{-1} to pregnancy values of 3.5, 3.3 and 3.1 mmol l^{-1}, respectively. Familiarity with these changes is vital, because values considered normal in non-pregnant women may signify decreased renal function in pregnancy. As a rough guide, values of plasma creatinine of 75 μmol l^{-1} and urea of 4.5 mmol l^{-1} should alert the clinician to assess renal function further. It should be remembered, however, that caution is necessary when serially assessing renal function on the basis of plasma creatinine levels alone, especially in the presence of renal disease. Even when up to 50% of renal function has been lost, it is still possible to have a plasma creatinine level of less than 130 μmol l^{-1}. If renal function is more severely compromised, however, a small decrement in GFR causes a marked rise in plasma creatinine and, under these conditions, creatinine excretion is diminished.

Creatinine clearance in clinical practice. To overcome such problems as 'washout' from changes in urine flow, 24-hour urine samples should be used for clearances (as discussed earlier) in an attempt to avoid difficulties caused by diurnal variations (Edwards et al, 1969); see Table 2. Many methods of determining creatinine in plasma also measure non-creatinine chromogens, leading to overestimates, that must be taken into account when calculating creatinine clearances (Davison and Hytten, 1974; Davison and Noble, 1981). In addition, recent intake of cooked meat can increase plasma creatinine levels by up to 16 μmol l^{-1} (because cooking converts preformed creatine into creatinine), and awareness of this influences the timing of blood sampling during a clearance period (Jacobsen et al, 1980).

Formulae have been devised to calculate a value for GFR from plasma creatinine level, taking into account the patient's age, height, weight and sex (Morrison et al, 1987). As discussed earlier, it is erroneous to use any such approach in pregnancy where body weight or size does not reflect functional renal mass.

Renal dysfunction and its implications. Many women with renal disease will remain symptom-free until GFR has decreased to less than 25% of its original level. Conceiving and sustaining a viable pregnancy is related to the degree of functional impairment rather than to the underlying renal lesion. Nature adds a helping hand by blunting fertility as renal function falls, and when plasma creatinine and urea levels before conception exceed 275 μmol l^{-1} and 10 mmol l^{-1} respectively, normal pregnancy is rare. These issues are further discussed in Chapter 9.

Urate handling

From the clinical viewpoint it is of interest that plasma urate concentration and renal absorption are significantly higher in pregnancies complicated by pre-eclampsia or intrauterine growth retardation (Dunlop et al, 1978). Above a critical blood level of 350 μmol l^{-1} there is significant perinatal mortality in hypertensive patients, and serial measurements can be used to monitor progress in pre-eclampsia (Redman et al, 1976). It must be remembered, however, that physiological variability is such that some healthy women have high plasma levels without problems, and that single random measurements are of no use clinically (Lind et al, 1984).

Glucose handling

The excretion of glucose increases soon after conception and may exceed non-pregnancy values (20–100 mg in 24 hours) by a factor of ten. The glycosuria can vary dramatically within any 24-hour period and from day to day, with an intermittency that is unrelated to either blood sugar concentration or stage of pregnancy (Davison and Hytten, 1975). One week after delivery, non-pregnant glucose excretion patterns are re-established (Davison and Love-dale, 1974).

Glycosuria of pregnancy reflects an alteration in renal function, rather than an alteration in carbohydrate metabolism. The testing of random urine samples during pregnancy is unhelpful in the diagnosis or control of diabetes mellitus, and unrepresentative as to the degree of glycosuria present.

Recent studies raise the possibility that women with more than usual glycosuria in pregnancy may have sustained renal tubular damage from earlier, untreated urinary tract infections, although no longer bacteriuric when pregnant (Davison et al, 1984). Why infection might cause an alteration in the renal handling of glucose is not known. Certainly infection can impair distal tubular function, as evidenced by reduced urine-concentrating ability, a manifestation of tubular dysfunction that is reversed once infection is eradicated. With the renal handling of glucose, however, if distal tubular sites are affected by infection, full recovery may not occur.

Protein excretion

Urine flow normally varies over a wide range from moment to moment so that the protein concentration of a random specimen can give only a semiquantitative appraisal of the degree of proteinuria. Although this estimate (which is recorded on a scale of 'pluses' or as an approximate concentration) is valuable, a more accurate quantitation is needed. Proteinuria should not be considered abnormal until it exceeds 300 mg in 24 hours.

Currently there is debate about the independent effect of normal pregnancy on long-term renal function, using microalbuminuria to detect any damage (Davison and Hytten, 1987; Wright et al, 1987a, 1987b). As mentioned earlier, the consensus is that pregnancy does not damage the kidney; and in any case, better markers are needed than albumin excretion, however corrected. This is discussed further in Chapter 2, and the significance and interpretation of urinary protein excretion in chronic renal disease and pre-eclampsia are discussed in Chapters 9 and 12.

SUMMARY

In human pregnancy, effective renal plasma flow and glomerular filtration rate increase to levels 50–80% above non-pregnant values. The increments occur shortly after conception, persist throughout the second trimester and reduce slightly in late pregnancy. The hyperfiltration of pregnancy does not seem to be a potentially damaging process. The increased excretion of glucose and other nutrients, as well as uric acid and protein, is related in part to altered tubular function. Renal physiology is altered so much in pregnancy that non-pregnant norms cannot be used in antenatal care.

REFERENCES

Assali NS, Dignam WJ & Dasgupta K (1959) Renal function in human pregnancy. II. Effects of venous pooling on renal hemodynamics and water, electrolyte and aldosterone excretion during normal gestation. *Journal of Clinical and Laboratory Medicine* **54:** 395–408.
Assali NS, Rauramo L & Peltonen T (1960) Measurement of uterine blood flow and uterine metabolism. VIII. Uterine and fetal blood flow and oxygen consumption in early human pregnancy. *American Journal of Obstetrics and Gynecology* **79:** 86–98.
Atherton JC, Bobinski H & Davison JM (1987) Renal fluid handling and plasma atrial natriuretic peptide in human pregnancy. *Journal of Physiology* **387:** 90P.
Atkins AJF, Watt JM, Milan P, Davies P & Selwyn Crawford J (1981a) A longitudinal study of cardiovascular dynamic changes throughout pregnancy. *European Journal of Obstetrics, Gynecology and Reproductive Biology* **12:** 215–224.

Atkins AJF, Watt JM, Milan P, Davies P & Selwyn Crawford J (1981b) The influence of posture upon cardiovascular dynamics throughout pregnancy. *European Journal of Obstetrics, Gynecology and Reproductive Biology* **12**: 357–372.

Baylis C (1980a) Glomerular filtration rate and plasma volume in the pregnant rat. *Journal of Physiology* (London) 305: 64P.

Baylis C (1980b) The mechanism of the increase in glomerular filtration rate in the twelve-day pregnant rat. *Journal of Physiology* (London) **305**: 405–414.

Baylis C (1982) Glomerular ultrafiltration in the pseudopregnant rat. *American Journal of Physiology* **243**: F300–F305.

Blake S, Bonar F, McCarthy C & MacDonald D (1983) The effect of posture on cardiac output in late pregnancy complicated by pericardial constriction. *American Journal of Obstetrics and Gynecology* **146**: 865–867.

Blake S, O'Neill H & MacDonald D (1982) Haemodynamic effects of pregnancy in patients with heart failure. *British Heart Journal* **47**: 495–496.

Bosch JP, Saccaggi A, Lauer A, Ronco C, Belledonne M & Glabman S (1983) Renal functional reserve in humans. Effect of protein intake on glomerular filtration rate. *American Journal of Medicine* **75**: 943–950.

Bosnes RW & Lange WA (1950) Inulin clearance during pregnancy. *Federation Proceedings* **9**: 154.

Brandstetter F & Schüller E (1956) Die Clearanceuntersuchung in der Gravidität. Ein Beitrag zur Physio-Pathologie der Niere und Leber in der Schwangerschaft. *Fortschritte der Geburtshilfe und Gynäkologie Bibliotheca Gynaecologica* **14(IV)**: 1–99.

Brenner BM, Baylis C & Deen WM (1976) Transport of molecules across renal glomerular capillaries. *Physiological Reviews* **56**: 502–534.

Brenner B, Meyer TW & Hostetter T (1982) Dietary protein intake and the progressive nature of kidney disease: the role of hemodynamically mediated glomerular injury in the pathogenesis of progressive glomerular sclerosis in aging, renal ablation and intrinsic renal disease. *New England Journal of Medicine* **307**: 652–659.

Brenner BM, Troy JL & Daugharty TM (1971). The dynamics of glomerular ultrafiltration in the rat. *Journal of Clinical Investigation* **50**: 1776–1780.

Brenner BM, Troy JL, Daugharty TM, Deen WM & Robertson CR (1972) Dynamics of ultrafiltration in the rat. II. Plasma-flow dependence of GFR. *American Journal of Physiology* **223**: 1184–1190.

Brøchner-Mortensen J (1971) The effect of glucose on the glomerular filtration rate in normal man. A preliminary report. *Acta Medica Scandinavica* **189**: 109–111.

Brøchner-Mortensen J (1973) The glomerular filtration rate during moderate hyperglycemia in normal man. *Acta Medica Scandinavica* **194**: 31–37.

Brod J & Sirota JH (1948) The renal clearance of endogenous 'creatinine' in man. *Journal of Clinical Investigation* **27**: 645–654.

Bucht H (1951) Studies on renal function in man with special reference to glomerular filtration and renal plasma flow in pregnancy. *Scandinavian Journal of Clinical and Laboratory Investigation* 3(Suppl): 1–64.

Buttermann K (1958) Clearance-Untersuchungen in der normalen und pathologischen Schwangerschaft. Zugleich eine kritische Beurteilung des Verfahrens. *Archiv für Gynäkologie* **190**: 488–492.

Chesley LC (1960) Renal functional changes in normal pregnancy. *Clinical Obstetrics and Gynecology* **3**: 349–363.

Chesley LC & Sloan DM (1964) The effect of posture on renal function in late pregnancy. *American Journal of Obstetrics and Gynecology* **89**: 754–759.

Chesley LC & Williams LO (1945) Renal glomerular and tubular function in relation to the hyperuricemia of pre-eclampsia and eclampsia. *American Journal of Obstetrics and Gynecology* **59**: 367–375.

Clarke RW & Smith HW (1932) Absorption and excretion of water and salts by the elasmobranch fishes. III. The use of xylose as a measure of the glomerular filtrate in *Squalus acanthias*. *Journal of Cellular and Comparative Physiology* **1**: 131–143.

Crawford JS, Lewis M & Weaver JB (1987) Hypertension in the puerperium. *Lancet* ii: 693–694.

Davison JM (1985) The effect of pregnancy on kidney function in renal allograft recipients. *Kidney International* **27**: 74–79.

Davison JM (1987) Hypertension in pregnancy. In Sharp F & Symonds EM (eds) *Proceedings of the Sixteenth Study Group of the Royal College of Obstetricians and Gynaecologists*, pp 92–95 New York: Perinatology Press.

Davison JM & Dunlop W (1980) Renal hemodynamics and tubular function in normal human pregnancy. *Kidney International* **18;** 152–161.

Davison JM & Dunlop W (1984) Changes in renal hemodynamics and tubular function induced by normal human pregnancy. *Seminars in Nephrology* **4:** 198–207.

Davison JM, Dunlop W & Ezimokhai M (1980) 24-hour creatinine clearance during the third trimester of normal pregnancy. *British Journal of Obstetrics and Gynaecology* **87:** 106–109.

Davison JM & Hytten FE (1974) Glomerular filtration during and after pregnancy. *Journal of Obstetrics and Gynaecology of the British Commonwealth* **81:** 588–595.

Davison JM & Hytten FE (1975) The effect of pregnancy on the renal handling of glucose. *Journal of Obstetrics and Gynaecology of the British Commonwealth* **82:** 374–381.

Davison JM & Hytten FE (1987) Can normal pregnancy damage your health? *British Journal of Obstetrics and Gynaecology* **94:** 385–386.

Davison JM & Lovedale C (1974) The excretion of glucose during normal pregnancy and after delivery. *Journal of Obstetrics and Gynaecology of the British Commonwealth* **81:** 30–34.

Davison JM & Noble MCB (1981) Serial changes in 24-hour creatinine clearance during normal menstrual cycles and the first trimester of pregnancy. *British Journal of Obstetrics and Gynaecology* **88:** 10–17.

Davison JM, Sprott MS & Selkon JB (1984) The effect of covert bacteriuria in schoolgirls on renal function at 18 years and during pregnancy. *Lancet* **ii:** 651–655.

De Alvarez RR (1958) Renal glomerulotubular mechanisms during normal pregnancy. I. Glomerular filtration rate, renal plasma flow and creatinine clearance. *American Journal of Obstetrics and Gynecology* **75:** 931–944.

Deen WM, Robertson CR & Brenner BM (1972) A model of glomerular ultrafiltration in the rat. *American Journal of Physiology* **223:** 1191–1200.

Deen WM, Troy JL, Robertson CR & Brenner BM (1973) Dynamics of glomerular ultrafiltration in the rat. IV. Determination of the ultrafiltration coefficient. *Journal of Clinical Investigation* **52:** 1500–1508.

Dignam WJ, Titus P & Assali NS (1958) Renal function in human pregnancy. I. Changes in glomerular filtration rate and renal plasma flow. *Proceedings of the Society for Experimental Biology and Medicine* **97:** 512–514.

Dill LV, Isenhour CE, Cadden JF & Schaffer NK (1942) Glomerular filtration and renal blood flow in the toxemias of pregnancy. *American Journal of Obstetrics and Gynecology* **43:** 32–42.

Dunlop W (1976) Investigations into the influence of posture on renal plasma flow and glomerular filtration rate during late pregnancy. *British Journal of Obstetrics and Gynaecology* **83:** 17–23.

Dunlop W (1981) Serial changes in renal haemodynamics during normal human pregnancy. *British Journal of Obstetrics and Gynaecology* **88:** 1–9.

Dunlop W (1982a) Changes in renal haemodynamics induced by human pregnancy. PhD thesis, University of Newcastle upon Tyne.

Dunlop W (1982b) Altered renal response to intravenous saline during human pregnancy: results of serial studies. *Clinical and Experimental Hypertension* B1(2–3): 325.

Dunlop W & Davison JM (1977) The effect of normal pregnancy upon the renal handling of uric acid. *British Journal of Obstetrics and Gynaecology* **84:** 13–21.

Dunlop W, Furness C & Hill LM (1978) Maternal haemoglobin concentration, haematocrit and renal handling of urate in pregnancy ending in births of small-for-dates infants. *British Journal of Obstetrics and Gynaecology* **85:** 938–940.

Edwards OM, Bayliss RIS & Miller S (1969) Urinary creatinine excretion as an index of the completeness of 24-hour urine collections. *Lancet* **ii:** 1165–1166.

Ezimokhai M, Davison JM, Philips PR & Dunlop W (1981) Non-postural serial changes in renal function during the third trimester of normal human pregnancy. *British Journal of Obstetrics and Gynaecology* **88:** 465–471.

Gylling T (1961) Renal haemodynamics and heart volume in normal pregnancy. *Acta Obstetricia et Gynaecologica Scandinavica* **49** (suppl. 5): 1–68.

Hakim RM, Goldszer RC & Brenner BM (1984) Hypertension and proteinuria: long-term sequelae of uninephrectomy in humans. *Kidney International* **25:** 930–936.

Hamilton HFH (1949) The cardiac output in normal pregnancy. *Journal of Obstetrics and Gynaecology of the British Empire* **56:** 548–552.

Hendricks CH & Barnes AC (1955) Effect of supine position on urinary output in pregnancy. *American Journal of Obstetrics and Gynecology* **69:** 1225–1232.

Hostetter TH (1986) Human renal response to a meat meal. *American Journal of Physiology* **250:** F613–F618.

Hytten FE (1954) Clinical and chemical studies in human lactation. VI. The functional capacity of the breast. *British Medical Journal* **1:** 912–915.

Hytten FE & Leitch I (1971) *Physiology of Human Pregnancy*, 2nd edn, pp 144–145. Oxford: Blackwell Scientific.

Hytten FE & Paintin DB (1963) Increase in plasma volume during normal pregnancy. *Journal of Obstetrics and Gynaecology of the British Commonwealth* **70:** 402–407.

Jacobsen FK, Christensen CK, Mogensen CE & Heilskow HSC (1980) Evaluation of kidney function after meals. *Lancet* **i:** 319.

Joliffe N & Chasis H (1933) The filtration and secretion of exogenous creatinine in man. *American Journal of Physiology* **104:** 677–680.

Kariher DH & George RH (1943) Toxemias of pregnancy and the inulin-Diodrast clearance tests. *Proceedings of the Society of Experimental and Biological Medicine* **52:** 245–247.

Kerr MG, Scott DB & Samuel E (1964) Studies of the inferior vena cava in late pregnancy. *British Medical Journal* **1:** 532–533.

Kjeldsen J (1979) Haemodynamic investigations during labour and delivery. *Acta Obstetricia et Gynecologica Scandinavica* **89**(suppl): 144–153.

Klopper A (1964) Changes in renal function in late pregnancy. *Lancet* **ii:** 565–566.

Kurtzman NA & Pillay VKG (1973) Renal reabsorption of glucose in health and disease. *Archives of Internal Medicine* **131:** 901–904.

Lanz R & Hochuli E (1955) Über die Nierenclearance in der normalen Schwangerschaft und bei hypertensiven Spättoxikosen, ihre Beeinflussung durch hypotensive Medikamente. *Schweizerische Medizinische Wochenschrift* **17:** 395–400.

Lees MM, Taylor SH, Scott DB & Kerr MG (1967) A study of cardiac output at rest throughout pregnancy. *Journal of Obstetrics and Gynaecology of the British Commonwealth* **74:** 319–328.

Lind T, Godfrey KA, Otun H & Philips PR (1984) Changes in serum uric acid concentrations during normal pregnancy. *British Journal of Obstetrics and Gynaecology* **91:** 128–132.

Lindheimer MD & Katz AI (1975) Renal changes during pregnancy: their relevance to volume homeostasis. *Clinics in Obstetrics and Gynaecology* **2:** 345–346.

Lindheimer MD & Katz AI (1986) The kidney in pregnancy. In Brenner BM & Rector FD (eds) *The Kidney*. Philadelphia: WB Saunders.

Lopez-Espinoza I, Dhar H, Humphreys S & Redman CWG (1986) Urinary albumin excretion in pregnancy. *British Journal of Obstetrics and Gynaecology* **93:** 176–181.

MacGillivray I, Rose GA & Rowe B (1969) Blood pressure survey in pregnancy. *Clinical Science* **37:** 395–407.

McLennan FM, Haites NE & Rawles JM (1987) Stroke and minute distance in pregnancy: a longitudinal study using Doppler ultrasound. *British Journal of Obstetrics and Gynaecology* **94:** 499–506.

Marshall EK & Grafflin AL (1932) The function of the proximal convoluted segment of the renal tubule. *Journal of Cellular and Comparative Physiology* **1:** 161–176.

Mogensen CE (1971) Kidney function and glomerular permeability to macromolecules in early juvenile diabetes. *Scandinavian Journal of Clinical and Laboratory Investigation* **28:** 79–90.

Morrison RBI, Davison JM & Kerr DNS (1987) In Weatherall DJ, Ledingham JGG & Warrell DA (eds) *Oxford Textbook of Medicine*, pp 18.1–18.17. Oxford: Oxford University Press.

Newman B, Derrington C & Dore C (1983) Cardiac output and the recumbent position in late pregnancy. *Anaesthesia* **38:** 322–335.

Pesce AJ & First MR (1979) *Proteinuria: An Integrated Review*, pp. 5–31. New York: Marcel Dekker.

Pippig L (1969) Clinique des affections rénales pendant la grossesse. *Médecine et Hygiène* **859:** 181–191.

Pritchard JA, Barnes AC & Bright RH (1955) The effect of the supine position on renal function in the near-term pregnant woman. *Journal of Clinical Investigation* **34:** 777–781.

Rawles JM, Schneider KTM, Huch R & Huch A (1987) The effect of position and delay on stroke and minute distance in late pregnancy. *British Journal of Obstetrics and Gynaecology* **94:** 507–511.

Redman CWG, Beilin LJ, Bonnar J & Wilkinson R (1976) Plasma urate measurements in predicting fetal death in hypertensive pregnancy. *Lancet* **i:** 1370–1373.

Rehberg PB (1926) Studies on kidney function. I. The rate of filtration and reabsorption in the human kidney. *Biochemistry* **20:** 447–460.

Robertson CR, Deen WM, Troy JL & Brenner BM (1972) Dynamics of glomerular ultrafiltration in the rat. III. Hemodynamics and autoregulation. *American Journal of Physiology* **223:** 1191–1200.

Robertson EG & Cheyne GA (1972) Plasma biochemistry in relation to oedema of pregnancy. *Journal of Obstetrics and Gynaecology of the British Commonwealth* **79:** 769–776.

Robson SC, Hunter S, Boyes R & Dunlop W (1987a) Serial measurement of maternal haemodynamics over conception and during the first trimester of pregnancy. *British Journal of Obstetrics and Gynaecology* (in press).

Robson SC, Dunlop W, Moore M & Hunter S (1987b) Cardiac output during labour. *British Medical Journal* **295:** 1169–1172.

Robson SC, Dunlop W & Hunter S (1987c) Haemodynamic changes during the early puerperium. *British Medical Journal* **294:** 1065.

Robson SC, Hunter S, Moore M & Dunlop W (1987d) Haemodynamic changes during the puerperium: a Doppler and M-mode echocardiographic study. *British Journal of Obstetrics and Gynaecology* **94:** 1028–1039.

Robson SC, Hunter S & Dunlop W (1987e) Left atrial dimension during early puerperium. *Lancet* **ii:** 111–112.

Rutherford AJ, Anderson JV, Elder MG & Bloom SR (1987) *Lancet* **i:** 928–929.

Schwarz R (1964) Das Verhalten des Kreislaufs in der normalen Schwangerschaft. I. Der arterielle Blutdruck. *Archiv für Gynäkologie* **199:** 549–570.

Shannon JA (1934) Absorption and excretion of water and salts by the elasmobranch fishes. IV. The secretion of exogenous creatinine by the dogfish, *Squalus acanthias. Journal of Cellular and Comparative Physiology* **4:** 211–220.

Shannon JA (1935) The renal excretion of creatinine in man. *Journal of Clinical Investigation* **14:** 403–410.

Shannon JA, Joliffe N & Smith HW (1932) The excretion of urine in the dog. VI. The filtration and secretion of exogenous creatinine. *American Journal of Physiology* **102:** 534–550.

Shannon JA & Smith HW (1935) The excretion of inulin, xylose and urea by normal and phlorizinized man. *Journal of Clinical Investigation* **14:** 393–401.

Shemesh O, Golbetz H, Kriss JP & Myers BD (1985) Limitations of creatinine as a filtration marker in glomerulopathic patients. *Kidney International* **28:** 830–838.

Sims EA & Krantz KE (1956) Serial studies of renal function throughout pregnancy and the puerperium in the normal woman. *Clinical Research Proceedings* **4:** 142.

Sims EAH & Krantz KE (1958) Serial studies of renal function during pregnancy and the puerperium in normal women. *Journal of Clinical Investigation* **37:** 1764–1774.

Smith HW (1951) *The Kidney. Structure and Function in Health and Disease*, p 161. New York: Oxford University Press.

Sohar E, Scadron E & Levitt MF (1956) Changes in renal hemodynamics during normal pregnancy. *Clinical Research Proceedings* **4:** 142.

Steegers EAP, Hein PR, Groeneveld EAM, Jongsma HW, Tan ACITL & Benraad TJ (1987) Atrial natriuretic peptide concentrations during pregnancy. *Lancet* **i:** 1267.

Thomsen K & Olesen VO (1984) Renal lithium clearance as a measure of the delivery of water and sodium from the proximal tubule in humans. *American Journal of Medical Sciences* **288:** 158–161.

Ueland K, Novy MJ, Petersen EN & Metcalf J (1969) Maternal cardiovascular dynamics. IV. The influence of gestational age on the maternal cardiovascular response to posture and exercise. *American Journal of Obstetrics and Gynecology* **104:** 856–864.

Ullrich KJ, Fromter E, Hinton BT, Rumrich G & Kleinzeller A (1976) Specificity of sugar transport across the brush border of rat proximal tubule. *Current Problems in Clinical Biochemistry* **6:** 256–261.

Vorys N, Ullery JC & Hanusek GE (1961) The cardiac output changes in various positions in pregnancy. *American Journal of Obstetrics and Gynecology* **82:** 1312–1321.

Walker EW, McManus M & Janney JC (1934) Kidney function in pregnancy. II. Effect of posture on diuresis. *Proceedings of the Society for Experimental and Biological Medicine* **31:** 392–397.

Walters WAW, MacGregor WG & Hills M (1966) Cardiac output at rest during pregnancy and the puerperium. *Clinical Science* **30:** 1–11.

Walters WAW & Lim YL (1975) Blood volume and haemodynamics in pregnancy. *Clinics in Obstetrics and Gynaecology* **2:** 301–320.

Walters BJN, Thompson ME, Lee A & de Swiet M (1986) Blood pressure in the puerperium. *Clinical Science* **71:** 589–594.

Walters BJN & Walters T (1987) Hypertension in the puerperium. *Lancet* **ii:** 330.

Warren JV, Brannon ES & Merrill AJ (1944) A method of obtaining renal venous blood in unanesthetized persons with observations on the extraction of oxygen and sodium para-amino hippurate. *Science* **100:** 108–110.

Welsh CA, Wellen I & Taylor HC (1942) The filtration rate, effective renal blood flow, tubular excretory mass and phenol red clearance in normal pregnancy. *Journal of Clinical Investigation* **21:** 57–61.

Welsh GW & Sims EAH (1960) The mechanisms of renal glucosuria in pregnancy. *Diabetes* **9:** 363–375.

Wright A, McIntosh C, Steele P, Bennett J & Polak A (1987a) Urinary albumin excretion during normal pregnancy in women of low and high parity: evidence for albumin leakage after prolonged hyperfiltration. *Abstracts of Xth International Congress of Nephrology*, p 513, London.

Wright A, Steele P, Bennett JR, Watts G & Polak A (1987b) The urinary excretion of albumin in normal pregnancy. *British Journal of Obstetrics and Gynaecology* **94:** 408–412.

Young DB & Rostorfer HH (1973) Blood flow and filtration rate responses to alterations in renal arterial osmolarity. *American Journal of Physiology* **225:** 1003–1008.

Young M, Davis M, Richardson MC & Dennis KJ (1984) Urinary protein excretion in normal pregnancy. *Proceedings of IVth World Congress of International Society for the Study of Hypertension in Pregnancy*, p 192A.

2

Glomerular filtration and volume regulation in gravid animal models

CHRISTINE BAYLIS

Gestational increases in glomerular filtration rate have been described in a number of animal species, including the dog, rabbit, sheep and rat (Conrad, 1987). Much of our information on the general physiology of the kidney has been obtained from studies in animals, particularly the male rat. The gravid rat also provides an excellent animal model for study of the gestational changes that occur not only in renal but also in systemic haemodynamics (see below). This chapter discusses the information that has been derived, mainly from studies in the rat, about the mechanisms that control the altered kidney function of normal pregnancy. Perception and control of extracellular fluid volume in pregnancy is also discussed. Finally, recent studies are described that provide insight into possible long-term effects of pregnancy on the maternal kidney.

SOME CHARACTERISTICS OF PREGNANCY IN THE RAT

Gestation in the rat lasts for approximately 22 days and the normal litter size ranges between 5 and 15 pups per litter. The female rat becomes sexually mature at about 8–10 weeks old, when the regular oestrus cycle begins. The female comes into oestrus (when she ovulates) once every 4–5 days; if environmental conditions are optimal, there is a high likelihood of conception and successful pregnancy occurring as a result of a fertile mating (Schwartz, 1973). The female will only permit mating to occur when she is in oestrus. Within hours of mating, the first of a series of diurnal pituitary prolactin surges begin (MacDonald, 1978; Smith and Neill, 1976). Prolactin is the luteotrophic hormone of the rat and maintains the corpus luteum so that progesterone levels are also elevated and remain high throughout the entire gestation period. The maternal pituitary prolactin provides the luteotrophic stimulus for the first 10 days of the pregnancy; thereafter, chorionic gonadotropins take over the luteotrophic role and the pituitary prolactin surges cease, with maternal prolactin levels remaining low until just before term. Oestrogen levels remain low throughout the entire gestation period until close to term (Garland et al, 1987; MacDonald, 1978; Smith and Neill, 1976: Schwartz, 1973).

There are also major alterations in the non-sex-related hormones during a normal pregnancy in the rat. As in the pregnant woman, plasma renin and aldosterone levels are increased in pregnancy (Garland et al, 1987). Plasma osmolality falls by 10 mosmol/kg plasma water, and both osmotic and volume-dependent control of antidiuretic hormone release is reset in the normal gravid rat (Lindheimer et al, 1987). These alterations are discussed in detail in Chapters 4 and 5.

RENAL HAEMODYNAMICS IN PREGNANCY

Time course and different experimental models

In elegant longitudinal studies in the conscious, chronically catheterized rat, Conrad has shown that an early rise in glomerular filtration rate (GFR) is evident by day 5 of pregnancy; by day 12, GFR has risen further and this maximum increment (of approximately 30% above the virgin value) is maintained until some time beyond day 16 (Figure 1(a)). Close to term (day 20), GFR is beginning to return towards the non-pregnant value (Conrad, 1984). This pattern of change closely resembles that seen in the normal pregnant woman (Davison and Dunlop, 1980).

Use of the conscious, chronically catheterized rat preparation provides an experimental model in which renal haemodynamics may be investigated in a setting uncomplicated by the stress that attends studies conducted under general anaesthesia and during acute surgical interventions. The rats can be trained to accept handling and the various non-invasive manoeuvres required by a renal function study, and are thus completely calm and unstressed by the procedure. Accurate measurement of GFR requires that a constant IV infusion of an isotonic solution containing inulin be administered, but it is possible to avoid significant alterations in extracellular fluid (ECF) volume status by maintaining a very low rate of infusion which matches the rate of urine output in this preparation.

The advantage of the conscious rat preparation is that measurements can be made in a completely undisturbed animal with a near-normal extracellular fluid volume status. The disadvantage, however, is that only whole kidney measurements can be made. In order to gain insight into the intrarenal mechanisms that control GFR during pregnancy, studies have been performed using the micropuncture technique, which permits sampling and measurements in the superficial cortical structures of the rat kidney. Many of the experiments described here are micropuncture studies carried out in the gravid Munich–Wistar rat, a unique strain of rat that possesses glomerular capillaries on the immediately subcapsular surface of the renal cortex. Collection of tubular fluid in these rats allows measurement of single-nephron (SN) GFR; collection of preglomerular and postglomerular blood samples allows measurement of preglomerular and postglomerular protein concentrations, and thus of preglomerular and postglomerular plasma oncotic

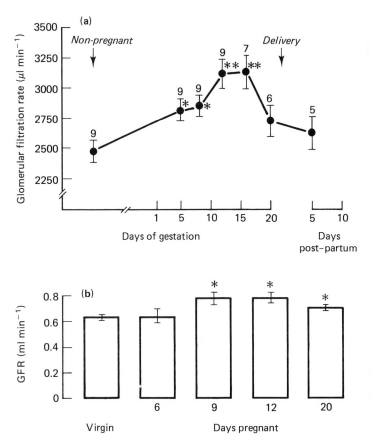

Figure 1. (a) Magnitude and time course of the gestational change in GFR (for both kidneys) measured in the conscious, chronically catheterized Long–Evans rat. From Conrad (1984) with permission. (b) GFR (left kidney) measured in the euvolaemic Munich–Wistar rat before and during pregnancy. From Baylis (1984). In both (a) and (b) data are shown as mean $\pm$ SE; a significant difference from the virgin value is denoted by * ($p < 0.05$) and ** ($p < 0.001$).

pressures; direct measurement of glomerular capillary blood pressure and hydrostatic pressure in the proximal tubule (equal to the pressure in Bowman's space) allows assessment of the hydrostatic pressure gradient across the wall of the glomerulus. Direct measurement of blood pressure in the postglomerular, efferent arterioles is also possible using these techniques. From these directly measurable variables it is possible to calculate single-nephron filtration fraction, glomerular plasma flow rate, preglomerular and postglomerular arteriolar resistances and the glomerular capillary ultra-filtration coefficient, K_f, the product of glomerular wall water permeability and available filtration surface area. Thus, all the haemodynamic determinants of glomerular ultrafiltration, as well as SNGFR itself, can either be directly measured or calculated by the glomerular micropuncture techniqu (Baylis, 1986).

The study of glomerular haemodynamic changes during pregnancy pre sents a challenge to the investigator, since by definition this invasive techniqu requires cross-sectional studies. It is necessary, during the glomerula micropuncture experiment, to preserve pre-existing differences in plasm volume between pregnant and virgin rats. Although not perfect, th 'euvolaemic' preparation is now used by many workers to provide a relativel undisturbed volume state during micropuncture experiments (Ichikawa et a 1978). A gestational increase in GFR can be detected in the gravic euvolaemic Munich–Wistar rat, which reaches a maximum by day 9 o pregnancy and begins to decline by close to term (day 20) (Figure 1(b)).

There have been many other studies in which gravid rats have bee subjected to extremes of extracellular fluid volume expansion or contractio as well as acute surgery, and in these settings the gestational rise in GFR ma be blunted or absent (Baylis, 1984). There is also evidence that late pregnan rats exhibit a different response to the acute stress of surgery and anaesthesi compared to virgin controls (Baylis and Collins, 1986). For these reasons, th following discussion on glomerular haemodynamics in pregnancy concen trates mainly on data derived from studies in the euvolaemic, anaesthetize preparation and in the normovolaemic, conscious rat.

Determinants of glomerular filtration in pregnancy

The single-nephron (SN) GFR, and therefore the GFR, is controlled by fou determinants:

1. Glomerular plasma flow rate.
2. The hydrostatic pressure gradient across the wall of the glomerulus (th difference between the hydrostatic pressure of the glomerular blood and o Bowman's space fluid).
3. The oncotic pressure of the plasma arriving at the glomerulus (due to th plasma proteins.
4. The glomerular capillary ultrafiltration coefficient, K_f, the product o glomerular wall water permeability and glomerular filtration surface are (Baylis, 1986).

In the normal, euvolaemic rat the net filtration pressure—the differenc between the transmural hydrostatic pressure gradient (favouring filtration o fluid) and the transmural oncotic pressure gradient (which opposes glomeru lar filtration)—averaged over the length of the glomerulus, is sufficiently hig that less than the maximum available filtration area is utilized. In other words the transmural oncotic pressure (which rises along the length of th glomerular capillary as protein-free glomerular filtrate is formed), has risen t a value that equals (and opposes) the transmural hydrostatic pressure gradien somewhere before the end of the glomerulus. This state is known as *filtratior pressure equilibrium*, and implies that filtration has ceased somewhere before the end of the glomerulus (Baylis, 1986).

In an animal at filtration pressure equilibrium, SNGFR is highly dependent on glomerular plasma flow rate, with a rise in plasma flow rate eliciting a proportional increase in filtration. SNGFR can also be increased, either by increasing glomerular blood pressure (and thus the transmural hydrostatic pressure gradient, which drives filtration of fluid) or by reducing the oncotic pressure of the plasma arriving at the glomerulus. At filtration equilibrium the glomerular capillary ultrafiltration coefficient is sufficiently high that further increases in this variable will not increase SNGFR (Baylis, 1986).

Micropuncture studies have been performed in the euvolaemic, midterm (12 day) pregnant Munich–Wistar rat, and have indicated that a substantial (approximately 30%) increase occurs in superficial cortical SNGFR (Baylis, 1980). This increase in filtration rate is the result exclusively of an increase in glomerular plasma flow rate, shown in the upper panel of Figure 2. As shown in the lower panel of Figure 2, there are no changes in hydrostatic and oncotic pressures at the glomerulus. As also shown here, pregnant rats remain at filtration pressure equilibrium, as indicated by the equality between the transmural hydrostatic pressure gradient (ΔP) and the immediately postglomerular arteriolar oncotic pressure (π_E). Although not shown, the arterial blood pressure is unaltered at midterm pregnancy compared to the virgin value, which together with the near-constancy of the glomerular capillary blood pressure implies that a uniform vasodilatation occurs at both the preglomerular and postglomerular arteriolar resistance vessels. Because midterm pregnant rats remain at filtration pressure equilibrium, the glomerular capillary ultrafiltration coefficient cannot be a factor in determining the increase in SNGFR (Baylis, 1986). The gestational increase in SNGFR is therefore the result exclusively of the increase in glomerular plasma flow rate.

In these same micropuncture experiments, measurements were also made of whole kidney GFR and renal plasma flow rate (RPF). The gestational increase in SNGFR was in parallel to the increase in GFR (both rising by approximately 30%), implying an evenly distributed rise in filtration rate in all populations of glomeruli in the kidney. Furthermore, the increase in glomerular plasma flow to the superficial cortical glomeruli was parallel to the rise in RPF, indicating an evenly distributed vasodilatation throughout the kidney. There are studies by others, however, which suggest that in the gravid rat, an intrarenal redistribution of filtration may occur with a shift towards increased filtration in the inner, juxtaglomerular nephrons (Garland and Green, 1982). A major concern with these latter studies relates to the abnormal volume status of the animals. These rats were receiving an IV saline infusion, at the rate of approximately 25% of their extracellular fluid volume per hour, for several hours prior to and throughout the experiment. Given the importance of extracellular fluid volume status in determining both systemic and renal haemodynamics, and given the likelihood that the vasculature of gravidas may respond to changes in plasma volume in a fundamentally different manner to that of non-gravid animals (see below), it is reasonable to give greater credence to observations performed in euvolaemic rather than volume expanded states.

Plasma protein concentrations, albumin to globulin ratio and thence the systemic oncotic pressure are constant throughout the first part of pregnancy

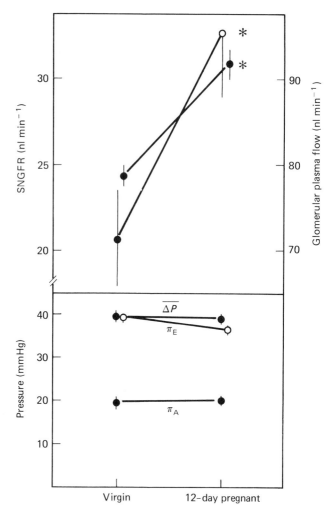

Figure 2. Determinants of glomerular filtration in the virgin and 12-day pregnant, euvolaemic Munich–Wistar rat. In the upper panel, single-nephron GFR (SNGFR) is represented by the solid circles and glomerular plasma flow rate by the open circles. The lower panel summarizes the mean ultrafiltration pressures; the mean transglomerular hydrostatic pressure difference (ΔP), the difference between glomerular capillary blood pressure and the hydrostatic pressure of the fluid in Bowman's space are represented by solid circles. The afferent and efferent oncotic pressures (π_A and π_E respectively) are represented by solid and open circles. Data shown as mean $\pm$ SE; * denotes a significant difference between virgin and 12-day pregnant rats, with $p < 0.05$. From Baylis (1980).

in the rat, although progressive reductions in plasma albumin concentration have been reported beyond about day 12 (Baylis, 1980; Beaton et al, 1961). This contrasts with the situation in women, in whom the plasma albumin

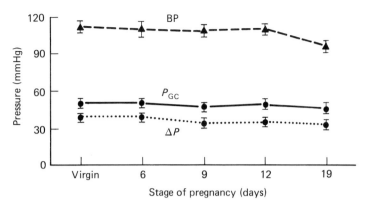

Figure 3. Glomerular blood pressures (P_{GC}), transglomerular hydrostatic pressure difference (ΔP) and arterial blood pressure (BP) measured in virgin, 6, 9, 12 and 20-day pregnant, euvolaemic Munich–Wistar rats. Data are shown as mean $\pm$ SE; * denotes a significant difference from the virgin value. Data shown here is taken from Baylis (1979/80, 1980, 1982, 1987a).

concentration (and thence total plasma protein concentration and systemic oncotic pressure) decreases early in pregnancy and remains low through to term (Lindheimer and Katz, 1985). This decline in systemic oncotic pressure should provide an additional mechanism by which GFR is increased in the normal pregnant woman; however, this mechanism is not predicted to produce very marked effects on GFR. Studies in the male rat have shown that reductions in plasma protein concentration much below the normal range lead to reductions in the glomerular capillary ultrafiltration coefficient, K_f, sufficient to produce filtration pressure disequilibrium and reduce GFR (Baylis, 1986). Thus, a fall in plasma protein concentration is predicted to result in two offsetting changes in the determinants of glomerular ultrafiltration, resulting in little net change in GFR.

Micropuncture studies have now been carried out early (day 6), at midterm (days 9 and 12) and late (days 19–20) in the euvolaemic Munich–Wistar rat (Baylis, 1979/80; 1980; 1982; 1987a). One significant finding from these studies is that no sustained rise occurs in glomerular capillary blood pressure during the gestation period, despite the renal vasodilatation of pregnancy (Figure 3). This has important consequences in regard to possible long-term effects of pregnancy on the maternal kidney, and is discussed in more detail later. The observations in the euvolaemic preparation contrast in some respects with the observations reported in one other study in the 16-day pregnant Munich–Wistar rat, studied under conditions of both mild volume contraction and marked ECF expansion (Dal Canton et al, 1982). In this study, significant increases in glomerular blood pressure and thus in transmural hydrostatic pressure have been reported, together with some fall in K_f. The SNGFR, however, did rise in association with marked increases in glomerular plasma flow rate. No obvious explanation is available for this disparity in experimental findings, although these latter studies were not conducted in the normal plasma volume condition. In any event it seems safe to conclude, from studies in the euvolaemic pregnant rat, that glomerular blood pressure and K_f are not influenced by normal pregnancy in any sustained manner.

Mechanism(s) of the initiation of the gestational rise in GFR

Under most physiologic conditions GFR does not change more than 10–15% (e.g. in response to postural changes and in diurnal rhythm (O'Connor, 1982)). There are only two physiologic situations that elicit large rises in GFR: one is a response to high-protein feeding, and the other is the large and sustained rise that occurs in response to normal pregnancy. Many workers have attempted to elucidate the stimulus responsible for the renal vasodilatation of pregnancy, but to date no one agent has been unequivocally shown to be responsible. However, animal studies have yielded much information in this area, and the following section describes what is known of the gestational vasodilatory stimulus.

The first question is to determine whether the renal vasodilatory stimulus in pregnancy arises from the mother or from feto-placental sources. This has been easy to study in the rat. The rat will readily become pseudopregnant when mated with a vasectomized male; pseudopregnancy is defined as cessation of the oestrus cycle (which may be confirmed by taking daily vaginal smears) with the female remaining in a state of continual dioestrus (exactly as occurs in pregnancy). Pseudopregnancy is also characterized by an accelerated rate of body weight gain (as occurs in pregnancy) and by twice daily prolactin surges which start within hours of mating and last for approximately 9 days. Plasma levels of progesterone are also elevated, as are the non-sex-related hormones including aldosterone and renin. Hormonally, the pseudopregnant rat appears identical to the pregnant rat for the first 10 days after mating (Garland et al, 1987; Schwartz, 1973).

Pseudopregnant rats (studied under euvolaemic conditions) have also been shown to exhibit rises in GFR and RPF similar to gravid animals studied at the same time period after mating. Glomerular micropuncture studies have revealed that the changes in outer cortical single-nephron function are identical in pregnant and pseudopregnant rats, studied on day 9 after mating. Further, the plasma volume expansion that attends normal pregnancy is also evident in pseudopregnant rats (Baylis, 1982). These studies strongly suggest that the feto-placental unit is not necessary for the increase in GFR, and indicate that some maternal stimulus initiates the gestational vasodilatation. Increased GFR has also been reported in volume-expanded Sprague–Dawley rats studied at days 5–6 and 10–11 of pseudopregnancy (Atherton et al, 1982). Serial studies in women during the first trimester of pregnancy have demonstrated a very early increase in GFR, which is also suggestive of a maternal rather than a feto-placental origin of the gestational vasodilatation (Davison and Noble, 1981).

There may, however, be some role of the placenta in the maintenance of the elevated GFR later in pregnancy. Early studies demonstrated that removal of the feto-placental unit on day 13 of pregnancy led to declines in GFR and RPF when renal function was measured on day 18. In contrast, 18-day pregnant rats and rats in whom the fetuses but not the placenta were removed on day 13, both showed increased GFR and RPF (Matthews and Taylor, 1960).

There are dramatic changes in the endocrine status of the female rat after mating, with a number of hormonal candidates as the possible initiators of the gestational vasodilatation. Progesterone levels increase within 24 hours after mating in the rat; however, neither acutely nor chronically administered progesterone has any effect on renal haemodynamic effects (Elkarib et al, 1983; Lindheimer et al, 1976; Matthews, 1963). Pituitary prolactin release is the primary hormonal response to mating in the rat (MacDonald, 1978; Smith and Neill, 1976). Acute prolactin administration has no renal haemodynamic effects in the rat (Elkarib et al, 1983; Baylis, 1984). When administered chronically to the rat, ovine prolactin (like progesterone) produces a chemical form of pseudopregnancy, characterized by cessation of the oestrus cycle and an accelerated rate of body weight gain. Several groups have demonstrated significant increases in GFR and SNGFR following chronic administration of ovine prolactin to female rats (Elkarib et al, 1983; Matthews, 1963; Walker and Garland, 1985). Studies from my laboratory have, however, disagreed with these observations. In micropuncture studies, neither GFR nor SNGFR or its determinants were different in euvolaemic, prolactin-induced pseudopregnant rats and sham injected controls. Prolactin-injected males also showed no renal or glomerular haemodynamic response to prolactin. Further, we failed to observe any difference in GFR or RPF between prolactin-induced pseudopregnant rats and their sham injected controls in longitudinal studies in the conscious rat (Baylis et al, 1985). We are unable to explain these differences between studies, although one general criticism that can be levelled at all these experiments is that ovine rather than rat prolactin was used. Recent work has investigated the renal haemodynamic effects of hyperprolactinaemia induced by grafting rat anterior pituitaries under the renal capsule of female and male rats; in both sexes, GFR rose in rats with pituitary allografts (Conrad et al, 1986; Garland and Milne, 1983). Anterior pituitary implants may produce elevated levels of other hormones apart from prolactin; although, as Conrad points out, since prolactin is under chronic inhibitory control by the hypothalamus (whereas secretion of other anterior pituitary hormones require hypothalamic stimulation) the implants secrete mainly prolactin (Conrad, 1987).

Another line of evidence indicating that native rat prolactin may produce an increase in GFR is the observations in lactation. During lactation, endogenous prolactin levels are extremely high, and the lactating rat exhibits an elevation in GFR above the virgin or late pregnant value, mainly because of increases in RPF (Arthur and Green, 1983). Thus, native prolactin may be the hormone responsible for causing the gestational rise in GFR (and lactation) although the nature of the relationship between hyperprolactinaemia and increased GFR is not yet clear.

It has also been suggested that prostaglandins mediate the renal vasodilatation of pregnancy. It is well documented that urinary prostaglandin (PG) levels rise in normal gravid women, rats and rabbits (Conrad and Colpoys, 1986; Pedersen et al, 1983; Venuto and Donker, 1982), and this has been generally assumed to reflect an increased renal synthesis of these renal

vasodilator hormones. Studies with acute cyclo-oxygenase inhibitors admir
istered to the pregnant rat have indicated that the PGs are not the ren?
vasodilators of pregnancy, since PG synthesis inhibition does not obliterat
the gestational rise in GFR in either anaesthetized rats or in the consciou:
chronically catheterized preparation (Baylis, 1987a; Conrad and Colpoy:
1986). Chronic administration of cyclo-oxygenase inhibitors to the pregnar
rabbit (for three days) similarly does not blunt the gestational rise in GFI
(Venuto and Donker, 1982). The cyclo-oxygenase inhibitors have a number c
other actions too, and interpretation of results using these drugs in intac
animals is therefore difficult. Accordingly, Conrad and Dunn recently use
another approach to study this issue, and compared PG production b?
isolated glomeruli, cortical and papillary slices from pregnant and virgin rat:
They report that PG production is not elevated in pregnancy in any of thes?
preparations, which provides a further indication that the PGs are not th?
renal vasodilators of pregnancy (Conrad and Dunn, 1987). It is interestin
that in their study they were able to document rises in urine PG excretion rat
in the gravid rats; these studies therefore challenge the notion that urinary P(
excretion provides a reflection of intrarenal PG synthesis. In general th?
weight of the evidence does not support a role for PGs in mediating th?
gestational rise in GFR; perhaps this is not surprising, since we previousl
found that when renal vasodilatory doses of PGs are administered to mal?
rats, no increase in GFR occurs despite marked rises in RPF, because of a?
offsetting fall in K_f (Baylis et al, 1976).

The renin–angiotensin II (AII) vasoactive hormone system is also modifie?
during pregnancy (Bay and Ferris, 1979), and could conceivably be involve?
in modulating the gestational renal vasodilatation. The changes that occur i?
the renin–AII system are complicated, and include increases in plasma reni?
activity with a decreased responsivity to vasopressor effects of administere?
AII (Gant et al, 1987; Paller, 1987). This reduced sensitivity to administere?
AII in pregnancy is likely to be the result of postreceptor changes, but whethe
this loss of sensitivity to the vasoconstrictor actions of AII extends to the rena
vasculature has never been directly investigated; this would be a fruitful are?
for further study. There is a suggestion, however, from an early paper that th?
blood vessels of the kidneys of gravidas may not share the gestational loss o
AII responsiveness that is demonstrated by the peripheral vasculature. It wa
shown that AII administration to the late-pregnant rat lowers GFR, while i?
virgins the same manoeuvre leaves GFR unaffected (Sicinska et al, 1971)
There is certainly evidence in the male rat to support the concept that rena
vascular AII receptors differ from those in the periphery (Caldicott et al
1981).

We further investigated the role of AII in the renal response to lat?
pregnancy (Baylis and Collins, 1986). Close to term, GFR begins to fall i?
normal women and in rats. Why this fall should occur is unclear, and migh
signal an increased renal sensitivity to AII late in the gestational period. W?
therefore investigated the renal haemodynamic consequences of acute AI
inhibition using either converting enzyme inhibitors or the AII recepto?
antagonist saralasin. We found that in the conscious, chronically catheterizec
rat, AII inhibition by either method had little effect on GFR or blood pressur?

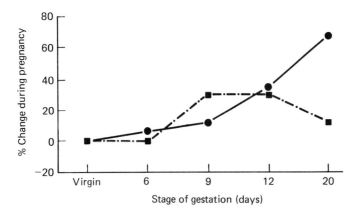

Figure 4. Time course and percentage change, compared to the virgin value, of the gestational increases in GFR (■) and plasma volume (●). These curves are derived from data published by Baylis (1979/80, 1980, 1982, 1987a) and Baylis and Collins (1985).

in late pregnancy. However, when rats were studied in the surgically stressed (but volume-replete, euvolaemic) condition, blood pressure in late-pregnant rats—but not in virgin rats—was highly dependent on AII, since AII inhibition by either method led to profound falls in blood pressure, sometimes to such low levels that renal autoregulation was impaired and GFR fell. We interpreted these data to indicate that the late-pregnant rat is very sensitive to surgical stress, for some currently unknown reason. In view of the lack of a renal response to acute AII inhibition in awake, late-pregnant rats we concluded that a preferential change in the renal responsivity to AII was not a contributing factor to the GFR fall of late pregnancy.

Influence of the plasma volume expansion on the gestational rise in GFR

It is well known that plasma volume expansion, in and of itself, will cause renal vasodilatation and increases in RPF and GFR in non-gravid rats, providing the volume expansion is of sufficient magnitude (Brenner et al, 1972). A slow and cumulative volume expansion occurs during pregnancy in both women and rats, such that close to term, plasma volume is enormously and maximally expanded—up to 70% above the non-pregnant value in the rat (Baylis, 1984; Lindheimer and Katz, 1985). Early in pregnancy, however, the plasma volume expansion is less pronounced even at a time when GFR has already reached its maximum value (Figure 4). Further, close to term when GFR is declining, plasma volume is at its maximum. There is thus a dissociation between the plasma volume increase and the GFR increase of pregnancy in both women and rats; this suggests that the plasma volume expansion of pregnancy is not the primary determinant of the gestational rise in GFR. We have also found, in currently unpublished studies, that when virgin female rats are acutely expanded with a volume of plasma equivalent to that accumulated by the 12-day pregnant rat, trivial and insignificant changes result in GFR, RPF and in outer cortical SNGFR and its determinants. This we take as further suggestive evidence that the gestational plasma volume expansion is not the cause of the rise in GFR seen in pregnancy. There may be an altered sensitivity of the renal vasculature of gravidas to the effects of volume expansion, so that the plasma volume expansion may play some role; but at present there is no information that directly addresses this point. There is, however, considerable evidence to suggest that the body's volume-sensor and control systems are markedly modified by pregnancy, and this is discussed in more detail below.

FUNCTIONAL CHARACTERISTICS OF THE RENAL VASCULATURE DURING PREGNANCY

Response to amino acid infusion and high dietary protein

As discussed above, the renal vasculature of gravid rats is chronically vasodilated compared to that of the virgin animal. It is of interest to determine how the renal vasculature of gravidas will respond to an additional vasodilatory signal, since this will give some insight into the precise nature of the gestational vasodilatation.

In normal, non-gravid humans and experimental animals, either a high-protein meal or an amino acid infusion has been shown to elicit substantial increases in GFR due to a renal vasodilatation with accompanying increases in RPF (Bosch et al, 1983; Castellino et al, 1986; Hostetter, 1984; Meyer et al, 1983). In micropuncture studies in the male rat, IV amino acid infusion was effective in producing rises in GFR and SNGFR which were exclusively the result of increases in RPF and glomerular plasma flow rate, respectively (Meyer et al, 1983). The techniques of amino acid infusion or acute protein loading have recently been used to assess the vasodilatory capacity of the kidney or the 'renal reserve', the ability of the kidney to raise its GFR and RPF due to an acute vasodilatory stimulus (Bosch et al, 1983, 1984; ter Wee et al, 1985). In recent studies in the normal midterm pregnant rat, exhibiting the maximal gestational renal vasodilatation and increases in GFR and RPF, administration of an acute amino acid infusion produced further substantial rises in GFR and SNGFR (Baylis, 1987b). These increments in filtration are exclusively the result of increases in RPF and glomerular plasma flow rate, respectively, due to proportional reductions in afferent and efferent arteriolar resistances with no change in glomerular blood pressure. With similar amino acid loads the percentage increase in GFR and SNGFR was similar in virgin and midterm pregnant rats, although the more vasodilated (pregnant) kidney might have been expected to have already exhausted some of its renal reserve.

In one preliminary report in the normal pregnant woman, a meal of meat protein, given in the third trimester, evoked a substantial acute rise in the endogenous creatinine clearance that was superimposed on the chronic gestational rise in GFR (Brendolan et al, 1985). These findings are in agreement with observations in the rat indicating a significant renal reserve in normal pregnancy, although they await confirmation using inulin clearances. In this regard, preliminary unpublished observations by Beilin, Barron and Lindheimer (personal communication) have suggested that inulin-*p*-amino-hippuric acid (PAH) clearances rise marginally, if at all, in their population of normal gravidas; we await confirmation of these studies.

Comparable experiments to those described above were also conducted in rats that had been chronically maintained on a high-protein dietary intake for 6 months prior to study (Baylis, 1987b). High-protein feeding is thought to present a chronic renal vasodilatory stimulus to the kidney. At the time of measurement of renal haemodynamics, GFR was statistically significantly higher in virgin rats maintained on the high-protein diet compared to those maintained on normal dietary protein. The response to amino acid infusion was blunted in these chronically high-protein fed rats, indicating that the renal reserve of these kidneys was reduced.

Ablation of renal mass is another manoeuvre leading to chronic renal vasodilatation, and observations in the uninephrectomized, non-gravid human have indicated that renal reserve (as assessed by a high-protein meal or amino acid infusion) was still present but blunted, provided that residual renal function was normal (Bosch et al, 1984; ter Wee et al, 1985). In the midterm pregnant rat, GFR was non-statistically significantly higher in midterm pregnant rats maintained on long-term, chronic high-protein feeding, compared to younger midterm pregnant rats maintained on a normal dietary protein intake. There is one preliminary observation in the normal pregnant woman that indicates that the endogenous creatinine clearance tends to be higher in women in whom the dietary protein intake is highest (Shiffman et al, 1987), although no statistics are given in this report, and this would also require confirmation using inulin clearance to measure GFR. Interestingly, the high-protein fed, mid-term pregnant rat exhibited substantial renal reserve to glycine, giving increases in GFR and SNGFR that were much greater than those seen in the high-protein fed virgin.

Pregnancy does seem to confer some unique vasodilatory character to the kidney. For example, in elegant human studies it has been shown that in normal, uninephrectomized women in whom residual renal function is normal, the superimposition of pregnancy evokes a significant gestational rise in GFR despite the underlying and long-term chronic vasodilatory stimulus of nephron loss (Davison et al, 1976). Even more remarkable is the observation that women who are renal transplant recipients also show a gestational rise in GFR providing that function in the transplanted kidney is good prior to conception (Davison, 1985). Given that these single kidneys are hypertro-phied, ectopic, receive at best an abnormal renal nerve supply, and were mostly derived from male donors, the ability to superimpose a gestational rise in GFR is remarkable. Taken together, these observations in gravid women and rats suggest that the hormonal milieu of pregnancy may induce changes that are actually beneficial to the kidney, at least in the short term. Long-term renal consequences of pregnancy are considered later in this chapter.

VOLUME REGULATION IN NORMAL PREGNANCY

Tubuloglomerular feedback in pregnancy

The tubuloglomerular feedback system may be viewed primarily as a volume sensing and regulatory mechanism. This feedback system provides a mechanism whereby the rate of delivery of fluid (or some constituent of tubular fluid) controls the rate of filtration (SNGFR) at the glomerulus of the same nephron (Blantz and Pelayo, 1984). When fluid delivery in the early distal nephron increases this is somehow sensed by the macula densa; a signal is sent to the parent glomerulus, which results in a vasoconstriction with a consequent reduction in SNGFR and restoration of early distal fluid delivery. In some states of chronic volume expansion in the non-gravid animal, tubuloglomerular feedback activity has been found to be suppressed such that very little feedback-evoked change in SNGFR is observed over a wide range of distal fluid flow rates (Blantz and Pelayo, 1984). This adaptive response presumably allows the volume-expanded organism to excrete efficiently the excess volume load.

Although the precise sensor at the macula densa has not yet been determined, it is possible to investigate experimentally the activity of the tubuloglomerular feedback system by varying the rate of fluid delivery to the macula densa. Using the micropuncture technique, a wax block is placed in a midproximal segment of the nephron while the last proximal segment (and thus the early distal segment) are artificially perfused at varying rates with a perfusion pump. The SNGFR at the parent glomerulus is measured by simultaneous micropuncture and collection of fluid from an early proximal segment of the same nephron. Such studies have been performed in the midterm pregnant rat, which exhibits a marked rise in GFR and a more moderate, but statistically significant increase in plasma volume.

As shown in Figure 5, reductions in SNGFR of approximately 30% are achieved in the virgin rat when nephron fluid flow rate is increased over the physiologic range from 10–20 nl min^{-1}. In the midterm pregnant rat, SNGFR is (as anticipated) higher than in the virgin studied under similar conditions. Over the same range of increasing nephron fluid flow rates, the tubuloglomerular feedback system evokes slightly greater than a 30% reduction in SNGFR in pregnant rats. Thus, the tubuloglomerular feedback system is not suppressed in normal pregnancy. These observations rule out the possibility that the gestational rise in GFR results from a 'permissive' increase in GFR secondary to feedback suppression. More importantly, these observations also indicate that the volume expansion of pregnancy (which is about 30% at midterm) does not elicit feedback suppression, whereas in non-gravid volume-expanded states, feedback suppression is generally seen (Baylis and Blantz, 1985).

Other volume-sensing systems in pregnancy

The entire nature of volume sensing and control in pregnancy appears to differ from that seen in non-gravid states. Osmoregulation by the antidiuretic

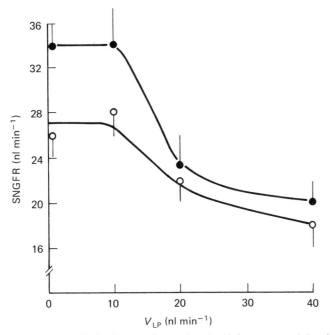

Figure 5. Tubuloglomerular feedback curves for euvolaemic, 12-day pregnant (●) and virgin (○) Munich–Wistar rats. V_{LP} gives the rate at which the late proximal tubule is artificially perfused, and SNGFR is the early proximal SNGFR for the same nephron. See text for details. Data shown as mean $\pm$ SE. From Baylis and Blantz (1985).

hormone system exhibits fundamental alterations in normal gravida which indicate that the expanded volume of pregnancy is sensed as normal—a subject that is dealt with in detail in Chapters 4 and 5. The renin–AII–aldosterone axis is another major volume-sensing and control system. In non-pregnant animals and humans, volume depletion is associated with increased levels of renin, AII and aldosterone, which lead to renal sodium retention and eventual volume repletion. Conversely, extracellular volume expansion is associated with suppression of the renin–AII system with subsequent reductions in the level of aldosterone, permitting increases in renal sodium excretion and eventual restoration of a normal plasma volume. In gravid animals, however, elevated levels of renin, AII and aldosterone co-exist with a plasma volume which in absolute terms is expanded; again indicative that the maternal volume receptor system which controls the renin–AII–aldosterone axis is sensing the plasma volume as either normal or even as contracted (Schrier and Durr, 1987). The renin–AII–aldosterone system in pregnancy is discussed further in Chapter 4.

Another system that has recently been implicated in normal volume homeostasis is the atrial natriuretic peptide system. Secretory granules are present in the left and right cardiac atria, which release a peptide hormone possessing numerous actions including the ability to produce a substantial and rapid natriuresis. In normal animals the synthesis of atrial peptide is directly related to sodium intake (Ballerman and Brenner, 1986). Several studies have so far attempted to evaluate the atrial peptide system in pregnancy. Studies in the rat by Kristensen and colleagues have indicated that the cardiac content of atrial peptide (when extracted, purified and assayed in test animals) is similar in virgin and in late-pregnant rats, despite an absolute increase in plasma volume of 70% above the virgin value (Kristensen et al, 1986). In additional experiments these workers also reported that the renal natriuretic (and peripheral vascular) responsiveness to administered, purified atrial peptides was similar in virgin and pregnant rats when the atrial peptides were administered in quantities calculated to produce equivalent increases in circulating atrial peptide concentrations. This similarity in response persisted over a wide dose range.

These observations differ from a preliminary report by Corwin and Solomon, which claimed that a blunting in the natriuretic effects of administered atrial peptides occurred in pregnant rats. In this latter study, however, atrial peptides were administered in a dose based on body weight; since the plasma volume expands at a disproportionally greater rate than the increase in body weight (after midterm), it is likely that these workers were studying gravid rats with lower atrial peptide concentrations compared to the virgins (Corwin and Solomon, 1985). In another preliminary report, atrial peptide levels in gravid rats and virgin rats, measured by sensitive radioimmunoassay, were found to be unchanged in early pregnancy (days 7–8), elevated at midterm (days 13–14) and returned to baseline in late pregnancy (days 18–19) when the absolute plasma volume was maximally expanded (Nadel et al, 1987).

Although there is not yet a clear picture of the performance of the atrial peptide system in normal pregnancy, most of the available data indicates that the response at late pregnancy, when the plasma volume is maximally expanded, differs from that seen in non-gravid, volume-expanded states. The fact that the majority of the sodium retained during pregnancy is apparently retained over the last part of the gestational period, when maternal plasma volume is at its greatest, is a further anomalous finding.

Taken in concert, the various volume-sensing and control systems discussed above seem to be dramatically altered in normal pregnancy. Despite clear evidence of a large expansion in the absolute value of the plasma volume, the body's volume-sensor systems apparently perceive the maternal plasma volume as normal or even slightly contracted. This raises the concept of 'effective', rather than absolute, vascular volume; in pathophysiologic states abnormal distributions of the intravascular contents might be at least one reason why volume control is deranged. In normal, physiologic pregnancy, the peripheral vasculature is markedly vasodilated; this is the only mechanism by which the elevated cardiac output of pregnancy could be accommodated without producing rises in arterial blood pressure. This vasodilatation of the arterial tree produces substantial pooling of blood in the venous side of the circulation, which would cause arterial volume receptor systems to sense the 'effective' blood volume as less expanded. The presence of an arterio–venous (AV) fistula causes renal sodium retention, suggesting that the 'effective' blood volume may be sensed as reduced (Epstein et al, 1953). As indicated in a recent rat study, the responses of the atrial peptide system in late pregnancy in the rat are consistent with the presence of an 'AV fistula' (the uteroplacental perfusion circuit), while the abrupt rise in atrial peptide levels immediately following parturition is consistent with closure of the same 'AV fistula' (Nadel et al, 1987). There are undoubtedly other reasons for the readjustment of the volume-sensing systems in pregnancy, that are as yet unknown.

The functional implications of all these alterations in volume control systems in pregnancy, together with a consideration of how the sodium retention and volume expansion of pregnancy are mediated, are dealt with in previous review articles (Barron, 1987; Baylis, 1984; Lindheimer and Katz, 1985) and are also considered in Chapters 1, 4 and 5.

THE CONSEQUENCES OF PREGNANCY ON THE MATERNAL KIDNEY

At the present time, nephrologists are concerned about the possibility that prolonged periods of increased single-nephron filtration may exert potentially damaging effects on the glomerulus. This hypothesis is based largely on experiments in male rats with either experimentally induced diabetic nephropathy or with extensive renal ablation, both conditions known to produce substantial increases in filtration, generally referred to as 'hyperfiltration', in the remnant nephrons (Hostetter et al, 1982). A prolonged, high-protein dietary intake is known to accelerate the progression of these glomerular diseases, while low-protein feeding is protective. Since a maintained high-protein intake is believed to lead to chronic renal vasodilatation and increases in renal plasma flow and GFR, the exacerbation due to high-protein feeding may result, at least partly, from the imposition of an additional hyperfiltration stimulus. The hyperfiltration theory holds that the primary damaging stimulus is, in fact, the prolonged increase in glomerular blood pressure that frequently attends renal vasodilatation (Hostetter et al, 1982). Use of converting enzyme inhibitors or dietary protein restriction, both manoeuvres that reduce glomerular blood pressure, confer considerable protection against the progression of new or established glomerular disease (Meyer et al, 1987; Zatz et al, 1987). In hypertensive states the degree of glomerular damage is directly related to glomerular blood pressure, determined largely by the afferent arteriolar tone (Olson et al, 1986: Dworkin et al, 1987).

Pregnancy is also a hyperfiltration state; although, unlike the studies cited above, it is a moderate, physiologic hyperfiltration which proceeds without loss of nephron number or underlying disease and is reversible. Also, as indicated above, there is no sustained increase in glomerular blood pressure during a single gestation period (see Figure 3), since the renal vasodilatation that attends pregnancy involves an even reduction in tone at both afferent and efferent arterioles.

Long-term renal effects of pregnancy when underlying renal function is normal

There are no clinical studies that have directly investigated the long-term effects on the maternal kidney of gestational hyperfiltration. However, we recently performed studies in the female rat to assess the renal consequences of five successive pregnancies and lactations (Baylis and Rennke, 1985). GFR is elevated for over half of the 22-day gestation period, and after parturition GFR will remain high provided the mother is allowed to lactate (Arthur and Green, 1983). Within 4–8 days after delivery the mother will postpartum mate even when lactating and will become pregnant with the next litter. Thus, five successive and closely spaced pregnancies and lactations will cause the mother to remain in a state of continuous nephron hyperfiltration for 6 months, which represents a very long period of hyperfiltration in the life of a rat. The acute studies to assess renal function were not performed until 4–6 weeks after the end of the last lactation, so that no short-term stimuli influenced the kidney. Throughout their lives these rats were chronically maintained on a normal (23%) dietary protein intake.

By the time these rats were acutely studied they were aged approximately 11–12 months, but despite their advancing age there was no evidence of either proteinuria or morphologic damage in repetitively pregnant or age-matched virgin rats (Baylis and Rennke, 1985). In the renal function experiments there was no evidence that repetitive pregnancies caused any reduction in GFR or adverse alterations in glomerular or renal haemodynamics. In particular, there was no elevation in glomerular blood pressure despite the prolonged period of renal vasodilatation. On the contrary, glomerular function seemed to be mildly better in repetitively pregnant rats compared to virgin rats, as assessed by significantly greater values of SNGFR in the breeders. Thus, pregnancy *per se* does not lead to any acceleration in the non-specific, age-dependent deterioration in renal function in animals whose kidneys were previously normal.

Effects of pregnancy when underlying renal function is compromised

There is evidence in the clinical literature that pregnancy in women with underlying renal disease can, on occasion, lead to a rapid worsening of the disease with acceleration in the rate of progression to end-stage renal failure (Becker et al, 1985). The consequence (both short-term and long-term) of pregnancy in women whose renal disease is not severe (i.e. those women exhibiting only mild or moderate impairment in renal function prior to conception) is a subject of controversy (Becker et al, 1985; Katz and Lindheimer, 1985; Hayslett, 1985). Also unknown is the mechanism (or mechanisms) by which pregnancy does aggravate renal function in those situations where a clear relationship between pregnancy and acceleration of underlying renal damage has been shown. There has been little experimental study of this issue in animal models; however, some preliminary observations in the rat are discussed below.

Short-term effects of pregnancy on experimentally induced glomerulonephritis

The glomerular haemodynamic consequences of experimentally induced, immune-mediated glomerulonephritis have been studied in the male rat by a number of workers. With specific antibodies it has been possible to create lesions of varying severity that can be characterized according to glomerular function, using micropuncture techniques (Wilson and Blantz, 1985). Irrespective of the antibody employed, all workers report a marked reduction in the value of the glomerular capillary ultrafiltration coefficient (K_f, the product of glomerular water permeability and filtration surface area). The magnitude of this fall in K_f is sufficient to produce filtration pressure disequilibrium in all animals. In addition, a substantial rise occurs in the glomerular capillary blood pressure in this lesion. Because the alterations in K_f and glomerular capillary blood pressure are offsetting in terms of their influence on glomerular filtration, the net change in SNGFR and GFR is determined by what happens to glomerular plasma flow rate. This varies with different lesions, and can be normal or low; thus SNGFR (and GFR) can remain unchanged or fall in various models of immune-mediated glomerulonephritis (Bohrer et al, 1978; Gushwa et al, 1984).

In recent studies in the rat we investigated the effects of superimposition of pregnancy, to midterm, on the glomerular functional alterations produced in a diffuse model of glomerulonephritis (Baylis and Wilson, 1985). This lesion was associated with a significant proteinuria, with urine protein excretion rising to approximately 15 times the control value by the third week after induction of the disease, and remaining fairly constant thereafter. At three weeks after the induction of the disease, 50% of the rats were mated with a male, and two weeks later (at day 12 of pregnancy), measurements were made of glomerular haemodynamics in both virgin and pregnant rats with glomerulonephritis. The glomerular haemodynamic changes in the virgin female with this model of glomerulonephritis were similar to those reported previously for the male, i.e. high glomerular capillary blood pressure and low K_f. Both SNGFR and GFR were maintained at near-normal values, since glomerular plasma flow rate and renal plasma flow (RPF) were slightly elevated. Of particular note is the finding that pregnancy did not worsen the increase in glomerular blood pressure due to the glomerulonephritis (Baylis and Wilson, 1985).

This constancy of glomerular blood pressure was particularly surprising since the kidneys of rats with glomerulonephritis did exhibit a gestational renal vasodilatation; an increase in GFR occurred in the pregnant rats due to an increase in RPF. It seems remarkable that, given such dramatic alterations in the values of glomerular capillary blood pressure and K_f due to the glomerulonephritis, there remains a capacity to produce further, moderate gestational increases in filtration. Not only does the maternal kidney retain its ability to increase GFR, but there is also no evidence of any exacerbation of the glomerular disease by pregnancy in the short term. The level of proteinuria and the glomerular morphology were similar in virgin and pregnant rats with glomerulonephritis, as were values of glomerular blood pressure and K_f. Although the model of glomerular disease studied here may be considered mild in that there was no net reduction in GFR, there were major alterations in glomerular haemodynamics and a moderately severe proteinuria. In clinical studies in women with underlying, mild to moderate renal disease of diverse origin, gestational increases in GFR were usually observed (Katz et al, 1980).

Long-term effects of pregnancy when superimposed on underlying nephron hyperfiltration

We have made preliminary observations in rats in which five successive pregnancy and lactation cycles were superimposed on the underlying nephron hyperfiltration stimuli of uninephrectomy plus high-protein feeding (40% protein) (Baylis and Collins, 1987). Rats were uninephrectomized and placed on a high-protein intake when they were weaned (at about 30 days old), and were studied at 10–11 months of age. The general time course of these studies was similar to that used in the repetitively pregnant rats with normal underlying renal function, discussed above. Urinary protein excretions were slightly elevated compared to two-kidney controls, but were similar in virgins and repetitively pregnant rats with one kidney and a high-protein diet. The values of K_f were also similar in both groups, and were not different from those of normal, two-kidney rats of the same age maintained on normal dietary protein intakes. The glomerular blood pressure was significantly elevated in rats subjected to the long-term hyperfiltration stimuli of uninephrectomy plus high-protein feeding, but was no higher in repetitively pregnant rats compared to virgins. Due to the cumulative long-term hyperfiltration stimuli that these kidneys were exposed to, SNGFR and glomerular plasma flow rates were higher than the values previously reported for two-kidney, age-matched controls (Baylis and Collins, 1987; Baylis and Rennke, 1985). The SNGFR and GFR were somewhat lower in repetitively pregnant rats compared to virgin rats subjected to uninephrectomy plus high-protein hyperfiltration; however, interestingly, the functional response to glycine was intact in repetitively pregnant rats whereas renal reserve was absent in the virgins (Baylis and Collins, 1987). One might expect the long-term hyperfiltration stimuli of uninephrectomy plus high-protein feeding to have produced a state of near-maximal renal vasodilatation so that the renal reserve capacity of the kidney was attenuated or exhausted; this appeared to occur in virgin rats. Although the repetitively pregnant rats exhibited lower SNGFRs in the control state compared to virgins, the presence of a substantial renal reserve suggests that these kidneys were not further damaged by the additional imposed gestation/lactation hyperfiltration stimuli. Perhaps the absence of glomerular hypertension in pregnancy is the reason for the lack of exacerbation of the underlying glomerular impairment due to long-term uninephrectomy plus high-protein feeding. Another factor to be borne in mind when comparing hyperfiltration due to pregnancy with other hyperfiltration states is that pregnancy occurs only in females! There is considerable evidence in both the human and rat literature that females are protected against the non-specific deterioration in renal function that occurs as part of the normal ageing process (Booker and Williams, 1981; Corman et al, 1985; Elema and Arends, 1975; Friedman and Friedman, 1957; Haley and Bulger, 1983; Morrison et al,

1987; Wesson, 1969). Further, the kidneys of male rats seem to be more at risk (compared to females) from the long-term effects of ablation plus high-protein induced hyperfiltration (Baylis, unpublished data).

SUMMARY

The gestational increase in glomerular filtration rate (GFR) that occurs in the normal rat is the result exclusively of an increase in plasma flow rate, and there is no sustained increase in glomerular capillary blood pressure during a normal pregnancy. The factor or factors that initiate the gestational renal vasodilatation (and plasma volume expansion) are maternal, not fetoplacental in origin. Apart from ruling out prostaglandins as an initiating agent, animal studies have not yet defined the precise nature of the initiating factors; it is unlikely that the gestational plasma volume expansion can be the sole cause of the increased GFR seen in pregnancy. The normal kidney in pregnancy exhibits substantial renal reserve to amino acid infusion, despite being already vasodilated by the gestational stimulus. The renal volume-sensing and control system of tubuloglomerular feedback is fully operative in pregnancy, and appears to be 'reset' to perceive the expanded plasma volume of pregnancy as normal. This observation agrees with many other indications that the sensors perceiving and controlling intravascular volume are reset during a normal pregnancy to enable the mother to accommodate the increased plasma volume without provoking a natriuretic response. Multiple pregnancies do not have any cumulative, long-term deleterious effects on renal function, either when the underlying function is normal or when it has been compromised by removal of renal mass plus high-protein feeding. In the short-term, pregnancy does not worsen kidney function when underlying glomerulonephritis is present. Therefore, the hyperfiltration of pregnancy does not appear to be a damaging entity, unlike other hyperfiltration states studied in the male rat. Still unknown is the mechanism by which pregnancy does worsen underlying glomerular disease in some women. The preliminary data in the rat, presented above, suggest that the exacerbating influence may be something other than the glomerular haemodynamic changes of pregnancy.

Acknowledgements

The support of NIH grant HL31933 is gratefully acknowledged.

REFERENCES

Arthur SK & Green R (1983) Renal function during lactation in the rat. *Journal of Physiology* **334**: 379–393.

Arthur SK & Green R (1986) Fluid reabsorption by the proximal convoluted tubule of the kidney in lactating rats. *Journal of Physiology* **371**: 267–275.

Atherton JC, Bulock D & Pirie SC (1982) The effect of pseudopregnancy on glomerular filtration rate and salt and water reabsorption in the rat. *Journal of Physiology* **324**: 11–20.

Ballerman BJ & Brenner BM (1986) Role of atrial peptides in body fluid homeostasis. *Circulation Research* **58:** 619–631.

Barron WM (1987) Volume homeostasis during pregnancy in the rat. *American Journal of Kidney Disease* **9:** 296–302.

Bay WH & Ferris TF (1979) Factors controlling plasma renin and aldosterone during pregnancy. *Hypertension* **1:** 410–415.

Baylis C (1979/1980) Effect of early pregnancy on glomerular filtration rate and plasma volume in the rat. *Renal Physiology* **2:** 333–339.

Baylis C (1980) The mechanism of the increase in glomerular filtration rate in the 12 day pregnant rat. *Journal of Physiology* **305:** 405–414.

Baylis C (1982) Glomerular ultrafiltration in the pseudopregnant rat. *American Journal of Physiology* **243:** F300–F305.

Baylis C (1984) Renal hemodynamics and volume control during pregnancy in the rat. *Seminars in Nephrology* **4:** 208–220.

Baylis C (1986) Glomerular filtration dynamics. In Lote CJ (ed.) *Advances in Renal Physiology*, pp 33–83. London: Croom Helm.

Baylis C (1987a) Renal effects of cyclooxygenase inhibition in the pregnant rat. *American Journal of Physiology* (in press).

Baylis C (1987b) Effect of amino acid infusion as an index of renal reserve in pregnancy in the rat. Submitted for publication.

Baylis C & Blantz RC (1985) Tubuloglomerular feedback activity in virgin and pregnant rats. *American Journal of Physiology* **249:** F169–F173.

Baylis C & Collins RC (1986) Angiotensin II inhibition on blood pressure and renal hemodynamics in pregnant rats. *American Journal of Physiology* **250:** F308–F314.

Baylis C & Collins R (1987) Glomerular hemodynamics and renal reserve in uninephrectomized (UNX), 40% casein fed (40%C) repetitively pregnant (RP) rats compared to virgins. *Kidney International* **31:** 419A.

Baylis C & Rennke HG (1985) Renal hemodynamics and glomerular morphology in repetitively pregnant aging rats. *Kidney International* **28:** 140–145.

Baylis C & Wilson CB (1985) Effects of midterm pregnancy, day 12 (12P) on glomerular hemodynamics in rats with pre-existing glomerulonephritis. *Clinical Research* **33:** 83A.

Baylis C, Deen WM, Myers B & Brenner BM (1976) Effects of some vasodilator drugs on transcapillary fluid exchange in renal cortex. *American Journal of Physiology* **230:** 1148–1158.

Baylis C, Badr KF & Collins R (1985) Effects of chronic prolactin administration on renal hemodynamics in the rat. *Endocrinology* **117:** 722–729.

Beaton GH, Selby AE & Vene MJ (1961) Starch gel electrophoresis of serum proteins. II Slow α_2-globulins and other serum proteins in pregnant, tumor bearing and young rats. *Journal of Biological Chemistry* **236:** 2005–2008.

Becker GJ, Fairley KF & Whitworth JA (1985) Pregnancy exacerbates renal disease. *American Journal of Kidney Disease* **6:** 266–272.

Blantz RC & Pelayo JC (1984) A functional role for the tubuloglomerular feedback mechanism. *Kidney International* **25:** 739–746.

Bohrer MP, Baylis C, Humes HJ, et al (1978) Permselectivity of the glomerular capillary wall. Facilitated filtration of circulating polycations. *Journal of Clinical Investigation* **62:** 72–78.

Booker B & Williams R (1981) Glomerular hemodynamics in aged rats. *Kidney International* **19:** 195A.

Bosch JP, Saccaggi A, Lauer A et al (1983) Renal functional reserve in humans: effect of protein intake on glomerular filtration rate. *American Journal of Medicine* **75:** 943–950.

Bosch JP, Lauer A & Glabman S (1984) Short term protein loading in assessment of patients with renal disease. *American Journal of Medicine* **77:** 873–897.

Brendolan A, Bragantini L, Chiaramonte S et al (1985) Renal functional reserve in pregnancy. *Kidney International* **28:** 232A.

Brenner BM, Troy JL, Daugharty TM, Deen WM & Robertson CR (1972) Dynamics of glomerular ultrafiltration in the rat. II Plasma flow dependence of GFR. *American Journal of Physiology* **223:** 1184–1190.

Caldicott WJH, Taub KJ, Margulies SS & Hollenberg N (1981) Angiotensin receptors in glomeruli differ from those in renal arteries. *Kidney International* **19:** 687–693.

Castellino P, Coda B & DeFronzo RA (1986) Effect of amino acid infusion on renal hemodynamics in humans. *American Journal of Physiology* **251:** F132–F140.

Conrad KP (1984) Renal hemodynamics during pregnancy in chronically catheterized conscious rats. *Kidney International* **26:** 24–29.

Conrad KP (1987) Possible mechanisms for changes in renal hemodynamics during pregnancy: studies from animal models. *American Journal of Kidney Disease* **9:** 253–259.

Conrad KP & Colpoys MC (1986) Evidence against the hypothesis that prostaglandins are the vasodepressor agents of pregnancy. *Journal of Clinical Investigation* **77:** 236–245.

Conrad KP & Dunn MJ (1987) Renal synthesis and urinary excretion of eicosinoids during pregnancy in the rat. *American Journal of Physiology* (in press).

Conrad KP, Brinck-Johnsen T & Adler RA (1986) Evidence that chronic hyperprolactinemia increases renal hemodynamics. *Clinical Research* **34:** 695A.

Corman B, Pratz J & Poujeol P (1985) Changes in anatomy, glomerular filtration and solute excretion in ageing rat kidney. *American Journal of Physiology* **248:** R282–R287.

Corwin E & Solomon S (1985) Atrial natriuretic factor in pregnancy. *Federation Proceedings* **44:** 815A.

Dal Canton A, Conte G, Esposito C et al (1982) Effects of pregnancy on glomerular dynamics: micropuncture study in the rat. *Kidney International* **22:** 608–612.

Davison JM (1985) The effect of pregnancy on kidney function in renal allograft recipients. *Kidney International* **27:** 74–79.

Davison JM & Dunlop W (1980) Renal hemodynamics and tubular function in normal human pregnancy. *Kidney International* **18:** 152–161.

Davison JM & Noble MCB (1981) Serial changes in 24h creatinine clearance during normal menstrual cycles and during the first trimester of pregnancy. *British Journal of Obstetrics and Gynaecology* **88:** 10–17.

Davison JM, Uldall PR & Walls J (1976) Renal function after nephrectomy in renal donors. *British Medical Journal* **1:** 1050–1052.

Dworkin LD, Feiner HD & Randazzo J (1987) Glomerular hypertension and injury desoxycorticosterone-salt rats on antihypertensive therapy. *Kidney International* **31:** 718–724.

Elema JD & Arends A (1975) Focal and segmental glomerular hyalinosis and sclerosis in the rat. *Laboratory Investigation* **33:** 554–561.

Elkarib AO, Garland HO & Green R (1983) Acute and chronic effects of progesterone and prolactin on renal function in the rat. *Journal of Physiology* **337:** 389–400.

Epstein FH, Post RS & McDowell RM (1953) Effects of arteriovenous fistula on renal hemodynamics and electrolyte excretion. *Journal of Clinical Investigation* **32:** 233–240.

Friedman SM & Friedman CL (1957) Salt and water balance in ageing rats. *Gerontology* **1:** 107–121.

Gant NF, Whalley PJ, Everett RB, Worley RJ & MacDonald PC (1987) Control of vascular reactivity in pregnancy. *American Journal of Kidney Disease* **9:** 303–307.

Garland HO & Green R (1982) Micropuncture study of changes in glomerular filtration rate and ion and water handling by the rat kidney during pregnancy. *Journal of Physiology* **329:** 389–409.

Garland HO & Milne CM (1983) Altered renal function in chronically hyperprolactinemic rats – effects of ovariectomy. *Proceedings of the International Union of Physiological Sciences* **15:** 506A.

Garland HO, Atherton JC, Baylis C, Morgan MRA & Milne CM (1987) Hormone profiles for progesterone, estradiol, prolactin, plasma renin activity, aldosterone and corticosterone during pregnancy and pseudopregnancy in two strains of rats; correlation with renal studies. *Journal of Endocrinology* (in press).

Gushwa LC, Wilson CB & Blantz RC (1984) Chronic effects of concomitant hypertension on glomerular hemodynamics in a model of antiglomerular basement membrane nephritis. *Clinical Research* **32:** 533A.

Haley DP & Bulger RE (1983) The ageing male rat: structure and function of the kidney. *American Journal of Anatomy* **167:** 1–13.

Hayslett JP (1985) Pregnancy does not exacerbate primary glomerular disease. *American Journal of Kidney Disease* **6:** 273–277.

Hostetter TH (1984) Human renal response to a meat meal. *American Journal of Physiology* **250,** F613–F618.

Hostetter TH, Rennke HG & Brenner BM (1982) The case for intrarenal hypertension in the initiation and progression of diabetic and other glomerulopathies. *American Journal of Medicine* **72:** 375–380.

Ichikawa I, Maddox DA, Cogan MC & Brenner BM (1978) Dynamics of glomerular ultrafiltration in euvolemic Munich–Wistar rats. *Renal Physiology* **1,** 121–131.

Katz AI & Lindheimer MD (1985) Does pregnancy aggravate primary glomerular disease. *American Journal of Kidney Disease* **6:** 261–265.

Katz AI, Davison JM, Hayslett JP, Singson E & Lindheimer MD (1980) Pregnancy in women with kidney disease. *Kidney International* **18:** 192–206.

Kristensen CG, Nakagawa Y, Coe FL & Lindheimer MD (1986) Effect of atrial natriuretic factor in rat pregnancy. *American Journal of Physiology* **250:** R589–R594.

Lindheimer MD & Katz AI (1985) Renal physiology in pregnancy. In Seldin DW & Geibisch G (eds), *The Kidney: Physiology and Pathophysiology,* vol. 2, pp 2017–2042. New York: Raven Press.

Lindheimer MD, Koeppen B & Katz AI (1976) Renal function in normal and hypertensive pregnant rats. In Lindheimer MD, Katz AI & Zuspan FP (eds) *Hypertension in Pregnancy,* pp 217–274. New York: John Wiley.

Lindheimer MD, Barron WM, Durr JA & Davison JM (1987) Water homeostasis and vasopressin release during rodent and human gestation. *American Journal of Kidney Disease* **9:** 270–275.

MacDonald GJ (1978) Factors involved in maintenance of pregnancy in the rat: the temporal need for estrogen, prolactin and the ovary. *Biology of Reproduction* **19:** 817–823.

Matthews BM (1963) Effect of hormones, placental extracts and hypophysectomy on inulin and para-aminohippurate clearances in the anesthetized rat. *Journal of Physiology* **165:** 1–9.

Matthews BM & Taylor DW (1960) Effects of pregnancy on inulin and para-aminohippurate clearances in the anesthetized rat. *Journal of Physiology* **151:** 385–389.

Meyer TM, Ichikawa I, Zatz R & Brenner BM (1983) The renal hemodynamic response to amino acid infusion in the rat. *Transactions of the Association of American Physicians* **96:** 76–83.

Meyer TW, Anderson S, Rennke HG & Brenner BM (1987) Reversing glomerular hypertension stabilizes glomerular injury. *Kidney International* **31:** 752–759.

Morrison RBI, Davison JM & Kerr DNS (1987) Clinical physiology of the kidney: tests of renal function and structure. In Weatherall DJ, Ledingham JGG & Warrell DA (eds) *Oxford Textbook of Medicine,* pp 18.17. Oxford: Oxford University Press.

Nadel AS, Ballerman BJ, Anderson S, Troy JL & Brenner BM (1987) Adaptation of intravascular volume during normal pregnancy. *Kidney International* **31:** 281A.

O'Connor WJ (1982) *Normal Renal Function.* London: Croom Helm.

Olson JL, Wilson SK & Heptinstall RH (1986) Relation of glomerular injury to pre-glomerular resistance in experimental hypertension. *Kidney International* **29:** 849–857.

Paller MS (1987) Decreased pressor responsivity in pregnancy: studies in experimental animals. *American Journal of Kidney Disease* **9:** 308–311.

Pedersen EB, Christensen NJ, Christensen P et al (1983) Preeclampsia – a state of prostaglandin deficiency? Urinary prostaglandin excretion, the renin-aldosterone system, and circulating catecholamines in preeclampsia. *Hypertension* **5:** 105–111.

Schrier RW & Durr JA (1987) Pregnancy: an overfill or underfill state. *American Journal of Kidney Disease* **9:** 284–289.

Schwartz NB (1973) Mechanisms controlling ovulation in small mammals. In Greep RO & Astwood EB (eds), *Handbook of Physiology,* Endocrinology II, Part 1, pp 125–146. Baltimore: Waverly Press.

Shiffman R, Tejani N, Verma U & McNerney R (1987) Renal function and dietary protein intake in pregnancy. *Kidney International* **31:** 426A.

Sicinska J, Bailie MD & Rector FC (1971) Effects of angiotensin on blood pressure and renal function in pregnant and non pregnant rats. *Nephron* **8:** 375–381.

Smith MS & Neill JD (1976) Termination at midpregnancy of two daily surges of prolactin initiated by mating in the rat. *Endocrinology* **98:** 696–701.

ter Wee PM, Geerlings W, Rosman JB, Sluiter WJ, van der Geest S & Donker AJM (1985) Testing renal reserve filtration capacity with an amino acid solution. *Nephron* **41:** 193–199.

Venuto RC & Donker AJM (1982) Prostaglandin E$_2$, plasma renin activity and renal function throughout rabbit pregnancy. *Journal of Laboratory and Clinical Medicine* **99:** 239–246.

Walker J & Garland HO (1985) Single nephron function during prolactin-induced pseudopregnancy in the rat. *Journal of Endocrinology* **107:** 127–131.

Wesson LJ (1969) *Physiology of the Human Kidney*, pp 96–108. New York: Grune & Stratton.

Wilson CB & Blantz RC (1985) Editorial: Nephroimmunopathology and pathophysiology. *American Journal of Physiology* **248:** F319–F331.

Zatz R, Anderson S, Meyer TW, Dunn BR, Rennke HG & Brenner BM (1987) Lowering of arterial blood pressure limits glomerular sclerosis in rats with renal ablation and in experimental diabetes. *Kidney International* **31:** suppl. 20, S-123–129.

3

Renal tubular function in the gravid rat

J. C. ATHERTON
R. GREEN

It is generally accepted that the increase in glomerular filtration rate, detected early in gestation in the rat and human, is maintained for most of the gestational period (see Chapters 1 and 2). Such increases are large enough (20–40% in rats and 50–100% in women) to result in increases in ultrafiltrable solutes delivered to the nephron, even for solutes such as sodium whose concentration in plasma decreases as pregnancy advances (Durr et al, 1981). These dramatic increases in filtered load would lead to severe, rapid wasting of essential solutes and to volume depletion unless accompanied by parallel changes in tubular reabsorption and/or significant increases in food and fluid intake. In fact, one characteristic feature of pregnancy is that it is associated not with loss of electrolytes and water but with their net retention to such an extent that extracellular fluid volume is expanded (see Chapters 4 and 5).

This chapter is concerned with alterations in tubular handling of solutes and water during normal pregnancy in the normotensive rat. The limited data available for gravid, spontaneously hypertensive rats are also included. Much of the data has come from experiments in which the kidney has been treated as a 'black box', and hence many of the changes in reabsorption relate to the whole kidney; information on the underlying mechanisms and nephron sites involved is sparse. Micropuncture and microperfusion experiments have been reported and have made invaluable contributions to our understanding of altered function. However, since such experiments, of necessity, are per-formed in anaesthetized animals that have undergone extensive surgery, the possibility of different responses to surgical intervention between virgins and animals at different stages of pregnancy cannot be ignored (Davison and Lindheimer, 1980).

The recent suggestion (Thomsen, 1984) that the clearance of administered lithium can be used as a measure of fluid (sodium and water) passing from the proximal tubules into loops of Henle, if correct, provides new and exciting possibilities for investigation of salt and water reabsorption in proximal tubules and in distal nephron segments (which include the loop of Henle, distal convoluted tubule and collecting duct) of conscious animals and humans. However, it must be emphasized that unequivocal validation of this method is still awaited, although values for outflow of fluid from the proximal tubule using this method are more realistic than those using other markers of

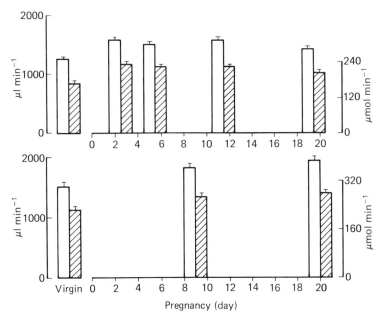

Figure 1. Reabsorption of water (□) and sodium (▦) by the whole kidney in virgin controls and rats at various stages of pregnancy. Data are mean values ± SEM. The upper panel presents data from anaesthetized rats infused with 0·9% saline and is calculated from Atherton and Pirie (1981). The lower panel presents data from conscious rats infused with 2.5% dextrose (Atherton et al, 1988).

proximal tubular function (urea—Goldstein et al, 1969; uric acid and phosphate—Gallery and Gyory, 1979; free water clearance—Seldin and Rector, 1973). Critical appraisals of the method and the experimental conditions in which it appears to be of value are presented in a number of recent publications (Thomsen, 1984; Thomsen and Leyssac, 1986a, 1986b; Atherton et al, 1987; Navar and Schafer, 1987; Skøtt et al, 1987).

SALT AND WATER REABSORPTION

Whole kidney studies

Although enhanced, whole-kidney reabsorption of salt and water is recognized as a consistent feature of normal pregnancy in rats, the exact stage of the gestational period when changes can be detected is controversial. Increased reabsorption has been reported as early as two to three days after mating (Atherton and Pirie 1981) and during the second week of gestation (Atherton and Pirie, 1981; Bishop and Green, 1981; Garland and Green, 1982; Atherton, 1983; Conrad, 1984; Atherton et al, 1988) (Figure 1). In contrast, others (Lichton, 1963; Lindheimer and Katz, 1971) did not detect changes in early and mid-gestation. Controversy also exists concerning changes close to term;

some reports suggest increased reabsorption (Atherton and Pirie, 1981; Atherton, 1983; Atherton et al, 1988; Hutchinson, 1987) (Figure 1) while others show no significant change from amounts reabsorbed by virgins (Arthur and Green, 1983, 1986; Churchill et al, 1982; Conrad, 1984). Observations of increased reabsorption at both mid-gestation and late gestation in New Zealand spontaneously hypertensive rats (Hutchinson, 1987) are also at variance with data in Wistar Kyoto spontaneously hypertensive rats (Lindheimer et al, 1983).

When reabsorption is expressed as a fraction of the filtered load it was found to be increased throughout pregnancy in animals infused with saline (Lichton, 1963; Lindheimer and Katz, 1971; Atherton and Pirie, 1981; Garland and Green, 1982; Atherton, 1983; Hutchinson, 1987) including New Zealand hypertensive late-pregnant rats (Hutchinson, 1987). In contrast, unaltered fractional reabsorption was observed at 9 and 20 days of pregnancy in animals infused with 2.5% dextrose to induce and maintain a steady-state water diuresis (Atherton et al, 1988); even reduced fractional reabsorption was seen throughout pregnancy when Ringer's solution was infused at 10 μl min^{-1} 100 g^{-1} body weight (Conrad, 1984).

Many possibilities could be advanced to account for these discrepant observations in whole-kidney reabsorption; but it is significant that changes in absolute reabsorption were dependent on changes in glomerular filtration. Thus the important question is why there are differences in glomerular filtration rate at various stages of pregnancy.

To account for the lack of difference in glomerular filtration rate (and presumably reabsorption) between virgin and 8–10 day pregnant rats, Davison and Lindheimer (1980) suggested that the differences others had observed at mid-gestation were perhaps artefacts arising from the administration of large fluid loads. This now appears not to be the case; although alterations in *fractional* reabsorption may be related to the infusion protocol (see above), increases in *absolute* reabsorption at mid-gestation have been demonstrated using a wide variety of infusion rates and infusates.

Anaesthesia and (more relevant) surgical intervention have marked depressive effects on kidney function (Maddox et al, 1977; Thomsen and Olesen, 1980; Walker et al, 1983). In one study using term-pregnant anaesthetized animals that had been subjected to extensive surgery for micropuncture experiments, glomerular filtration rate and whole kidney reabsorption of salt and water were similar to values obtained in virgin controls (Churchill et al, 1982); a further study showed no change in glomerular filtration rate, a non-significant rise in absolute reabsorption but a significant rise in fractional reabsorption (Arthur and Green, 1983); a third study had no data on reabsorption but showed no significant increases in glomerular filtration rate with virgins (Arthur and Green, 1986); in the fourth study (Garland and Green, 1982) although glomerular filtration rate and reabsorption were significantly greater at term than in virgins, they were reduced compared to values earlier in gestation. These latter experiments were consistent with data from anaesthetized animals not prepared for micropuncture (Atherton and Pirie, 1981).

Conrad (1984), using conscious animals studied throughout the whole gestational period, also detected a fall in glomerular filtration rate at day 20 when absolute reabsorption returned towards pre-pregnancy values. Studies in our laboratory using conscious animals infused with either 0.9% saline (Atherton, 1983; Atherton and Hutchinson, 1987) or 2.5% dextrose (Atherton et al, 1988) (Figure 1) failed to demonstrate such a preterm fall and are thus comparable to those reported by Davison and Lindheimer (1980). However, in our studies both glomerular filtration and reabsorption might have risen after the ninth day of pregnancy with a subsequent fall to term.

Conrad's experiments (1984) raise another possible cause of these differences, i.e. that the exact day prior to parturition on which the studies were undertaken could be of importance. Days of pregnancy are usually counted from the morning on which a plug of cervical mucus appears on the cage floor; mating could have occurred 12–24 hours earlier. In our laboratory this is designated as day 0 whereas others (Conrad, 1984) designate it as day 1. Thus, there may be up to two days difference in dates at which studies were performed. Immediately after parturition, glomerular filtration rate and reabsorption are comparable to virgin controls (Arthur and Green, 1983, 1986). When does the decline from raised values in pregnancy occur? Is it a consequence of the major upheaval in whole body haemodynamics and fluid volume *at* parturition, or does it start *prior* to parturition? If the latter, then differences in counting the days of pregnancy might be important.

In spite of differences prior to term, the consensus of opinion is that whole-kidney absolute reabsorption is increased at certain, if not all, stages of gestation in the rat. Do these changes represent a direct renal adaptation to pregnancy which contributes to expansion of extracellular fluid volume, or are they just a passive consequence of volume expansion and consequent changes in the filtered loads at the glomeruli? Expansion of extracellular fluid volume implies that there is an imbalance between the intake of salt and water and their excretion. Metabolic balance studies (Churchill et al, 1980; Atherton et al, 1982b) have clearly demonstrated that increases in food and water intake are not matched by parallel increases in salt and water output during the second half of gestation. Since, in all studies, the output of solutes and water increased (see Figure 4 for calcium, magnesium, urate and urea), expansion of extracellular fluid volume must be primarily related to increased intake. Thus, the increased renal reabsorption prevents volume depletion rather than making a direct contribution to volume expansion. Data from infusion studies are also consistent with this interpretation. Salt and water output in conscious, pregnant animals are *usually* higher than or equal to values in virgin controls, although this may reflect a response to the infusion rather than a renal adaptation to pregnancy.

Sodium and water reabsorption in the proximal tubule

The increase in whole-kidney reabsorption of salt and water in pregnant rats is so great that increased reabsorption in the proximal tubule would be expected to contribute significantly. Direct experiments in rats, measuring sodium and water reabsorption by the rate of shrinkage of droplets of sodium chloride

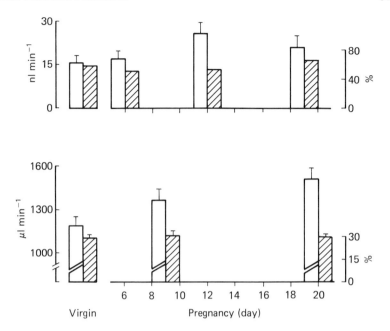

Figure 2. Fluid handling by the proximal tubule in virgin controls and rats at various stages of pregnancy. Data represent mean (±SEM) absolute fluid reabsorption (□) and fractional fluid excretion (▨) from the proximal tubules obtained using micropuncture techniques in 0.9% saline-infused rats (upper panel, from Garland and Green, 1982) and using lithium clearance as a marker of fluid delivery from the proximal tubules to the loops of Henle in 2.5% dextrose-infused rats (lower panel, from Atherton et al, 1988).

solution between oil blocks in the proximal convoluted tubule (split-drop experiments) showed that the rate of reabsorption per unit area was not altered in pregnancy (Garland and Green, 1982). In other words, the intrinsic reabsorptive capacity of the tubule is not increased. Thus, if the proximal tubule reabsorbs more in pregnancy, it must do so because of its increased length (Garland et al, 1978) or because reabsorption is flow-dependent. Reabsorption from the proximal tubule is dependent on the rate of fluid flow along the nephron in male and female virgin rats (Green et al, 1981; Häberle and Von Baeyer, 1983; Garland et al, 1984); but in pregnancy, at least in 12-day pregnant rats, reabsorption is no longer flow dependent (Walker, 1983; Garland et al, 1984).

That there is increased sodium and water reabsorption in the proximal tubule is certainly borne out by experiments in mid-gestation using either micropuncture techniques in anaesthetized rats infused with 0.9% saline (Garland and Green, 1982) or lithium clearance in conscious rats infused with 2.5% dextrose (Atherton et al, 1988); fractional reabsorption by the proximal tubules was unaltered (Figure 2). However, as shown in Figure 2, in late gestation there are differences between data obtained by these techniques. In micropunctured animals, absolute proximal fluid reabsorption had returned to values seen in virgin controls and fractional reabsorption was reduced (Garland and Green, 1982; Arthur and Green, 1986); whereas in conscious, Sprague-Dawley rats (Atherton et al, 1988) and New Zealand normotensive and spontaneously hypertensive rats (Hutchinson, 1987), absolute and fractional reabsorption were comparable to data obtained in mid-gestation in that fractional reabsorption is unaltered. Similar findings have been made in late pregnancy in humans (Atherton et al, 1988). Arthur and Green (1986) argued that reduced fractional reabsorption was not unexpected, since it is well known that extracellular fluid volume expansion decreases fractional reabsorption in proximal tubules (Landwehr et al, 1967). However, although this may be the case following acute volume expansion, it may not occur during chronic expansion (Daugherty et al, 1973). In addition, if volume homeostasis is reset during pregnancy (see Chapters 2 and 4), alterations in fractional reabsorption at the time of maximal extracellular fluid volume expansion might not be expected.

The reasons for these differences at term are not known. Several factors must be taken into consideration:

1. One of the assumptions on which interpretation of lithium clearance has been based is an equality between plasma and proximal tubular fluid concentrations of lithium. This has not been rigorously tested in pregnancy.
2. Micropuncture experiments measure reabsorption only to the end of the convoluted portion of the tubule, while the clearance of lithium measures reabsorption from the pars recta as well.
3. Micropuncture experiments measure only what happens in superficial tubules, whereas lithium clearance relates to all nephrons. There is some evidence (Garland and Green, 1982; Walker, 1983; Arthur and Green, 1986) that there is a significant redistribution of blood flow in pregnancy which would complicate the interpretation of the two sets of experiments.

Clearly, a satisfactory solution to account for these discrepancies must await the outcome of appropriate experiments to give more detailed information on lithium handling by the proximal tubule in pregnancy. However, it must be stressed that there is agreement except just prior to term.

Sodium and water reabsorption in distal nephron segments

Although sodium and water are reabsorbed together in the proximal tubules, their transport paths are to a large extent separate in distal nephron segments. In the loop of Henle, sodium enters and water leaves the descending limb, and sodium is reabsorbed by a variety of mechanisms in the ascending limb. Thus increased reabsorption of sodium relative to water implies alteration in the function of the loop and should result in a lower sodium concentration in the fluid delivered to early distal tubules.

In micropuncture studies, Garland and Green (1982) showed that the fraction of fluid delivered to the early distal tubule was similar in virgins and at all stages of pregnancy, even though different amounts of fluid escaped from the proximal tubule. This implies that there is increased reabsorption of fluid

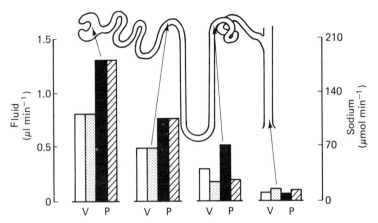

Figure 3. Total amount of fluid and sodium remaining at different points along nephrons in the kidneys of virgin and 12-day pregnant animals. □ indicates fluid and ▨ sodium in virgin animals (V), while ■ indicates fluid and ▨ sodium in pregnant animals (P). Scales are chosen such that equal height of the sodium and fluid columns indicates isotonicity. If the fluid column is higher then there is hypotonicity, while if the sodium column is higher the fluid is hypertonic. From Green (1986) with permission.

by the loop of Henle during pregnancy and particularly prior to term (Figure 3). This was confirmed directly by Green and Hatton (1987) even when the confounding influence of increased tubular flow rate had been eliminated.

Sodium concentration in early distal tubular fluid was much less in pregnant animals than in virgin controls (Figure 3) and this was taken as presumptive evidence that the loop of Henle reabsorbed more sodium in pregnancy. This was confirmed by perfusing loops of Henle; at 12 and 19 days of pregnancy 60% of the load was reabsorbed, whereas in virgins only 45% was reabsorbed (Green and Hatton, 1987). Unfortunately these experiments do not permit identification of the part of the loop (descending or ascending thin limb, thick ascending limb or even the proximal straight tubule) that is involved.

Distal convoluted tubules and/or collecting ducts also appear to increase the reabsorption of sodium and water in pregnancy (Garland and Green, 1982) (Figure 3), but direct experimental proof has yet to be obtained.

Studies using lithium clearance have also shown that nephron segments distal to the proximal tubule reabsorbed, in absolute terms, more sodium and water in pregnant, normotensive and hypertensive rats as well as in human pregnancy (Atherton et al, 1988; Hutchinson, 1987) but it is impossible to identify the site at which this occurs. However, if reabsorption is related to the amount of fluid or sodium presented to distal nephron segments (the so-called distal fractional reabsorption), differences in infusates cause different fractional reabsorption. In 0.9% saline-infused rats increased fractional reabsorption is apparent, whereas in 2.5% dextrose-infused animals fractional reabsorption is unaltered. In third-trimester women, distal fractional sodium and water reabsorption were increased (Atherton et al, 1988).

The mechanisms responsible for altered water and sodium handling by distal nephron segments remain to be elucidated. For sodium, many mechanisms can be suggested but no definite answer can be given. There may be redistribution of blood flow so that the medullary blood vessels have a greater blood flow which washes out the medullary gradient, thereby decreasing sodium entry into the descending limb and facilitating sodium loss from the ascending limb. This is consonant with a small reduction in medullary sodium concentration in pregnant rats (Al-Modhefer, 1984). Additionally there may be changes in the transport of sodium in the thick ascending limb or in the collecting duct, or perhaps changes in permeability.

While there is no increased medullary osmolality (Al-Modhefer, 1984) which would account for increased water reabsorption by the loop of Henle, the increased sodium reabsorption from the proximal straight tubule or the decreased entry into the descending thin limb of Henle's loop would mean that more of the osmotic equilibration was due to water movement than to sodium. However, this mechanism would be offset by the increased entry of urea (see below). It seems likely that increased water reabsorption—demonstrated in loop microperfusion experiments (Green and Hatton, 1987)—occurs in the proximal straight tubule. In distal tubules, since there is a reduced sodium concentration and a reduced osmolality, more water can be reabsorbed down its osmotic gradient.

The role of antidiuretic hormone (ADH) in more distal segments is uncertain. There are significant differences between plasma ADH concentrations in saline-infused and dextrose-infused virgin rats (Al-Jammaz, 1986) but, certainly in pregnant women, changes in plasma ADH concentration were not detected in spite of changes in plasma osmolality and extracellular fluid volume (see Chapters 4 and 5).

OTHER IONS AND SOLUTES

Potassium

Far less is known about the renal handling of potassium in pregnancy, but where data are available—Garland and Green (1982), using saline-infused anaesthetized rats; Al-Modhefer (1984), using 2.5% dextrose-infused conscious rats—an increase in reabsorption has been demonstrated in both mid-pregnant and late-pregnant rats. In fact, micropuncture experiments using early distal tubule collection sites (Garland and Green, 1982) revealed that not only was there an increase in the total amount reabsorbed, but also the percentage of filtered potassium remaining in the tubule at the puncture site was considerably reduced. Additional experiments involving microperfusion of short loops of Henle to clarify whether such changes were a proximal and/ or a loop phenomenon (Green and Hatton, 1987) revealed that potassium reabsorption was reduced, suggesting that in the earlier experiments proximal tubule potassium reabsorption must have been dramatically increased. Just why the loop reabsorbs less in pregnancy is not known. It is unlikely that there is inhibition of Na^+, K^+ and Cl^- reabsorption in the thick ascending limb of

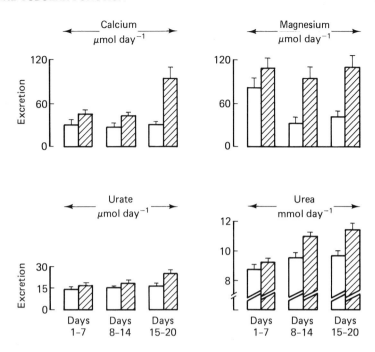

Figure 4. Excretion of calcium, magnesium, urate and urea (per 24 h) during the first, second and third weeks of pregnancy in rats (▨) and for equivalent periods of time in virgin controls (□). Data (mean ± SEM) for calcium are from Green and Hatton (1987), and for urea from Al-Modhefer (1984).

the loop of Henle, because sodium reabsorption was enhanced. Alternatively, a pregnancy-induced increase in normal recycling of potassium (Wright and Giebisch, 1978) with enhanced entry into the thin limb of the loop would be considered as reduced reabsorption. Whatever the reason for reduced reabsorption, it does not cause changes in medullary potassium concentration (Al-Modhefer, 1984).

Calcium and magnesium

In rats maintained in metabolic cages, daily calcium and magnesium excretion increased throughout pregnancy (Figure 4), with the increase being more pronounced in later stages (Green and Hatton, 1987); observations similar to those for calcium excretion in pregnant women (Pitkin, 1985). Attempts using anaesthetized animals to identify the renal mechanisms responsible for the raised calcium output have, to date, failed to confirm a raised output in pregnancy. In fact, reduced calcium excretion in the urine in pregnant rats is a consistent finding despite the normal, pregnancy-associated increase in glomerular filtration rate and unchanged ultrafiltrable calcium concentration in plasma (Hatton, unpublished observations) suggesting, therefore, that in the anaesthetized animal calcium reabsorption is increased. The reasons for this discrepancy between conscious and anaesthetized animals are not known. Clearance experiments in conscious virgin and pregnant animals may help to clarify this issue.

Chloride

Since altered handling of chloride in pregnancy is essentially similar to that of sodium at the whole-kidney level in conscious rats (Atherton, 1983; Al-Modhefer, 1984) and at the single nephron level in anaesthetized rats (Garland and Green, 1982; Green and Hatton, 1987) further comment is not included.

Urea

In pregnant and virgin rats maintained in metabolic cages, the daily output of urea was significantly higher throughout the second half of gestation (Al-Modhefer, 1984) (Figure 4). Unfortunately, in the absence of concurrent measurements of glomerular filtration rate and plasma urea concentration, it is impossible to know if this was the result of an increase in filtered load and/or a reduction in reabsorption. Medullary urea concentration was lower in 6-day and 20-day pregnant rats than in virgin controls (Al-Modhefer, 1984) suggesting that there is medullary washout of urea and/or increased secretion by the loop of Henle. In a separate series of experiments, plasma urea concentrations were lower in 9-day and 20-day pregnant conscious rats prior to the infusion of 2.5% dextrose, and the difference was maintained throughout a seven-hour infusion period; there were no differences in the filtered load despite the elevated glomerular filtration rate in pregnancy, but urinary urea output was not different from that in virgin controls (Al-Modhefer, 1984).

Differences between sodium and total solute handling by the proximal tubule and loop of Henle led to the suggestion that pregnancy was accompanied by an increase in urea secretion into the loop of Henle (Garland and Green, 1982). This has been confirmed subsequently in experiments in which short loops of Henle in 12-day and 19-day pregnant rats were perfused with urea-free solutions (Green and Hatton, 1987). In view of the fact that medullary urea concentration is reduced in pregnancy (Al-Modhefer, 1984) this could only have arisen from increases in the permeability of the loop of Henle.

Uric acid

In view of the importance of the renal handling of uric acid as a diagnostic tool in human pregnancy, it is surprising that so few studies have been undertaken. What is perhaps even more surprising is the distinct lack of information in the rat, although it is well known that the pregnant rat does not become hypertensive. Preliminary experiments in our laboratory (Green and Hatton, unpublished), in which rats were maintained in metabolic cages throughout pregnancy, clearly demonstrated that uric acid excretion is increased throughout the gestational period, although the increase was significant in only the third week of gestation (Figure 4). Subsequent clearance experiments in anaesthetized virgin controls and rats at 9 and 20 days of pregnancy confirmed these findings. In addition, in late-pregnant rats the increased uric acid excretion (and clearance) was more than could be accounted for by the increase in filtered load. In other words, fractional uric acid clearance was increased at 19 days of pregnancy but not at 9 days; these observations are consistent with those of Semple et al (1974) in late gestation in women, but at variance with others (Dunlop and Davison, 1977; Ezimokhai et al, 1981). The nephron sites responsible for the altered uric acid handling in pregnancy have not been identified. It might be predicted (Gallery and Gyory, 1979) that these data demonstrate reduced proximal fluid reabsorption (i.e. increased fractional excretion) late in pregnancy, thereby supporting observations in micropuncture experiments (Garland and Green, 1982). However, since uric acid excretion depends on the filtered load and at least two reabsorptive and secretory processes (Lang, 1981), such a conclusion is not yet justified.

Glucose

For many years it has been known that glucose excretion increases during human pregnancy. This also applies to rat pregnancy (Bishop and Green, 1980) and experiments have been undertaken to identify the nephron sites and investigate the mechanisms involved. Until recently it was thought that, at least in women, this arose from either an increase in the filtered load (Christiansen, 1958) or a reduction in the reabsorptive capacity of the proximal tubules (Welsh and Simms, 1960). However, in free flow micropuncture studies in rats, it was not possible to demonstrate defective glucose reabsorption in the proximal tubule. In fact, even when stressed by infusion of 5% glucose, the proximal convoluted tubules of pregnant rats reabsorbed more glucose than virgins; reduced amounts of glucose were passed on to the loops of Henle in pregnant animals (Bishop and Green, 1981, 1983). Direct experiments have shown reduced glucose reabsorption in the loop of Henle and collecting ducts in pregnant animals (Bishop and Green, 1983) which, for the loop of Henle when plasma glucose concentration is high, appears to be the result of an increase in leakage into the lumen (Bishop et al, 1981). Presumably this indicates a permeability change in the loop; whether a similar mechanism operates in the collecting duct is not known.

FACTORS RESPONSIBLE FOR ALTERED REABSORPTION

The control of salt and water reabsorption in normal kidney function is multifactorial. It is beyond the scope of this review to present a detailed assessment of each to the altered reabsorption of pregnancy; attention is focused here on factors that have been directly investigated in the rat. Some of these have already been considered:

1. The length of the proximal tubule is increased early in pregnancy, and by the end of the first week is 20–25% longer than in comparably aged virgin controls (Garland et al, 1978; Atherton and Pirie, 1981). Since proximal tubular diameter is not reduced, the increase in length is associated with an increase in surface area available for reabsorption. It is not known if other parts of the nephron alter in length, but since a general medullary hypertrophy has been described (Chang et al, 1978), this is a realistic possibility.

2. Normal flow-dependency of reabsorption in the proximal tubule is not evident in pregnancy (Walker, 1983). Reabsorption from the loop of Henle and other parts of the distal nephron is flow-dependent in non-pregnant animals (Landwehr et al, 1967) and may be important in the altered reabsorption in pregnancy.

3. The intrinsic reabsorptive capacity of the proximal tubule is unchanged in pregnancy (Garland and Green, 1982). Since the proximal tubule appears to reabsorb more, it must do so because it is longer.

4. Alteration in the distribution of filtration, favouring increased filtration in juxtamedullary salt-retaining nephrons, may be important (Garland and Green, 1982; Arthur and Green, 1986).

5. Alteration in the permeability of the loop of Henle, e.g. as suggested for urea and glucose (Green and Hatton, 1987) may be significant.

Hormonal effects

It has been suggested that changes in hormonal concentrations might also contribute to the changes in renal function in pregnancy. Removal of fetuses on day 14 of pregnancy in rats did not alter glomerular filtration rate at term, but complete hysterectomy reduced it to pre-pregnancy levels, thereby pointing to the importance of the placenta in maintaining renal changes (Matthews and Taylor, 1960). In early pregnancy, however, placental function is unlikely to be important for changes in salt and water reabsorption (and renal haemodynamics), since similar renal changes occur in pseudopregnant animals where the oestrous cycle is suspended but no fetus is present (Atherton et al, 1982a; Baylis, 1982). This suggests that maternal rather than fetal factors are important to the early changes and their maintenance in the first half of gestation. Since changes in maternal hormonal profiles in early pregnancy are comparable (Pepe and Rothchild, 1974; Smith and Neill, 1976; Garland et al, 1987), it has been suggested that changes in hormone secretion may be important in the genesis of renal changes (Atherton et al, 1982a). The experimental approach adopted to assess the importance of altered hormonal profiles has been to administer each hormone in amounts sufficient to raise plasma concentrations in male or female rats to values determined during pregnancy. It must be emphasized at the outset that so far there is no unequivocal evidence that any hormone has a *direct* involvement in changes in renal function during pregnancy. None of these approaches has been applied to segmental analysis of renal function.

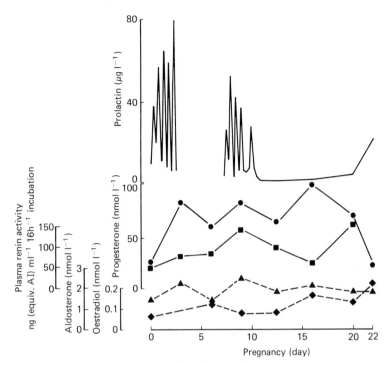

Figure 5. Changes in plasma concentration of oestradiol (♦), aldosterone (▲), renin (■) progesterone (●) and prolactin throughout pregnancy in the rat. Prolactin data for control and days 1–3 are from Smith et al (1976), those for days 7–11 from Smith and Neill (1976) and the remainder of prolactin and all other hormones from Garland et al (1987).

Oestrogens

Although chronic oestrogen administration to humans is associated with sodium retention, an effect on salt and water reabsorption in the rat is controversial. While some investigators observed a decrease in sodium excretion in oestrogen-treated rats (De Vries et al, 1972), others found little (Deming and Leutscher, 1950) or no (Dorfmann, 1949; Simpson and Tait, 1952) antinatriuretic action. The significance of these findings to renal changes in rat pregnancy is obscure since oestradiol concentrations remain low (apart from a transient surge at day 4 to 5) until day 18 of pregnancy, when they rise rapidly until parturition occurs (Yoshinaga et al, 1969; Garland et al, 1987) (Figure 5). Oestriol and other oestrogens have not been measured. Thus, although oestrogens may be implicated in salt and water retention in late pregnancy it seems unlikely that they are involved in the changes in early pregnancy.

Progesterone

Progesterone has a natriuretic effect in humans (Oelkers et al, 1974) which results from competitive inhibition of aldosterone (Ehrlich and Lindheimer,

1972) and possibly from its general vasodilator action on blood vessels (Oparil et al, 1975). However, a natriuretic action was not demonstrated following administration to rats (Lindheimer et al, 1976; El-Karib et al, 1983) although increased potassium retention did occur (El-Karib et al, 1983). Thus, although plasma progesterone concentrations increase in rat pregnancy (Pepe and Rothchild, 1974; Garland et al, 1987) (Figure 5) and no doubt contribute to some of the changes in maternal physiology, e.g. increased body weight and food intake (Hervey and Hervey, 1967; Garland, 1979), it is unlikely that this hormone has a significant role in enhanced sodium and water reabsorption, but it may be the potassium-sparing hormone of pregnancy (El-Karib, 1981).

Prolactin

Prolactin is concerned with volume and osmolal homeostasis in amphibians, birds and fish (Ensor, 1978), but there is controversy about a similar role in mammals. For example, some investigators report that acute administration of prolactin to conscious and anaesthetized rats reduced sodium and water excretion (Lucci et al, 1975; Bliss and Lote, 1982), while others showed effects (including increased potassium reabsorpion) following chronic but not acute administration (El-Karib et al, 1983; Mills et al, 1983). Subsequent studies have shown this to be a specific action of prolactin, rather than a response to general changes in maternal endocrinology through its luteotrophic action and induced state of pseudopregnancy. Thus, altered sodium and water reabsorption were detected in ovariectomized rats (Garland and Milne, 1983) and in hyperprolactinaemic male rats (Garland and Lewis, 1986). These effects might be mediated by a direct action on proximal tubular fluid reabsorption (Walker and Garland, 1985) and/or through an increase in proximal tubular length (Garland, 1979; El-Karib et al, 1983). Observations that prolactin levels rise early in pregnancy (Smith and Neill 1976; Garland et al, 1987) (Figure 5) have led to suggestions that this hormone may be important in accounting for some of the renal function changes in the pregnant rat (Garland et al, 1987). However, its actions could be through alterations in extracellular fluid volume—prolactin can act synergistically with angiotensin as a dipsogen (Kaufman, 1981)—rather than a direct effect on kidney function.

Renin–angiotensin–aldosterone

The role of the renin–angiotensin–aldosterone axis in normal control of salt and water balance is generally accepted. Renin is an enzyme that has no direct renal effects; its action is directed to the formation of angiotensin II which does have important renal actions. In low doses, angiotensin II caused sodium retention (Johnson and Malvin, 1977; Borresen et al, 1982). This is partly due to changes in renal haemodynamics consequent on the vascular actions of angiotensin II, but there is also a direct effect on the renal proximal tubule (Harris and Young, 1977); the latter observations have been confirmed by demonstrating increased proximal tubule fluid excretion in rats following the administration of angiotensin-converting enzyme inhibitors (Shirley et al,

1984). At higher doses, a direct inhibitory effect on proximal sodium reabsorption was reported (Harris and Young, 1977; Schuster et al, 1982). In addition, there are suggestions that angiotensin II might inhibit (Lowitz et al, 1969) or even increase (Johnson and Malvin, 1977) sodium reabsorption in the distal nephron by a direct effect on the tubular cells.

A very important action of angiotensin II is to evoke a prompt and sustained increase in aldosterone secretion from the adrenal cortex. Aldosterone is essential to normal sodium homeostasis in humans and animals through its control of sodium reabsorption and potassium secretion in distal convoluted tubules and collecting ducts (Schwartz and Burg, 1978; Wright and Giebisch, 1978) or even, perhaps, on the ascending limb of the loop of Henle (Sonnenblick et al, 1961) or proximal tubule (Stumpe and Ochwadt, 1968).

In rat pregnancy there is an increase in plasma renin and therefore, by inference, an increase in angiotensin II in early pregnancy and close to term (Whipp et al, 1978; Fowler et al, 1981; Garland et al, 1987) (Figure 5). In mid-gestation, plasma renin activity decreased (Garland et al, 1987). Plasma aldosterone levels are also raised in pregnancy (Whipp et al, 1978; Churchill et al, 1981; Garland et al, 1987), but the lack of correlation between plasma aldosterone and renin concentrations suggests that factors in addition to raised renin are responsible for the increased aldosterone levels (Mulrow and Schneider, 1976; Whipp et al, 1978; Garland et al, 1987) (Figure 5).

The exact role of the renin–angiotensin–aldosterone axis in normal pregnancy remains to be elucidated. Contributions to salt and water retention of pregnancy could be via the dipsogenic action of angiotensin (Epstein et al, 1970), by direct actions on proximal and distal reabsorption of sodium or by offsetting the potential natriuretic effect of progesterone. Indeed, there is a good correlation between progesterone and aldosterone concentrations throughout pregnancy and pseudopregnancy in the rat (Garland et al, 1987).

Antidiuretic hormone

It is generally accepted that the primary actions of ADH include increases in water permeability of certain nephron segments (Handler and Orloff, 1981), increases in urea permeability of the medullary collecting ducts (Rocha and Kokko, 1974) and increases in sodium reabsorption in the loop of Henle (Morel et al, 1981). In addition, ADH may have natriuretic activity (Balment et al, 1984), although others have failed to demonstrate this action (Al-Omar Azzawi and Shirley, 1983; Gellai et al, 1984), and a direct antikaliuretic action (Field et al, 1984).

Many of the changes of distal nephron function in pregnancy are consistent with these known actions of ADH. However, since plasma concentrations of the hormone do not increase in human and rat pregnancy (Durr et al, 1981; Davison et al, 1984) (see Chapters 4 and 5), the only way that ADH could have an effect would be through an increase in the responsiveness to the hormone; in view of the reduced vascular reactivity to ADH in pregnancy (Paller, 1984) this seems unlikely.

Other hormones

The plasma levels of many other hormones increase during human and rat pregnancy—prostaglandins, thyroxine, oxytocin, dopamine and atrial natriuretic peptide. However, the physiological significance of these changes to altered salt and water retention of pregnancy is uncertain. Indeed, in some instances (e.g. thyroxine, atrial natriuretic peptide and prostaglandins) there is no consensus of opinion as to their importance in the control of normal kidney function.

SUMMARY

Pregnancy in the rat is accompanied by enhanced reabsorption of salt and water throughout most, if not all, of the gestational period. Many mechanisms have been suggested but definitive answers are still awaited. The major area of controversy centres around the detection of changes at term. There is general agreement that, at least in mid-gestation, the increase in reabsorption can be attributed to increases in the proximal tubules, the loop of Henle and collecting duct. The contribution of the proximal tubule to the increased reabsorption at term is still uncertain. Enhanced salt and water reabsorption is demonstrated in distal nephron segments irrespective of the stage of gestation. Micropuncture and microperfusion experiments have identified increased reabsorption of water, sodium and chloride in the loop of Henle, but it appears that there is net addition of glucose, urea and potassium to the tubular fluid in this segment which, at least for potassium and glucose, offsets to some extent increased reabsorption by the proximal tubule. Altered renal handling of other solutes (uric acid, calcium and magnesium) also occurs throughout pregnancy but the mechanisms responsible and nephron sites involved remain to be investigated.

Attempts to attribute altered reabsorption to direct renal effects of changes in maternal hormones are inconclusive. Prolactin mimics some of the pregnancy-associated increases in reabsorption following chronic administration to male and non-pregnant female rats. These effects might be due to a direct renal action of the hormone or even to the volume expansion following its dipsogenic action.

REFERENCES

Al-Jammaz IAA (1986) Effect of Inactin anaesthesia on renal function in Sprague Dawley rats. PhD thesis, University of Manchester.
Al-Modhefer AKJ (1984) Renal function, osmoregulation and volume homeostasis during pregnancy in the conscious rat. PhD thesis, University of Manchester.
Al-Omar Azzawi S & Shirley DG (1983) The effect of vasopressin on renal blood flow and its distribution in the rat. *Journal of Physiology* **341:** 233–244.
Arthur SK & Green R (1983) Renal function during lactation in the rat. *Journal of Physiology* **334:** 379–393.
Arthur SK & Green R (1986) Fluid reabsorption by the proximal convoluted tubule of the kidney in lactating rats. *Journal of Physiology* **371:** 267–275.

Atherton JC (1983) Glomerular filtration rate and salt and water reabsorption during pregnancy in the conscious rat. *Journal of Physiology* **334:** 493–504.

Atherton JC & Hutchinson C (1987) Renal haemodynamics during pregnancy in the conscious rat. *Journal of Physiology* **391:** 107P.

Atherton JC & Pirie SC (1981) The effect of pregnancy on glomerular filtration rate and salt and water reabsorption in the rat. *Journal of Physiology* **319:** 153–164.

Atherton JC, Bullock D & Pirie SC (1982a) The effect of pseudopregnancy on glomerular filtration rate and salt and water reabsorption in the rat. *Journal of Physiology* **324:** 11–20.

Atherton JC, Dark JM, Garland HO et al (1982b) Changes in water and electrolyte balance, plasma volume and composition during pregnancy in the rat. *Journal of Physiology* **330:** 81–93.

Atherton JC, Green R, Hughes S et al (1987) Lithium clearance in man: effects of dietary salt intake, acute changes in extracellular fluid volume, amiloride and frusemide. *Clinical Science* **73:** 645–651.

Atherton JC, Bielinski A, Davison JM et al (1988) Sodium and water reabsorption in the proximal and distal nephron in conscious pregnant rats and third trimester women. *Journal of Physiology* (in press).

Balment RJ, Brimble MJ, Forsling ML & Musabayne CT (1984) Natriuretic response of the rat to plasma concentrations of arginine vasopressin within the physiological range. *Journal of Physiology* **352:** 517–526.

Baylis C (1982) Glomerular ultrafiltration in the pseudopregnant rat. *American Journal of Physiology* **234:** F300–F306.

Bishop JHV & Green R (1980) Effects of pregnancy on glucose handling by rat kidneys. *Journal of Physiology* **307:** 491–502.

Bishop JHV & Green R (1981) Effects of pregnancy on glucose reabsorption by the proximal convoluted tubule in the rat. *Journal of Physiology* **319:** 271–285.

Bishop JHV & Green R (1983) Glucose handling by distal portions of the nephron during pregnancy in the rat. *Journal of Physiology* **336:** 131–142.

Bishop JHV, Green R & Thomas S (1981) Glucose transport by short loops of Henle in the rat. *Journal of Physiology* **320:** 127–138.

Bliss DJ & Lote CJ (1982) Effect of prolactin on urinary excretion and renal haemodynamics in conscious rats. *Journal of Physiology* **322:** 399–407.

Borresen HC, Rorvik S, Gulduog I & Aakvaag A (1982) Angiotensin II and renal excretion of sodium and potassium in unanaesthetised dogs. *Scandinavian Journal of Clinical and Laboratory Investigation* **42:** 87–92.

Chang C, Pike RL & Clagett CO (1978) Progressive gross changes in renal medullary composition in pregnant rats. *Lipids* **13:** 167–173.

Christiansen PJ (1958) Tubular reabsorption of glucose during pregnancy. *Scandinavian Journal of Clinical and Laboratory Investigation* **10:** 364–371.

Churchill SE, Bengele HH & Alexander EA (1980) Sodium balance during pregnancy in the rat. *American Journal of Physiology* **239:** R143–R148.

Churchill SE, Bengele HH, Melby JC & Alexander EA (1981) Role of aldosterone in sodium retention in the rat. *American Journal of Physiology* **240:** R175–R181.

Churchill SE, Bengele HH & Alexander EA (1982) Renal function in the term-pregnant rat: a micropuncture study. *Renal Physiology* **5:** 1–9.

Conrad K (1984) Renal haemodynamics during pregnancy in chronically catheterised, conscious rats. *Kidney International* **26:** 24–29.

Daugherty TM, Ueki IF, Nicholas DP & Brenner BM (1973) Renal response to chronic intravenous salt loading in the rat. *Journal of Clinical Investigation* **52:** 21–31.

Davison JM & Lindheimer MD (1980) Changes in renal haemodynamics and kidney weight during pregnancy in the unanaesthetised rat. *Journal of Physiology* **301:** 129–136.

Davison JM, Gilmore EA, Durr JA, Robertson GL & Lindheimer MD (1984) Altered osmotic thresholds for vasopressin secretion and thirst in human pregnancy. *American Journal of Physiology* **246:** F105–F109.

Deming QB & Leutscher JA (1950) Bioassay of desoxycorticosterone-like material in urine. *Proceedings of the Society for Experimental Biology and Medicine* **73:** 171–175.

De Vries JR, Ludens JH & Fanestil DD (1972) Estradiol renal receptor molecules and estradiol-dependent antinatriuresis. *Kidney International* **2:** 95–100.

Dorfmann RI (1949) Influence of adrenal cortical steroids and related compounds on sodium metabolism. *Proceedings of the Society for Experimental Biology and Medicine* **72**: 395–398.

Dunlop W & Davison JM (1977) The effect of pregnancy on the renal handling of uric acid. *British Journal of Obstetrics and Gynaecology* **84**: 13–21.

Durr JA, Stamoutsos B & Lindheimer MD (1981) Osmoregulation during pregnancy in the rat. *Journal of Clinical Investigation* **68**: 337–346.

Ehrlich EN & Lindheimer MD (1972) Effect of administered mineralocorticoids on ACTH in pregnant women. *Journal of Clinical Investigation* **51**: 1301–1309.

El-Karib AO (1981) Effects of progesterone and prolactin on renal function in the rat. PhD thesis, University of Manchester.

El-Karib AO, Garland HO & Green R (1983) Acute and chronic effects of progesterone and prolactin on renal function in the rat. *Journal of Physiology* **337**: 389–400.

Ensor DM (1978) *Comparative Endocrinology of Prolactin.* London: Chapman & Hall.

Epstein AN, Fitzsimons JT & Rolls BJ (1970) Drinking induced by injection of angiotensin into the brain of the rat. *Journal of Physiology* **210**: 457–474.

Ezimokhai M, Davison JM, Philips PR & Dunlop W (1981) Non-postural serial changes in renal function during the third trimester of normal human pregnancy. *British Journal of Obstetrics and Gynaecology* **88**: 465–471.

Field MJ, Stanton BA & Giebisch G (1984) Influence of ADH on renal potassium handling: a micropuncture and microperfusion study. *Kidney International* **25**: 502–511.

Fowler WJ, Johnson JA, Kurz KD et al (1981) Role of renin-angiotensin system in maintaining arterial pressure in conscious rats. *Endocrinology* **109**: 290–295.

Gallery EDM & Gyory AZ (1979) Glomerular and proximal renal tubular function in pregnancy-associated hypertension: a prospective study. *European Journal of Obstetrics, Gynaecology and Reproductive Biology* **9**: 3–12.

Garland HO (1979) A role for prolactin in increasing proximal tubule length during pregnancy in the rat. *Journal of Endocrinology* **83**: 28P.

Garland HO & Green R (1982) Micropuncture study of changes in glomerular filtration rate and ion and water handling by the rat kidney during pregnancy. *Journal of Physiology* **329**: 389–409.

Garland HO & Lewis AG (1986) Altered renal function in chronically hyperprolactinaemic male rats. *Journal of Physiology* **371**: 257P.

Garland HO & Milne CM (1983) Altered renal function in chronically hyperprolactinaemic rats—effect of ovariectomy. *Proceedings of the International Union of Physiological Sciences,* **XV**: 506.

Garland HO, Green R & Moriarty RJ (1978) Changes in body weight, kidney weight and proximal tubular length during pregnancy in the rat. *Renal Physiology* **1**: 42–47.

Garland HO, Green R & Walker J (1984) Effect of alterations in perfusion rate on proximal tubule reabsorption in the pregnant rat. *Journal of Physiology* **346**: 102P.

Garland HO, Atherton JC, Baylis C, Morgan MRA & Milne CM (1987) Hormone profiles for progesterone, oestradiol, prolactin, plasma renin activity, aldosterone and corticosterone during pregnancy and pseudopregnancy in two strains of rat: correlation with renal studies. *Journal of Endocrinology* **113**: 435–444.

Gellai M, Silverstein JH, Hwang JC, La Rochelle FT & Valtin H (1984) Influence of vasopressin on renal haemodynamics in conscious Brattleboro rats. *American Journal of Physiology* **246**: R819–R827.

Goldstein MH, Lenz PR & Levitt MF (1969) Effect of urine flow rate on urea reabsorption in man: urea as a 'tubular marker'. *Journal of Applied Physiology* **26**: 594–599.

Green R (1986) Renal function in pregnancy. In Lote CJ (ed.) *Advances in Renal Physiology*, pp 297–329. London: Croom Helm.

Green R & Hatton TM (1987) Renal tubular function in gestation. *American Journal of Kidney Disease* **9**: 265–269.

Green R, Moriarty RJ & Giebisch G (1981) Ionic requirements of proximal tubular fluid reabsorption: flow dependence of transport. *Kidney International* **20**: 580–583.

Häberle DA & Von Baeyer H (1983) Characteristics of glomerular tubular balance. *American Journal of Physiology* **240**: F355–F366.

Handler JS & Orloff J (1981) Antidiuretic hormone. *Annual Review of Physiology* **43**: 611–624.

Harris PF & Young JA (1977) Dose dependent stimulation and inhibition of proximal tubular sodium reabsorption by angiotensin II in the rat kidney. *Pflügers Archiv* 367: 295–297.

Hervey E & Hervey GR (1967) The effects of progesterone on body weight and composition in the rat. *Journal of Endocrinology* 37: 361–384.

Hutchinson C (1987) Renal function in virgin and pregnant normotensive and spontaneously hypertensive conscious rats. PhD thesis, University of Manchester.

Johnson MD & Malvin RL (1977) Stimulation of renal sodium reabsorption by angiotensin II. *American Journal of Physiology* 232: F298–F306.

Kaufman S (1981) The dipsogenic activity in male and female rats. *Journal of Physiology* 310: 435–444.

Landwehr DM, Klose RM & Giebisch G (1967) Renal tubular sodium and water reabsorption in the isotonic sodium chloride-loaded rat. *American Journal of Physiology* 212: 1327–1333.

Lang F (1981) Renal handling of urate. In Greger R, Lang F & Silbernagl S (eds) *Renal Transport of Organic Substances*, pp 234–261. Berlin: Springer-Verlag.

Lichton IJ (1963) Urinary excretion of water, sodium and total solutes by the pregnant rat. *American Journal of Physiology* 201: 563–567.

Lindheimer MD & Katz AI (1971) Kidney function in the pregnant rat. *Journal of Laboratory and Clinical Medicine* 78: 633–641.

Lindheimer MD, Koeppen B & Katz AI (1976) Renal function in normal and hypertensive pregnant rats. In Lindheimer MD, Katz AI & Zuspan FP (eds) *Hypertension and Pregnancy*, pp 217–218. New York: John Wiley.

Lindheimer MD, Katz AI, Koeppen B, Ordonez NG & Oparil S (1983) Kidney function and sodium handling in the pregnant spontaneously hypertensive rat. *Hypertension* 5: 498–506.

Lowitz HD, Stumpe KD & Ochwadt B (1969) Micropuncture study of the action of angiotensin II on tubular sodium and water reabsorption in the rat. *Nephron* 6: 173–187.

Lucci MS, Bengele HH & Solomon S (1975) Suppressive action of prolactin on renal response to volume expansion. *American Journal of Physiology* 229: 81–85.

Maddox DA, Price DC & Rector FC (1977) Effects of surgery on plasma volume and salt and water excretion in rats. *American Journal of Physiology* 233: F600–F606.

Matthews BF & Taylor DW (1960) Effects of pregnancy on inulin and para-aminohippurate clearances in the anaesthetised rat. *Journal of Physiology* 151: 385–389.

Mills DE, Buckman MT & Peake GT (1983) Mineralocorticoid modulation of prolactin effect on renal solute excretion in the rat. *Endocrinology* 112: 823–828.

Morel F, Imbert-Teboul M & Charbardes D (1981) Distribution of hormone dependent adenylate cyclase in the nephron and its physiological significance. *Annual Review of Physiology* 43: 569–581.

Mulrow PJ & Schneider G (1976) Aldosterone regulation in the maternal and fetal rat kidney. *Perspectives in Nephrology and Hypertension* 5: 229–237.

Navar LG & Schafer JA (1987) Comments on 'Lithium clearance: a new research area'. *News in Physiological Sciences* 2: 34–35.

Oelkers W, Schoneshofer M & Blumel A (1974) Effects of progesterone and four synthetic progestogens on sodium balance and the renin–aldosterone system in man. *Journal of Clinical Endocrinology and Metabolism* 39: 882–890.

Oparil S, Ehrlich EN & Lindheimer MD (1975) Effect of progesterone on renal sodium handling in man: relation to aldosterone excretion and plasma renin activity. *Clinical Science and Molecular Medicine* 49: 139–147.

Paller MS (1984) Mechanism of decreased pressor responsiveness to ANG II, NE and vasopressin in pregnant rats. *American Journal of Physiology* 247: H100–H108.

Pepe GJ & Rothchild I (1974) A comparative study of serum progesterone levels in pregnancy and various types of pseudopregnancy in the rat. *Endocrinology* 95: 275–279.

Pitkin RM (1985) Calcium metabolism in pregnancy and the perinatal period: a review. *American Journal of Obstetrics and Gynecology* 151: 99–109.

Rocha AS & Kokko JP (1974) Permeability of medullary nephron segments to urea and water: effect of vasopressin. *Kidney International* 6: 379–387.

Schuster VL, Kokko JP & Jacobson HR (1982) Angiotensin II directly inhibits sodium reabsorption in the isolated perfused proximal tubule. *Clinical Research* 30: 462A.

Schwartz GJ & Burg MB (1978) Mineralocorticoid effects on cation transport by cortical collecting tubules *in vitro*. *American Journal of Physiology* 235: F576–F585.

Seldin DW & Rector FC (1973) Evaluation of clearance methods for localisation of site action of diuretics. In Lant AF & Wilson CM (eds) *Modern Diuretic Therapy in the Treatment of Cardiovascular and Renal Diseases*. Amsterdam: Excerpta Medica.

Semple PF, Carswell W & Boyle JA (1974) Serial studies of the renal clearance of urate and inulin during pregnancy and after the puerperium in normal women. *Clinical Science and Molecular Medicine* 47: 559–565.

Shirley DG, Skinner J & Walter SJ (1984) Effect of captopril on renal function in Brattleboro rats. *Journal of Physiology* 346: 107P.

Simpson SA & Tait JF (1952) A quantitative method for the bioassay of the effect of adrenal cortical steroids on mineral metabolism. *Endocrinology* 50: 150–161.

Skøtt P, Bruun NW, Giese J, Holstein-Rathlou NH & Leyssac PP (1987) What does lithium clearance measure during osmotic diuresis? *Clinical Science* 73: 126–127.

Smith MS & Neill JD (1976) Termination at mid-pregnancy of the two daily surges of plasma prolactin initiated by mating in the rat. *Endocrinology* 98: 696–701.

Smith MS, McLean BK & Neill JD (1976) Prolactin: the initial luteotrophic stimulus of pseudopregnancy in the rat. *Endocrinology* 98: 1370–1378.

Sonnenblick EH, Cannon PS & Laragh JH (1961) The nature of the action of intravenous aldosterone: evidence for a role of the hormone in urinary dilution. *Journal of Clinical Investigation* 40: 903–913.

Stumpe KD & Ochwadt B (1968) Wirkung von Aldosteron auf die Natrium- und Wasser resorption in proximalen Tubulus bei chronischer Koch saltzbelastung. *Pflügers Archiv* 300: 148–160.

Thomsen K (1984) Lithium clearance: a new method for determining proximal and distal tubular reabsorption of sodium and water. *Nephron* 37: 217–223.

Thomsen K & Leyssac PP (1986a) Acute effects of various diuretics on lithium clearance. *Renal Physiology* 9: 1–8.

Thomsen K & Leyssac PP (1986b) Effect of dietary sodium content on renal handling of lithium. *Pflügers Archiv* 407: 55–58.

Thomsen K & Olesen OV (1981) Effect of anaesthesia and surgery on urine flow and electrolyte excretion in different rat strains. *Renal Physiology* 4: 165–172.

Walker J (1983) Renal function in the female rat during various reproductive states. PhD thesis, University of Manchester.

Walker J & Garland HO (1985) Single nephron function during prolactin-induced pseudopregnancy in the rat. *Journal of Endocrinology* 107: 127–131.

Walker LA, Buscemi-Bergin M & Gellai M (1983) Renal haemodynamics in conscious rats: effects of anaesthesia, surgery and recovery. *American Journal of Physiology* 245: F67–F74.

Welsh GN & Simms EAH (1960) The mechanism of renal glycosuria in pregnancy. *Diabetes* 9: 363–369.

Whipp GT, Coghlan JP, Shulkes AA, Skinner SL & Wintour EM (1978) Regulation of aldosterone in the rat. Effect of oestrous cycle, pregnancy and sodium status. *Australian Journal of Experimental Biology and Medical Science* 56: 545–551.

Wright FS & Giebisch G (1978) Renal potassium transport: contributions of individual nephrons and populations. *American Journal of Physiology* 235: F515–F527.

Yoshinaga K, Hawkins RA & Stocker JF (1969) Estrogen secretion by the rat ovary *in vivo* during the estrous cycle and pregnancy. *Endocrinology* 85: 103–112.

4

Volume homeostasis in normal and hypertensive human pregnancy

EILEEN D. M. GALLERY
MARK A. BROWN

The concept of volume homeostasis was stated succinctly by Gauer and Henry (1976) as 'the continuous adjustment of blood volume to the changing size of the vascular bed so that at all times an adequate fullness of the blood stream is available to the left ventricle'.

Normal pregnancy is characterized by arteriolar and venous dilatation as well as by increasing needs for volume accumulation in fetal and placental tissues. Therefore, volume homeostatic mechanisms must be repeatedly readjusted throughout pregnancy. Many complex further alterations occur when hypertension complicates pregnancy, some being potentially harmful to mother and fetus, and some being compensatory and beneficial. It is the purpose of this review to examine available information concerning volume homeostatic mechanisms in normal pregnancy, and their derangement in women who have, or who develop, hypertension, with reference to both pathophysiology and significance for patient management.

BODY FLUID VOLUMES

In normal people in a steady state, extracellular fluid volume is maintained within narrow limits by a complicated interplay between factors sensing alterations in this volume and its composition and factors which translate these sensing mechanisms into appropriate retention or excretion of sodium and water. Extracellular fluid volume is primarily dependent on sodium content, and therefore regulation of renal sodium excretion is critical to its maintenance. Changes in extracellular fluid volume are sensed by stretch receptors in the atria, great vessels and perhaps in the interstitial space, and by arterial baroreceptors (Ganong, 1983). Changes in solute concentrations (measured indirectly by plasma osmolality) are also sensed by osmoreceptors in the anterior hypothalamus.

As specific factors involved in the control of plasma osmolality and renal water excretion are discussed fully in Chapter 5, they will be mentioned only briefly here, and in relation to the control of sodium balance.

Pregnancy is not a steady state. There is progressive weight gain, of which 6–8 kilograms represent expansion of the extracellular fluid volume (Hytten and Leitch, 1971), both interstitial and plasma volumes being increased (Chesley, 1944; Gallery et al, 1979a, 1981). There is much inter-individual variation in both the rate and extent of this weight gain. The plasma volume is demonstrably greater than non-pregnant values by 6 weeks of amenorrhoea (Lund and Donovan, 1967), reaching and being maintained at values of 30–40% above non-pregnant values by the third trimester (Gallery et al, 1979a). Animal data suggest that this new level is clearly recognized as normal, a reduction of less than 10% resulting in antidiuretic hormone release (Barron et al, 1984). This volume expansion has significant physiological correlates:

1. There is a highly significant close relationship between the extent of plasma volume expansion and fetal growth. This is true for both normotensive women and those with chronic hypertension (Pirani et al, 1973; Gallery et al, 1979b; Goodlin et al, 1983).
2. In pregnancies complicated by intrauterine growth retardation, plasma volume expansion is less than normal (Gibson et al, 1973).
3. There is a significant reduction in plasma volume in women with pregnancy-associated hypertension (pre-eclampsia) a reduction which often precedes the development of the clinical syndrome (Gallery et al, 1979a).

As the principal determinant of such extracellular and plasma volume expansion is sodium, regulation of its excretion will be considered in some detail.

CONTROL OF SODIUM EXCRETION

Normal pregnancy is characterized by the accumulation of about 900 millimoles of sodium. This represents retention of only 3–4 mmol/day, the result of a fine balance between factors promoting sodium excretion and those enhancing sodium retention (Table 1). It must be emphasized that normal pregnancy is a dynamic state with progressive changes in many of these factors, and any understanding of sodium control in pregnancy must take into account the stage of gestation under consideration.

Glomerular filtration rate (GFR)

One of the early threats to sodium accumulation in pregnancy is the rise in GFR. This increases as early as at 6 weeks of amenorrhoea (Davison and Noble, 1981) and reaches 50% of non-pregnant values by the end of the first trimester. This alone provides an additional 10 000 mmol/day of sodium which the renal tubules must absorb in order to prevent net loss of sodium. It is evident from the data of cross-sectional studies that this tubular adaptation occurs at somewhere between 5 (Weir et al, 1976) and 11 (Brown et al, 1987a) weeks gestation, probably in parallel with the changes in filtered sodium.

Table 1. Factors governing sodium excretion during pregnancy.

Natriuretic factors	Uncertain or variable factors	Anti-natriuretic factors
GFR	Angiotensin II	Aldosterone
Progesterone	AVP	Desoxycorticosterone
	Filtration fraction	Oestrogen
	Prostaglandins	Supine and/or upright posture
	Prolactin	
	Human placental lactogen	
	Cortisol	
	Placental 'shunting'	
	Kinins	
	Glucagon	
	Calcitonin	
	'Natriuretic hormones'	
	Atrial natriuretic peptide	
	Sympathetic nervous system	
	Renin	

Progesterone

At the same time as the rise in glomerular filtration rate, plasma progesterone concentrations begin to rise. This hormone can cause natriuresis by at least two mechanisms: (1) antagonism of the action of mineralocorticoids (Landau and Lugibihl, 1958), for which there is direct tissue receptor evidence (Sharp et al, 1966), or (2) increasing proximal tubular sodium rejection (Oparil et al, 1975). It has been claimed that there is a causal relationship between its increased production and the parallel increase in aldosterone production. We have recently examined the interrelationship of aldosterone and progesterone more closely during pregnancy under normal conditions and in response to changes in salt intake. With unrestricted salt intake, both progesterone and aldosterone increased in parallel throughout pregnancy, but the rates of increase in these two hormones within individuals were poorly correlated (Brown et al, 1986). While plasma aldosterone was stimulated or suppressed appropriately by changes in salt intake in these pregnant women, no significant alterations were seen in plasma progesterone (Table 2).Thus, while progesterone may have a background effect on sodium excretion in pregnancy, it is not involved in the acute regulation of sodium excretion, nor is it intimately related to changes in aldosterone production.

Prostaglandins

The vasodilator prostaglandins, particularly PGE_2 and prostacyclin, have received considerable attention in pregnancy as they appear to be produced in greater amounts (Spitz et al, 1984) than in the non-pregnant state, a phenomenon which could explain the vascular refractoriness to the pressor effects of infused angiotensin II (Gant et al, 1973). These compounds are natriuretic, independent of their effects on renal blood flow, and promote the excretion of free water (Levenson et al, 1982) but these actions have not been

Table 2. Plasma aldosterone and progesterone concentrations in response to dietary sodium manipulations during and after pregnancy.

		High-salt diet			Low-salt diet		
	Day	Second trimester	Third trimester	Post partum	Second trimester	Third trimester	Post partum
n		20	20	7	20	20	7
Plasma aldosterone	0	1127 ± 156	2156 ± 241	684 ± 231	1333 ± 153	2472 ± 321	502 ± 166
concentration	7	$840\pm105*$	$1152\pm117†$	$163\pm26‡$	$2694\pm328†$	$3846\pm319†$	871 ± 226
(fmol/ml)							
Progesterone	0	247 ± 16	667 ± 82	—	242 ± 17	419 ± 34	—
(nmol/l)	7	$248+18$	673 ± 82	—	267 ± 22	484 ± 30	—

* $P<0.005$, day 0 versus day 7.
† $P<0.001$, day 0 versus day 7.
‡ $P<0.01$, day 0 versus day 7.
From Brown and Gallery (1986), with permission.

specifically studied in pregnancy. In theory these compounds should contribute towards natriuresis, but the added property of stimulating renin release, particularly by prostacyclin, may offset this effect (Patrono et al, 1982).

Intrarenal haemodynamics

Just as the production of various hormones alters throughout pregnancy, so too do renal haemodynamics. Davison and Dunlop (1984) have shown from serial studies that renal blood flow rises slightly more than GFR early in pregnancy, but unlike GFR, falls slightly in the last few weeks of pregnancy. This means that the filtration fraction (GFR/effective renal plasma flow (ERPF)) is lowered in mid-pregnancy and increased in the last trimester. Changes in the filtration fraction affect peritubular colloid osmotic pressure and are therefore related positively to proximal tubular sodium reabsorption (Seely and Levy, 1981). This cannot be measured *directly* in human pregnancy and at present such a relationship between filtration and sodium excretion remains completely unstudied. It is likely that these changes in renal haemodynamics would favour sodium loss in mid-pregnancy and sodium retention in late pregnancy.

Antidiuretic hormone

The antidiuretic hormone, arginine vasopressin (AVP), has many actions other than its water-retaining property, including the ability to promote sodium excretion in pregnancy. In the 1960s there were reports of both a natriuretic (Torres et al, 1966) and an antinatriuretic (Assali et al, 1960) effect of infused AVP in normal pregnancy. As the latter study involved the administration of high doses of AVP, which may have caused a reduction in

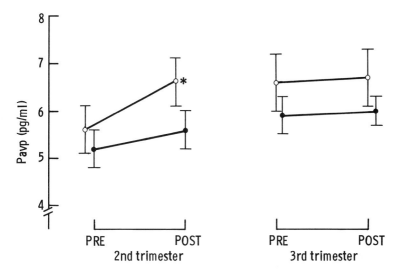

Figure 1. Plasma arginine vasopressin (plasma AVP) levels before and after dietary sodium manipulations. ○, high-salt diet; ●, low-salt diet; *P < 0.005, day 0 versus day 7. From Brown and Gallery (1986), with permission.

GFR, these results are likely to be incorrect. The results of the former study indicated a more marked natriuretic effect in mid-pregnancy than in late pregnancy. To examine this issue further we have measured plasma concentrations of AVP in primigravidas during mid- and late pregnancy, before and after dietary sodium loading or deprivation (Brown and Gallery, 1986). Plasma AVP rose in salt-loaded subjects during the second trimester but not during the third trimester and was unchanged by salt depletion (Figure 1). The rise in plasma AVP could not be explained by changes in plasma sodium, plasma volume or blood pressure. These results give support to the earlier suggestion of Torres et al (1966) that AVP facilitates natriuresis, particularly in mid-pregnancy. Although basal values for plasma AVP were slightly higher in third trimester subjects than second trimester subjects, the difference was not significant. These data are therefore compatible with those of Davison et al (1986) who observed similar basal plasma AVP measured prior to conception, early in pregnancy, in the third trimester and 10–12 weeks postpartum.

Atrial natriuretic peptide

Recent research interest has focused upon the potential effects on renal sodium excretion of atrial natriuretic peptide (ANP). This peptide, secreted by atrial cells in response to increased arterial pressure/volume, is capable of causing vasodilatation, hypotension, natriuresis and inhibition of the renin–angiotensin system (Cuneo et al, 1986). Circulating levels appear to be slightly increased late in normal pregnancy (Jackson et al, 1987). Prospective studies examining sequential alterations in human pregnancy are lacking. One study presently in progress suggests in the subhuman primate a reduction in early pregnancy, with values rising through the normal range to elevated values in late pregnancy (Phippard et al, 1987). These results, if confirmed in the human, would suggest relative underfilling of the circulation in early pregnancy with recognition of the volume-expanded state as normal in late pregnancy. The high levels of ANP seen in some patients at this stage of pregnancy therefore may represent an appropriate physiological response to prevent further volume expansion, although clearly much work remains to be done in this area.

Sodium potassium ATPase

The ouabain-sensitive sodium/potassium ATPase-dependent pump is the major pathway by which sodium and potassium electrochemical gradients are maintained across most cell membranes, and in the kidney this enzyme is involved in achieving sodium reabsorption. There is general agreement that pregnancy is associated with increased numbers of enzyme sites both on circulating cells and in kidney (Lindheimer and Katz, 1971; Rubython and Morgan, 1983; Aronson et al, 1984; Gallery et al, 1986). Increased function of the enzyme has also been demonstrated associated with a fall in intracellular sodium and a rise in intracellular potassium (Gallery et al, 1986), but the extent of increase in enzyme function appears to be significantly less than that in enzyme numbers (10-15% above non-pregnant values compared with a 65-75% increase), suggesting relative enzyme inhibition (Rubython and Morgan 1983; Gallery et al, 1986). Whether this is due to the elaboration of functionally inactive sites, to autoregulation by reduction in intracellular sodium, or to a circulating inhibitor is uncertain at the present time. In the non-pregnant state, volume expansion by sodium loading has been found to result in the elaboration of a circulating inhibitor of erythrocyte sodium/potassium ATPase (Boero et al, 1985; Weissberg et al, 1985), and as pregnancy is a state of chronic volume expansion, this situation might apply. In response to 7 days of dietary sodium loading, no change in either the number of erythrocyte sodium/potassium ATPase sites, or their intrinsic function, as measured in artificial media, was found in a recent study from our laboratory (Gallery et al, 1987a). A comparison of erythrocyte sodium/potassium ATPase in normotensive women in the third trimester with and without oedema, however, suggested that although there was no difference in enzyme function as measured in artificial medium, incubations in plasma resulted in inhibition of some 20% of ATPase function in the oedematous women, while there was no inhibition of enzyme function in the non-oedematous women (Gallery et al, 1987b). It would appear therefore, that this enzyme system and at least some of its control mechanisms are involved in volume homeostasis in normal pregnancy. The extent or clinical significance of this involvement is at present conjectural, and this too will undoubtedly be an area of further investigation.

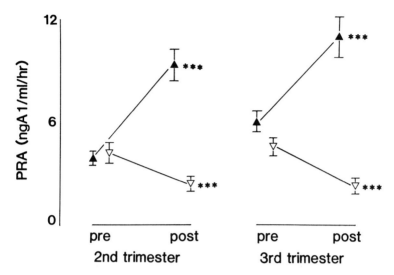

Figure 2. Plasma renin activity (PRA) response to changing sodium intake during both trimesters. (▲ = low salt diet; ▽ = high salt diet; ***$P < 0.001$). From Brown et al (1987d), with permission.

Renin–angiotensin–aldosterone axis

It is widely recognized that production of renin and its substrate is markedly increased in normal pregnancy (Helmer and Judson, 1967; Weinberger et al, 1976). The former arises predominantly from maternal kidney, but with an extrarenal, probably uteroplacental, component (Weir et al, 1975; Craven et al, 1983), and the latter (predominantly an oestrogen effect) arises from the maternal liver. Earlier disagreement about the extent of increase in plasma renin activity can be explained by methodological factors, as both acid- and cold-activatable portions of inactive renin are increased in human pregnancy (Lumbers, 1971; Rowe et al, 1979) and by variable sodium intake at the time of study. Aldosterone production is also increased presumably in response to the high angiotensin II levels that result from increased renin production, although as stated earlier, there may be a background direct progesterone effect that is also operative.

It is clear that there are two distinct components of renin production in pregnancy—one responsive and one unresponsive to alterations in sodium balance. There is no doubt, as has been shown by many authors (Gordon et al, 1973; Bay and Ferris, 1979; Vallotton et al, 1982; Brown et al, 1987d), that in normal pregnancy plasma renin activity (PRA) is appropriately stimulated by sodium depletion and suppressed by sodium loading (Figure 2). In addition, PRA at any given level of sodium intake is higher than in the non-pregnant state. Some of this high baseline may represent a physiological resetting geared to sodium retention, particularly in the second trimester, as is suggested by our finding that an increment of sodium intake in the order of 50 mmol/day is necessary to produce renin suppression (Brown et al, 1987d). From a recent study conducted in our laboratory, it is also clear that a

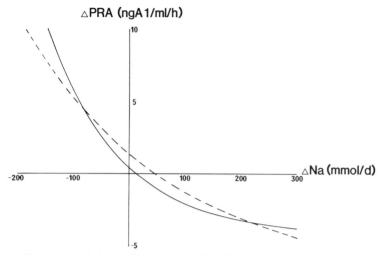

Figure 3. Exponential relationship between change in sodium excretion from baseline (△Na) and corresponding change in plasma renin activity (△PRA). These equations are △PRA = 8.6e$^{-0.0037\triangle Na}$ − 7.2, and △PRA = 4.8e$^{-0.0075 \triangle Na}$ − 4.3 for the second (– – – –) and third (———) trimesters respectively. From Brown et al (1986), with permission.

proportion of the high PRA levels is quite independent of maternal sodium intake. Even with a combination of dietary sodium loading followed by intravenous sodium loading, suppression to a minimum of 2.5 ng angiotensin 1 (A1)/ml/h was the most that could be achieved in both the second and third trimesters of pregnancy, compared with values below 0.4 ngA1/ml/h in the same subjects postpartum (Brown et al, 1986).

These studies have also shown that the relationship between acute changes in sodium intake and PRA is altered progressively in pregnancy (Figure 3). In non-pregnant subjects, the regression line describing this relationship over 7 days of altered sodium intake passed through the origin (i.e. no change in PRA occurred if there was no change in sodium intake). In second-trimester subjects however, there was a 25% increase in PRA following the 7 days of altered sodium intake *independent* of the sodium-related alteration. These findings are certainly compatible with the hypothesis that the second trimester of pregnancy—a time of increasing volume expansion with maximal arteriolar vasodilatation—is a stage when effective volume depletion is sensed and avid sodium retention must occur to maintain volume homeostasis and promote further elevation of plasma volume. Although PRA was slightly higher again in the third trimester, its relationship with sodium intake was reset back towards the non-pregnant state, suggesting that sodium balance was no longer perceived as under threat.

In addition to these alterations of renin–sodium relationships, there is some dissociation of the usually close nexus between renin and aldosterone in normal pregnancy. In the first trimester, aldosterone production increases before that of renin (Brown et al, 1987a), and by the third trimester the proportional increase in aldosterone far exceeds that of renin (Weinberger et

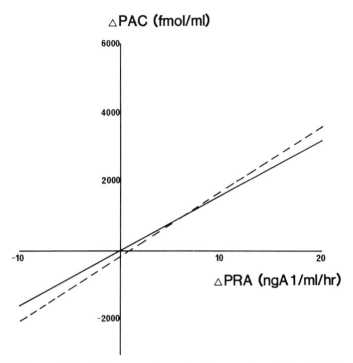

Figure 4. Linear relationship between change in plasma renin activity (ΔPRA) and the corresponding change in plasma aldosterone concentration (ΔPAC) following dietary sodium manipulations. These equations are ΔPAC = −178 + 189 ΔPRA, and ΔPAC = 29 + 159 ΔPRA for the second (- - - -) and third (———) trimesters respectively. From Brown et al (1987d), with permission.

al, 1976; Brown et al, 1987d). There is no doubt that the relationship is very close under acute conditions, for example following changes in sodium intake (Figure 4), throughout pregnancy, but clearly other background stimuli to aldosterone production are operative (such as progesterone, mentioned above).

Because of the marked increase in production of renin and its substrate, circulating levels of angiotensin II are elevated in normal pregnancy, though the vessels of the normal pregnant woman are refractory to its pressor effects. While considerable attention has been paid to these effects of angiotensin II in pregnancy, little has been diverted towards the influence of this peptide upon sodium excretion. In the non-pregnant subject angiotensin II directly affects tubular sodium excretion and also alters renal haemodynamics (Hollenberg et al, 1984).

One of the authors (Brown et al, 1987a) has recently shown that, following a saline load, both pregnant and non-pregnant women exhibited a dose-dependent reduction in sodium excretion in response to intravenously administered angiotensin II (over a range of 2–16 ng/kg/min). Sodium retention was achieved by (1) reduction in filtered sodium, (2) stimulation of aldosterone release (and distal nephron sodium reabsorption), and (3) enhancement of proximal tubular reabsorption (Brown et al, 1987a). In addition, it appeared that the sensitivity to these effects in normal pregnancy was increased when compared with non-pregnant subjects, in contrast to the refractoriness to the pressor effects of this peptide.

Desoxycorticosterone

Desoxycorticosterone (DOC) is another potent mineralocorticoid, produced intra- and extra-adrenally from progesterone, whose activity depends predominantly upon both renal and hepatic sulphation (Casey and MacDonald, 1982). DOC is produced in increased amounts in pregnancy (Ehrlich et al, 1976), much of the increment resulting from extra-adrenal 21-hydroxylation of progesterone (Winkel et al, 1980), potentially allowing a fine balance between the opposing actions of these two hormones on renal sodium excretion. DOC does not appear to be closely involved in short-term regulation of sodium excretion as plasma levels do not alter following changes in dietary sodium intake (Ehrlich et al, 1976). This may be explained by the lack of change of plasma progesterone in this situation, but in general little is known about the physiological role of DOC in pregnancy.

Oestrogen

The increased oestrogen production of normal pregnancy also promotes sodium retention, both by direct renal action and by increasing hepatic production of renin substrate, though it is not clear how closely involved this hormone is in sodium regulation in pregnancy. In addition, oestrogen may be responsible for the increase in mucopolysaccharide ground substance present in many women in the second half of pregnancy in skin and subcutaneous tissue, which in turn allows these tissues to retain fluid more than in the non-pregnant state (Fekete, 1954).

Posture

Finally, the supine posture has been shown to be a potent antinatriuretic position in pregnancy, irrespective of changes induced in filtered sodium, probably by enhancing proximal tubular reabsorption when changing from lateral recumbency to the supine posture (Lindheimer and Weston, 1969).

REGULATION OF THE PLASMA VOLUME

The individual factors discussed above must act in concert to regulate sodium excretion according to the body's needs for sodium and thereby maintain a constant extracellular fluid volume. We have noted previously that in normal pregnancy the plasma volume is maintained within a narrow range in the short term, despite large increments or reductions in sodium intake (Brown et al, 1987d). It is clear that this response is at least as efficient during pregnancy as in the non-pregnant state. However, significant changes in body weight occur, indicating changes in interstitial fluid volume. Hence, in normal pregnancy, as in non-pregnant subjects (Gauer and Henry, 1976), the plasma volume is maintained within a narrow range both by regulation of sodium excretion and by fluid 'buffering' from or into the interstitial fluid volume.

Evidence is accumulating that the conflicting stresses on sodium balance may result in difficulty for the pregnant woman to meet acute demands upon sodium excretory mechanisms. Although Bay and Ferris (1979) stated that both pregnant and non-pregnant subjects assumed sodium 'balance' (where intake equals output) over a few days in response to a 10 mmol/day sodium diet, Lindheimer (1980) reinterpreted their data to show that 'balance' may not have been achieved by the pregnant women, as the obligatory need to retain sodium should have led to a lower sodium excretion than that observed. We have extended these findings by examining sodium excretion following a 20 mmol/day sodium intake over a week in 60 primigravidas during the second trimester, 30 of these again in the third trimester and 9 postpartum. By the end of the week of study, sodium excretion fell to 28 and 27 mmol/day respectively during second and third trimesters and to 14 mmol/day postpartum, all groups having similar sodium intake prior to the study. The pregnant women not only lost the same weight (1.2 kg) as in their postpartum state but failed to increase their weight by the expected 0.4 kilograms at these stages, indicating that the reduced sodium intake resulted in significant extracellular fluid volume loss. These findings would support the hypothesis that pregnant women do have greater difficulty in adapting to sodium depletion than in their non-pregnant state.

In summary, clearly there is progressive resetting of volume controls in normal pregnancy, so that significant accumulation of sodium and water is accomplished and perceived as normal. There is some evidence that the physiological response to extremes of sodium intake is a little blunted in mid-pregnancy. This may put the pregnant woman at some risk of sodium depletion at this time, when it would appear that continuing positive volume accumulation is sensed as desirable. Hypertensive pregnancy, in contrast to the normal state can be complicated by several disturbances in volume homeostasis and by alterations in response to manipulation of sodium and volume.

PREGNANCY-ASSOCIATED HYPERTENSION (PAH)

Many women who develop pregnancy-associated hypertension (pre-eclampsia) also experience rapid weight gain, oedema and decrements in urine volume. In early studies, administered sodium was shown to be retained more avidly by these women than by normotensive subjects (Chesley et al, 1958; Sarles et al, 1968). Accordingly, the decreased plasma renin concentration and activity and aldosterone concentration in this condition were considered to be secondary to sodium retention. Subsequent recognition that this disorder is accompanied by plasma volume contraction (Blekta et al, 1970) led to a re-evaluation of traditional views of sodium regulation in PAH.

Prior to the development of the clinical syndrome, the plasma volume is reduced (Gallery et al, 1979a) and the sensitivity to angiotensin II is increased (Gant et al, 1973). Plasma levels of renin and aldosterone are not different from continuously normotensive subjects (Gallery et al, 1980), although the relationship between renin activity and sodium intake may be altered (Brown et al, 1987c). Sodium excretion following intravenous saline loading is not impaired, with, if anything, a tendency to more rapid excretion than in normal pregnant women (Gallery and Brown, 1987). Following development of the established syndrome, the findings are somewhat different. We have recently examined sodium excretory patterns in women with PAH, both with and without proteinuria (500 mg/24 h) on ad-libitum sodium intake in comparison to values from normotensive third trimester primigravidas eating either high, low or ad-libitum salt intake. All subjects were administered an intravenous saline infusion of 3 mmol/kg (Brown et al, 1987b). Non-proteinuric hypertensive subjects had sodium excretion similar to that of normotensives on unrestricted salt diets, while subjects with proteinuria retained sodium to the same degree as the sodium-deplete normotensive group. These hypertensive women had a reduced plasma volume, and a sodium-retaining response therefore appeared appropriate in this setting. However the sodium retention was effected by a decrease in GFR, and tubular sodium reabsorption was in fact less than that of salt-deplete normal control subjects. This may be explained in part by the very low PRA and plasma aldosterone concentrations in the women with severe (proteinuric) PAH, the normotensive sodium deplete group having stimulated their aldosterone system markedly and maintained their plasma volume at a near normal level.

These findings suggest that the sodium retention of PAH is a physiological renal response to volume contraction, aimed at maintenance of plasma volume. In this situation it is clear that tubular sodium reabsorptive mechanisms are defective, as is the response of the renin–aldosterone system. These two abnormalities may be causally linked. Perhaps juxtaglomerular cell damage may be an early feature of PAH, resulting in diminished ability to sense or respond to the volume contraction developing early in the course of the syndrome. Perhaps interstitial fluid volume is a more important determinant of renin release and sodium retention than is plasma volume.

There is no doubt that in PAH the (infrequently measured) changes in interstitial fluid volume are of great significance. Plasma volume expansion by administration of colloid solutions is accompanied by a shift of fluid from the interstitial to the intravascular compartment, with accompanying natriuresis and weight loss, despite a fall in blood pressure and an increase in plasma volume (Gallery et al, 1981, 1984). Clearly the interrelationship of these intercompartmental shifts of fluid and the control of renin and aldosterone release needs further clarification, particularly in the early stages of the development of PAH.

The place of atrial natriuretic peptide and sodium/potassium ATPase have not been closely assessed in the development of PAH. Atrial natriuretic peptide, which is increased late in normal pregnancy, has been estimated at both low and high levels in patients with established PAH (Andoh et al, 1986; Hirai et al, 1986). Low levels might be expected because of the volume contraction, but of greater potential interest in understanding the pathophysiology would be findings around the time of development of the syndrome. This will require sequential measurements in a sufficiently large number of normotensive women to pick up the 10–15% at risk, and such a study has not yet been performed.

Sodium/potassium ATPase, as mentioned earlier, is the principal enzyme involved locally in active sodium reabsorption across the renal tubular cell. Defective tubular sodium reabsorption could therefore be due to insufficient increase in the amount of this enzyme in PAH or suppression of this function by a circulating inhibitor, as has been suggested for chronic essential hypertension (de Wardener and MacGregor, 1983). To examine the possibility that such an inhibitor is present in PAH, we are presently conducting a study of sodium/potassium ATPase activity in erythrocytes from women with PAH in the presence and absence of their own plasma, compared to normotensive third-trimester women. Preliminary results suggest no inhibition of erythrocyte sodium/potassium ATPase by autologous plasma in women with PAH without peripheral oedema, and although those with peripheral oedema have a tendency towards lower levels of enzyme function in their own plasma ($n = 10$; 90% of values assayed in buffer), the amount of suppression is less than in normal pregnant women with peripheral oedema. To date therefore, these results do not suggest a central role for a sodium/potassium ATPase inhibitor in the genesis of PAH.

CLINICAL IMPLICATIONS

Many of these physiological studies have relevance to clinical care. In normal pregnancy it is clear that short-term maintenance of plasma volume can be achieved over a wide range of salt intakes. However, there is no doubt that the pregnant woman has greater difficulty in coping with severe sodium restriction than during her postpartum state, and this manoeuvre should be avoided during pregnancy, which is, after all, a sodium-retaining state. Accordingly, we do not advise pregnant women to ingest a blanket 'ideal' sodium intake, but rather to continue eating the same amount of salt as prior to pregnancy.

Prophylactic restriction of salt intake in pregnant women does not reduce the incidence of PAH (Campbell and MacGillivray 1975)—not surprisingly in view of the similar sodium excretory capacity of these subjects to normal women prior to the clinical development of this disorder. The recognition that the established disorder is characterized by plasma volume reduction and perhaps by inadequate tubular sodium reabsorption makes it clear that diuretic and salt restriction have no place in the management of PAH and may in fact aggravate the clinical manifestations (Palomaki and Lindheimer, 1970; Chesley, 1981). Clinicians have worried for years about the development of oedema in pregnancies complicated by PAH, but Chesley (1978) has demonstrated this to be a good prognostic feature, perhaps reflecting some success at maintenance of an adequate plasma volume.

The maintenance of volume homeostasis in pregnancy is determined by a complicated interplay of many factors regulating sodium excretion, vascular tone and capillary permeability, and poorly understood abnormalities in all of these factors occur in women with, or destined for, PAH. These physiological and pathophysiological relationships need further clarification and will undoubtedly be a subject of close scrutiny and investigation in the near future.

SUMMARY

In this chapter are outlined the many factors involved in the regulation of sodium and volume homeostasis in normal human pregnancy and their interrelationships. New developments concerning the role of sodium/potassium ATPase, atrial natriuretic peptide, arginine vasopressin and angiotensin II as regulatory forces are outlined, together with a review of earlier work. Abnormalities found in women with, or destined for, PAH are described and their significance is discussed.

REFERENCES

Andoh A, Tamura H, Igarashi M et al (1986) Atrial natriuretic peptide and the renin–aldosterone system in normal pregnancy and preeclampsia. *Abstracts of the 5th International Congress, (International Society for the Study of Hypertension in Pregnancy Nottingham, England)*, p. P3.

Aronson GK, Moore MP, Redman CWG & Harper C (1984) Erythrocyte cation transport receptor numbers and activity in pregnancies complicated by essential hypertension and pre-eclampsia. *British Medical Journal* **288:** 1332–1334.

Assali NS, Dignam WJ & Longo L. (1960) Effects of antidiuretic hormone (ADH) on renal hemodynamics and water and electrolyte excretion near term and postpartum. *Journal of Clinical Endocrinology* **20:** 581–592.

Barron WM, Stamoutsos BA & Lindheimer MD (1984) Role of volume in the regulation of vasopressin secretion during pregnancy in the rat. *Journal of Clinical Investigation* **73:** 923–932.

Bay WH & Ferris TF (1979) Factors controlling plasma renin and aldosterone during pregnancy. *Hypertension* **1:** 410–415.

Blekta M, Hlavaty V, Trnkova M, et al (1970) Volume of whole blood and absolute amount of serum protein in the early stage of late toxaemia of pregnancy. *American Journal of Obstetrics and Gynecology* **106:** 10–13.

Boero R, Quarello F, Guarena C, Rosati C & Picolli G (1985) Effects of an intravenous sodium load on erythrocyte sodium transport and normal human subjects. *Clinical Science* **69:** 709–712.

Brown MA, Broughton-Pipkin F & Symonds EM (1987a) The effects of intravenous angiotension II upon sodium and urate excretion in human pregnancy. Submitted for publication.

Brown MA & Gallery EDM (1986) Sodium excretion in human pregnancy: a role for arginine vasopressin. *American Journal of Obstetrics and Gynecology* **154:** 914–919.

Brown MA, Gallery EDM, Ross MR & Esber RP (1987b) Sodium excretion in normal and hypertensive pregnancy: a prospective study. Submitted for publication.

Brown MA, Nicholson E & Gallery EDM (1987c) Sodium–renin–aldosterone relationships in normal and hypertensive human pregnancy. Submitted for publication.

Brown MA, Nicholson E, Ross MR, Norton HE & Gallery EDM (1987d) Progressive re-setting of sodium-renin-aldosterone relationships in human pregnancy. *Clinical and Experimental Hypertension (B)* in press.

Brown MA, Sinosich MJ, Saunders DM & Gallery EDM (1986) Potassium regulation and progesterone-aldosterone interrelationships in human pregnancy. A prospective study. *American Journal of Obstetrics and Gynecology* **155**: 349–353.

Campbell DM & MacGillivray I (1975) The effect of a low calorie diet or a thiazide diuretic on the incidence of pre-eclampsia and on birth weight. *British Journal of Obstetrics and Gynaecology* **82**: 572–577.

Casey ML & Macdonald PC (1982) Metabolism of deoxycorticosterone and deoxycorticosterone sulphate in men and women. *Journal of Clinical Investigation* **70**, 312–319.

Chesley LC (1944) Weight changes and water balance in normal and toxic pregnancy. *American Journal of Obstetrics and Gynecology* **48**: 565–593.

Chesley LC (1978) *Hypertensive Disorders in Pregnancy*. New York: Appleton-Century Crofts.

Chesley LC (1981) The control of hypertension in pregnancy. *Obstetrics and Gynecology Annual* **10**: 69–106.

Chesley LC, Valenti C & Rein H (1958) Excretion of sodium loads by non-pregnant and pregnant normal hypertensive and pre-eclamptic women. *Metabolism* **7**: 575–588.

Craven DJ, Warren AY & Symonds EM (1983) Generation of angiotensin I by tissues of the human female genital tract. *American Journal of Obstetrics and Gynecology* **154**: 749–751.

Cuneo R, Espiner EA, Nicholls MG et al (1986) Renal hemodynamic and hormonal responses to atrial natriuretic peptide infusions in normal man, and effect of sodium intake. *Journal of Clinical Endocrinology and Metabolism* **63**: 946–953.

Davison JM & Dunlop W (1984) Changes in renal hemodynamics and tubular function induced by normal human pregnancy. *Seminars in Nephrology* **4**: 198–207.

Davison JM & Noble MCB (1981) Serial changes in 24 hour creatinine clearance during normal menstrual cycles and the first trimester of pregnancy. *British Journal of Obstetrics and Gynaecology* **88**: 10–17.

Davison JM, Shiells EA, Phillips PR, Barron WM & Lindheimer MD (1988) Serial studies of vasopressin release and thirst in human pregnancy: the role of human chorionic gonodotrophin in the osmoregulatory changes of gestation. *Journal of Clinical Investigation* (in press).

De Wardener HE & MacGregor GA (1983) The relation of a circulating sodium transport inhibitor (the natriuretic hormone) to hypertension. *Medicine* **62**: 310–326.

Ehrlich EN, Nolten WE, Oparil S & Lindheimer MD (1976) Mineralocorticoids in normal pregnancy. In Lindheimer MD et al (eds) *Hypertension in Pregnancy*, pp 189–201. New York: John Wiley.

Fekete S. (1954) Significance of mucopolysaccharides in pathogenesis of toxaemias of pregnancy. *Acta Medica Academica Scientiarum Hungaricae* **5**: 293–308.

Gallery EDM & Brown MA (1987) Control of sodium excretion in human pregnancy. *American Journal of Kidney Diseases* (in press).

Gallery EDM, Hunyor SN & Gyory AZ (1979a) Plasma volume contraction: a significant factor in both pregnancy-associated hypertension (pre-eclampsia) and chronic hypertension in pregnancy. *Quarterly Journal of Medicine* **48**: 593–602.

Gallery EDM, Saunders DM, Hunyor SN & Gyory AZ (1979b) Randomised comparison of methyldopa and oxprenolol for treatment of hypertension in pregnancy. *British Medical Journal* **i**: 1591–1594.

Gallery EDM, Stokes GS, Gyory AZ, Rowe J & Williams J (1980) Plasma renin activity in normal human pregnancy and in pregnancy-associated hypertension, with reference to cryoactivation. *Clinical Science* **59**: 49–53.

Gallery EDM, Delprado W & Gyory AZ (1981) Antihypertensive effect of plasma volume expansion in pregnancy-associated hypertension. *Australian and New Zealand Journal of Medicine* **11**: 20–24.

Gallery EDM, Mitchell MDM & Redmon CWG (1984) Fall in blood pressure in response to volume expansion in pregnancy-associated hypertension (pre-eclampsia). Why does it occur? *Journal of Hypertension* **2**: 177–182.

Gallery EDM, Rowe J, Brown MA et al (1986) Erythrocyte electrolyte transport in normal and hypertensive pregnancy. *Abstracts of the 5th International Congress of the International Society for the Study of Hypertension in Pregnancy*, p. 8.

Gallery EDM, Rowe J & Hawkins M (1988) Methods of assessment of erythrocyte Na^+ K^+ ATPase function in normal and hypertensive pregnancy. In Stokes GS & Marword JF (eds) *Progress in Biochemical Pharmacology-Sodium Transport Inhibitors*. Basel: Karger.

Ganong WF (1983) *Review of Medical Physiology*, 11th edn, pp 405–425. Los Angeles, California: Lange Medical.

Gant NF, Daley GL, Chand S, Whalley PJ & MacDonald PC (1973) A study of angiotensin II pressor response throughout primigravid pregnancy. *Journal of Clinical Investigation* **52**: 2682–2689.

Gauer OH & Henry JP (1976) Neurohormonal control of plasma volume. In Guyton AC & Cowley AW (eds) *Cardiovascular Physiology II* (International Review of Physiology Volume 9), pp 145–190. Baltimore: University Park Press.

Gibson HM (1973) Plasma volume and glomerular filtration rates in pregnancy and their relation to differences in fetal growth. *Journal of Obstetrics and Gynaecology of the British Commonwealth* **81**: 1067–1074.

Goodlin RC, Dobry CA, Anderson JC, Woods RE & Quaife M (1983) Clinical signs of normal plasma volume expansion during pregnancy. *American Journal of Obstetrics and Gynecology* **145**: 1001–1007.

Gordon RD, Symonds EM, Wilmshurst EG & Pawsey CGK (1973) Plasma renin activity plasma angiotensin and plasma and urinary electrolytes in normal and toxaemic pregnancy, including a prospective study. *Clinical Science and Molecular Medicine* **45**: 115–127.

Helmer OM & Judson WE (1967) Influence of high renin substrate levels on renin–angiotensin system in pregnancy. *American Journal of Obstetrics and Gynecology* **99**: 9–17.

Hirai N, Yamaji T, Ishibashi M, Yanairhara T & Nakayama T (1986) Alpha-human atrial natriuretic polypeptide in women during pregnancy. *Abstracts of the 5th International Congress (International Society for the Study of Hypertension in Pregnancy)*, p. 24.

Hollenberg NK (1984) The renin–angiotensin system and sodium homeostasis. *Journal of Cardiovascular Pharmacology* **6**: S176–S183.

Hytten FE & Leitch I (1971) *The Physiology of Human Pregnancy*, 2nd edn. Oxford: Blackwell Scientific.

Jackson B, Hodsman GP, Allen PS & Johnston CI (1987) Atrial natriuretic factor: plasma concentrations in normal pregnancy. *Kidney International* (in press).

Landau RL & Lugibihl K (1958) Inhibition of the sodium-retaining influence of aldosterone by progesterone. *Journal of Clinical Endocrinology and Metabolism* **18**: 1237–1245.

Levenson DJ, Simmons CE & Brenner BM (1982) Arachidonic acid metabolism, prostaglandins and the kidney. *American Journal of Medicine* **72**: 354–374.

Lindheimer MD (1980) Hypertension during pregnancy. In Hunt JC (ed.) *Hypertension Update* pp. 92–93. Bloomfield: Health Learning Systems.

Lindheimer MD & Katz AI (1971) Kidney function in the pregnant rat. *Journal of Laboratory and Clinical Medicine* **78**: 633–641.

Lindheimer MD & Weston PV (1969) Effect of hypotonic expansion on sodium, water and urea excretion in late pregnancy: the influence of posture on these results. *Journal of Clinical Investigation* **48**: 947–956.

Lumbers ER (1971) Activation of renin in human amniotic fluid by low pH. *Enzymologia* **40**: 329–336.

Lund CJ & Donovan JC (1967) Blood volume during pregnancy. *American Journal of Obstetrics and Gynecology* **98**: 393–403.

Oparil S, Ehrlich EN & Lindheimer MD (1975) Effect of progesterone on renal sodium handling in man: relation to aldosterone excretion and plasma renin activity. *Clinical Science and Molecular Medicine* **49**, 139–147.

Palomaki JF & Lindheimer MD (1970) Sodium depletion simulating deterioration in a toxemic pregnancy. *New England Journal of Medicine* **262**: 88–89.

Patrono C, Pugliese F, Ciabattoni G et al (1982) Evidence for a direct stimulatory effect of prostacyclin on renin release in man. *Journal of Clinical Investigaiton* **69**: 231–239.

Phippard AF, Hodsman GP, Horvath JS et al (1987) Sequential studies on atrial natriuretic peptide in pregnant and non-pregnant baboons. *Kidney International* (in press).

Pirani BBK, Campbell DM & MacGillivray I (1973) Plasma volume in normal first pregnancy *Journal of Obstetrics and Gynaecology of the British Commonwealth* **80**: 884–887.

Rowe J, Gallery EDM & Gyory AZ (1979) Cryoactivation of renin in plasma from pregnant and non-pregnant subjects, and its control. *Clinical Chemistry* **25**: 1972–1974.

Rubython J & Morgan DB (1983) The effect of pregnancy and pregnancy-induced hypertension on active sodium transport in the erythrocyte. *Clinica Chimica Acta* **132:** 91–99.

Sarles HE, Hill SS, LeBlanc et al (1968) Sodium excretion pattern during and following intravenous sodium chloride loads in normal and hypertensive pregnancies. *American Journal of Obstetrics and Gynecology* **102:** 1–7.

Seely JF & Levy M (1981) Control of extracellular fluid volume. In Brenner BM & Rector FC (eds) *The Kidney*, vol. I, pp 371–407. Philadelphia: WB Saunders.

Sharp GW, Komack CL & Leaf A (1966) Studies on the binding of aldosterone in the toad bladder. *Journal of Clinical Investigation* **45:** 450–459.

Spitz B, Deckmyn H, van Assche FA & Vermylen J (1984) Prostacyclin in pregnancy. *European Journal of Obstetrics, Gynaecology and Reproductive Biology* **18:** 303–308.

Torres C, Schewitz LJ & Pollak VE (1966) The effect of small amounts of antidiuretic hormone on sodium and urate excretion in pregnancy. *American Journal of Obstetrics and Gynecology* **94:** 546–558.

Vallotton MB, Davison JM, Riondel AM & Lindheimer MD (1982) Response of the renin–aldosterone system and antidiuretic hormone to oral water loading and hypotonic saline infusion during and after pregnancy. *Clinical and Experimental Hypertension (B)* **1:** 385–400.

Weinberger MH, Kramer NJ, Petersen LP, Cleary RE & Young PCM (1976) Sequential changes in the renin–angiotensin–aldosterone systems and plasma progesterone concentration in normal and abnormal human pregnancy. In Lindheimer MD, Katz AI & Zuspan FP (eds) *Hypertension in Pregnancy*, pp 263–269. New York: John Wiley.

Weir RJ, Brown JJ, Fraser R et al (1975) Relationship between plasma renin, renin substrate, angiotensin II, aldosterone and electrolytes in normal pregnancy. *Journal of Clinical Endocrinology and Metabolism* **40:** 108–115.

Weir RJ, Doig A, Fraser R et al (1976) Studies of the renin–angiotensin–aldosterone system, cortisol, DOC, and ADH in normal and hypertensive pregnancy. In Lindheimer MD et al (eds) *Hypertension in Pregnancy*, pp 251–261. New York: John Wiley.

Weissberg PL, West MJ, Kendall MJ, Ingram M & Woods KL (1985) Effect of changes in dietary sodium and potassium on blood pressure and cellular electrolyte handling in young normotensive subjects. *Journal of Hypertension* **3:** 475–480.

Winkel CA, Milewich L, Parker R et al (1980) Conversion of plasma progesterone to deoxycorticosterone in men, non-pregnant and pregnant women, and adrenal-ectomized subjects: evidence for steroid 21-hydroxylase activity in non-adrenal tissues. *Journal of Clinical Investigation* **66:** 803–812.

5

Water metabolism and vasopressin secretion during pregnancy

WILLIAM M. BARRON

Alterations in water handling and osmoregulation are among the earliest and most striking physiologic changes that occur during pregnancy. This chapter reviews these alterations, emphasizing changes in the control of secretion of the antidiuretic hormone, arginine vasopressin (AVP). In addition, polyuria complicating pregnancy is discussed, focusing on possible aetiologies of this interesting clinical problem.

GESTATIONAL ALTERATIONS IN BODY FLUID VOLUMES

Total body water, as measured by the deuterium oxide technique, increases by 7–8 litres by gestational week 36–38 and an additional 0.5–1.0 litre is probably added by term (Hytten, 1980). These average values, determined in non-oedematous women, may be exceeded by 1–2 litres in otherwise normal gravidas with generalized oedema. The added water is distributed approximately equally between maternal and fetal-placental compartments, and in the former, more than 75% of the fluid increment is retained within the extracellular space. This marked plasma and interstitial volume expansion and the accompanying sodium retention is discussed in further detail in Chapters 2 and 4. This chapter focuses on the striking gestational alteration in the concentration of solutes (particularly sodium) in body water: that is, the marked decrease in body tonicity characteristic of normal human pregnancy.

OSMOREGULATION

Prior to a discussion of alterations in water metabolism during gestation, a brief review of the physiology of osmoregulation is appropriate. Under normal circumstances sodium and its attendant anions (primarily chloride and bicarbonate) account for more than 90% of the osmotic activity of the extracellular fluid; hence, plasma sodium concentration determines plasma osmolality. The 'effective' osmolality of body fluids is a function of those solutes that do not readily permeate cellular membranes and thereby generate osmotic pressure, i.e. a concentration gradient for water across a membrane. Thus, sodium and its attendant anions, which are in much lower concentration in the intracellular than extracellular compartment, are the major osmotically 'effective' solutes, while urea, which is highly membrane permeable, is 'ineffective'.

In non-pregnant adults plasma osmolality (P_{osm}), which ranges from 280 to 300 mosmol kg^{-1}, varies but a few milliosmoles in any individual. The maintenance of P_{osm} within a very narrow range is due to a tightly regulated balance between water excretion, determined by the antidiuretic action of the posterior pituitary hormone (AVP) on the collecting duct of the distal nephron, and water intake, governed by the thirst mechanism. AVP, a nonapeptide synthesized in the magnocellular neurons of the supraoptic and hypothalamic nuclei, normally circulates at picogram levels. The potency of the hormone is demonstrated by the fact that in its absence urine osmolality (U_{osm}) may be as low as 40 mosmol kg^{-1}, and solute-free water may be excreted at rates as high as $1 \, 1 \, h^{-1}$. In contrast, an increase in levels of plasma AVP (P_{AVP}) to 5–7 pg ml^{-1} produces near-maximal urinary concentration of 1000–1200 mosmol kg^{-1} and may reduce urinary flow rates to 20 ml h^{-1} (Robertson and Berl, 1986).

Both osmotic and nonosmotic factors affect AVP secretion, but under normal circumstances plasma tonicity is the major determinant of hormone release. For instance, a decrease in total body water of but 1%, which increases P_{osm} only 2–3 mosmol kg^{-1}, will stimulate a 1 pg ml^{-1} rise in P_{AVP}. On the other hand, in normally hydrated individuals, a decrease in plasma tonicity of 1–2% (2–4 mosmol kg^{-1}) will suppress P_{AVP} to undetectable levels, resulting in a brisk water diuresis (Robertson and Berl, 1986).

There is debate whether the AVP-secretory mechanism exhibits true threshold behaviour or functions in a continuous manner. Nonetheless, there is a P_{osm} below which P_{AVP} is usually undetectable and U_{osm} minimal, and above which secretion is stimulated. In the latter circumstance, the AVP-osmolality relationship can be represented by a linear regression relating P_{AVP} to P_{osm}. Using such methodology, the slope of the regression ($\Delta P_{AVP}/\Delta P_{osm}$) represents the sensitivity of the system, while the x-axis intercept defines the set point or apparent osmotic threshold for AVP secretion (Figure 1).

Alterations in blood volume and/or hormone release are the most important non-osmotic factors regulating vasopressin release. Both hypovolaemia and hypotension stimulate secretion; however, in contrast to osmotic stimuli, no increase in P_{AVP} occurs until volume or pressure has been reduced by 5–10%. Beyond this, hormone levels rise exponentially and may reach concentrations capable of producing vasoconstriction, and hence of supporting blood pressure (Figure 1). In contrast, hypervolaemia and/or hypertension may suppress AVP secretion. These haemodynamic stimuli do not eliminate the effect of osmotic stimuli on vasopressin secretion: rather, they appear to alter the osmotic sensitivity and/or set of the system (Schrier et al, 1979; Robertson and Berl, 1986). For example, acute and chronic reductions in intravascular volume have been shown to lower the osmotic threshold for AVP secretion in both humans and animals (Dunn et al, 1973;

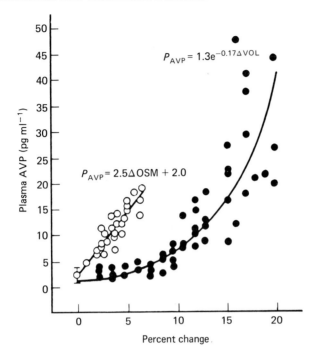

Figure 1. The relationship of P_{AVP} to percentage increase in plasma osmolality (○) and decrease in blood volume (●) in the rat. P_{osm} was increased by the IP injection of hypertonic saline while blood volume was decreased by IP injection of polyethylene glycol. The x-axis intercept of the regression of P_{AVP} on P_{osm} defines the apparent osmotic threshold for AVP secretion (i.e. the set of the system) while the slope defines the sensitivity, i.e. the change in P_{AVP} in response to alteration in plasma osmolality. From Dunn et al (1973) with permission.

Robertson, 1983), a circumstance that may have relevance to the pregnant state (see below).

As noted previously, thirst is another important determinant of body tonicity. The brain centres controlling thirst and AVP release are located in close proximity in the paraventricular anterior hypothalamus. Moreover, factors which alter the osmotic threshold of one usually alter the other in a similar fashion. This is important, for without appropriate activation or suppression of water ingestion, plasma tonicity could not be maintained with a narrow normal range regardless of changes in P_{AVP} (Robertson and Berl, 1986).

Alterations in body tonicity and AVP secretion in pregnancy

During gestation P_{osm} decreases by 8–10 mosmol kg^{-1} below values measured in the non-pregnant state (Davison et al, 1981). This decrement starts shortly after conception and becomes significant by gestational week 5; values reach a nadir by week 10 of pregnancy and thereafter remain unchanged until term

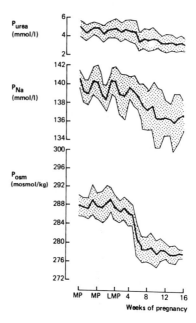

Figure 2. Mean values (±SD) for plasma urea (P_{urea}), sodium (P_{Na}), and osmolality (P_{osm}) measured at weekly intervals from before conception through the first trimester in nine healthy women with a normal pregnancy outcome. MP and LMP are menstrual and last menstrual period, respectively. From Davison et al (1981) with permission.

(Figure 2). Of importance is that only about 1.5 mosmol kg^{-1} of this decrease is due to alterations in plasma levels of urea; most of the decrement is due to a decline in the concentrations of sodium and its attendant anions. Thus, pregnancy is characterized by a true decrease in 'effective' osmolality.

If a similar decrease in the tonicity of body fluids were to occur in a non-pregnant individual, secretion of antidiuretic hormone would be suppressed and a large, continuous water diuresis similar to that in patients with diabetes insipidus would ensue. However, pregnant women are not polyuric; 24-hour urine volumes during gestation average no more than several hundred millilitres above those observed in non-gravid subjects (Parboosingh and Doig, 1973; Davison et al, 1984). Furthermore, pregnant subjects maintain their new P_{osm} within a narrow range, and water loading or fluid restriction leads to appropriate dilution and concentration of the urine (see below). Such data indicate that the osmotic set point or threshold for both thirst and vasopressin secretion are lowered during normal pregnancy – a hypothesis that has been verified by studies in both rodents and humans.

We began studies of AVP secretion during pregnancy using a rodent model for two reasons. First, rat gestation mimics human pregnancy in that it is accompanied by an 8–10 mosmol kg^{-1} decline in P_{osm} (Lindheimer et al, 1985), due primarily to decreases in plasma sodium. Secondly, placentae of gravid women (and other primates), but not those of rodents, produce a

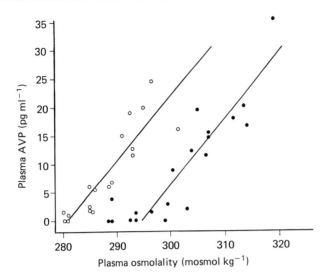

Figure 3. Relationship between P_{osm} and P_{AVP} in rats when blood tonicity was altered by IP injection of saline solutions ranging from 200–1200 mosmol kg^{-1}. Open circles represent gravid ($r=0.90$, slope of regression$=1.13$) and solid circles represent virgin controls ($r=0.91$, slope$=1.16$). From Dürr et al (1981) with permission.

cystine aminopeptidase (vasopressinase) which in vitro inactivates nanogram quantities of AVP (Tuppy, 1968; Rosenbloom et al, 1975); and until we perfected methods of instantaneously inactivating the enzyme during blood sampling, we were unable to measure plasma AVP meaningfully during human pregnancy (see below).

In 1981 Dürr and colleagues demonstrated that despite the marked decrement in tonicity during rodent pregnancy, basal P_{AVP} in near-term, gravid Sprague–Dawley rats averaged about 2 pg ml^{-1}, levels similar to those observed in virgin controls. Furthermore, basal U_{osm} was similar—and over 1400 mosmol kg^{-1}—in both groups. Following oral water loading, pregnant and virgin animals both suppressed P_{AVP} to undetectable levels and the urine became maximally dilute. In response to increments in P_{osm}, evoked by intraperitoneal hypertonic saline, P_{AVP} increased significantly in both pregnant and control animals. Construction of highly significant regressions of P_{AVP} on P_{osm} demonstrated that the apparent osmotic threshold for AVP secretion, defined by the x-axis intercept, was more than 10 mosmol kg^{-1} lower in the pregnant rats, while the slope or sensitivity of the response was unaltered (Figure 3).

Studies were also performed in Brattleboro rats, homozygous for congenital central diabetes insipidus. These animals produce no circulating AVP; nevertheless, P_{osm} in near-term rats was 16 mosmol kg^{-1} lower than levels in control virgins, while U_{osm} remained near maximally dilute. These observations indicated that the osmotic threshold for drinking also decreased in pregnancy (Barron et al, 1985).

Table 1. Basal values and effects of dehydration followed by water loading during and after pregnancy.

	Basal values			12 h Fluid deprivation			Water loading		
	Pregnant	Non-pregnant	P	Pregnant	Non-pregnant	P	Pregnant	Non-pregnant	P
P_{osm} (mosmol kg⁻¹)	280.9±2.0	289.4±2.1	<0.001	286.1±1.7	294.2±2.2	<0.001	277.2±1.8	284.3±2.1	<0.001
P_{urea} (mmol l⁻¹)	3.5±1.0	4.8±0.9	<0.05	4.0±1.1	5.5±1.2	<0.05	3.0±0.9	4.4±1.3	<0.05
$P_{glucose}$ (mmol l⁻¹)	4.7±0.9	5.6±1.1	NS	4.9±0.8	5.8±1.0	NS	4.7±0.9	5.6±1.1	NS
P_{Na} (mmol l⁻¹)	135.7±2.6	140.0±1.7	<0.01	136.8±2.1	141.1±1.9	<0.01	135.5±2.0	140.1±2.2	<0.01
Hct (%)	34.2±4.8	39.9±4.1	<0.05	35.1±4.7	39.9±5.0	NS	34.0±5.1	38.3±4.2	NS
P_{AVP} (pg ml⁻¹)	1.39±0.56	1.25±0.62	NS*	2.25±0.81	2.89±1.19	NS*	<0.5	<0.5	NS*
U_{osm} (mosmol kg⁻¹)	598±82	609±101	NS	779±121	784±102	NS	78±52	80±38	NS
Urinary volume (ml 24 h⁻¹)	1383±332	1292±287	NS	—	—	—	—	—	—

±SD, $n=8$;
* Non-significant when pregnant compared to non-pregnant values, however, both during and after pregnancy P_{AVP} increased significantly ($P<0.01$) in response to water deprivation and decreased significantly ($P<0.001$) after water loading. From Davison et al, 1984, with permission.

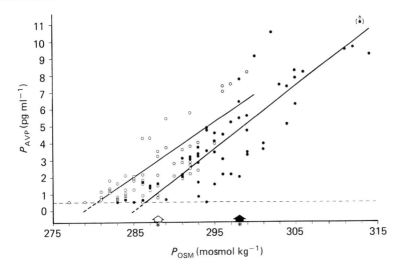

Figure 4. Relationship between P_{osm} and P_{AVP} during a 2-hour infusion of 5% saline in human pregnancy. O =data obtained during the third trimester ($P_{AVP} = 0.32$ ($P_{osm} - 279$); $r = 0.79$). ● =data for the same women 8–10 weeks postpartum ($P_{AVP} = 0.38$ ($P_{osm} - 285$); $r = 0.86$). Arrows represent thirst thresholds. From Davison et al (1984), with permission.

Following the development of a methodology for the rapid inactivation of vasopressinase, Davison and colleagues (1984) studied eight healthy women during their third trimester and again 8–10 weeks postpartum. Each was evaluated after 12 hours water deprivation, following oral water loading and during a 2-hour infusion of 5% saline. Despite a basal P_{osm} 8.5 mosmol kg^{-1} lower in the gravid subjects, P_{AVP} levels were similar during and after gestation (Table 1). In response to water deprivation, P_{osm}, U_{osm} and P_{AVP} increased similarly in pregnant and postpartum subjects. Following water loading, P_{osm} declined significantly and vasopressin levels became undetectable in both groups. During the administration of hypertonic saline P_{osm} increased from 281 ± 2 to 293 ± 4 mosmol kg^{-1}, while postpartum the same infusion resulted in increments from 289 ± 2 to 303 ± 6 mosmol kg^{-1}. Baseline P_{AVP}, similar in pregnant (1.4 ± 0.6 pg ml^{-1}) and non-pregnant (1.3 ± 0.7 pg ml^{-1}) women, increased to 4.1 ± 2.5 pg ml^{-1} in the former and to 7.0 ± 3.6 pg ml^{-1} in the postpartum studies. As in the rodent studies, the abscissal intercepts of the relationship of P_{AVP} to P_{osm} demonstrated that the apparent osmotic threshold for AVP release was significantly decreased during gestation (Figure 4). In addition, during the hypertonic saline infusions volunteers noted when a desire to drink first appeared; the value of this osmotic threshold for thirst was approximately 10 mosmol kg^{-1} lower during pregnancy than following pregnancy. Thus, osmoregulation during gestation in both humans and rodents is similar to that observed in non pregnant individuals, except that it occurs around a new set point which is 6–10 mosmol kg^{-1} lower.

The above data permit speculation as to how P_{osm} decreases during gestation. An initial lowering of the osmotic threshold for thirst stimulates an increase in water intake and dilution of body fluids. The decrease in osmotic threshold for AVP release permits continued secretion of antidiuretic hormone and retention of water. P_{osm} continues to decline until it falls below the new thirst threshold, at which point a new steady state is established. It is important to note that the comparable decrements in the osmotic thresholds for thirst and AVP secretion play an important role in the maintenance of the new steady-state level of body tonicity. If the AVP secretory threshold alone decreased, P_{osm} would remain unchanged despite considerable AVP secretion, since the gravid woman would not be stimulated to ingest additional fluid. On the other hand, if the thirst threshold alone declined, hormone secretion would be suppressed after a small decrement in P_{osm} and severe polydipsia would be required to maintain even a small degree of plasma hypotonicity. In essence, it is the parallel decrement in the osmotic thresholds for both thirst and AVP secretion that permits the gravid woman or rat to maintain a new steady-state P_{osm} within a narrow range without an alteration in urinary volume. Recent preliminary data (Davison and Lindheimer, unpublished observations) suggest that the decline in osmotic threshold for thirst may actually precede that of AVP release by several weeks. This is supported by observation of a transient increase in urinary volume during the first five to eight gestational weeks.

Metabolic clearance of AVP during pregnancy

Close inspection of Figure 4 reveals a subtle decrease in the slope of the relationship between P_{AVP} and P_{osm} in pregnant subjects. Although not significant in these original studies, further experiments (Davison and Lindheimer, unpublished observations) have demonstrated a statistically significant decrement. This apparent decrease in the sensitivity of the P_{AVP} response to osmotic stimulation could be explained by a reduced hypothalamic–pituitary responsiveness or by a increase in the metabolic clearance rate (MCR) of AVP during gestation. To investigate the latter, Davison et al (1987) measured the MCR of AVP during steady-state infusions in 14 healthy gravidas in late gestation and again 8–10 weeks postpartum. Mean clearance in the pregnant subjects, approximately $3 \, l \, min^{-1}$, was more than four times greater than values postpartum, $0.67 \, l \, min^{-1}$. In addition, MCR was similar in two gravidas with multiple gestation and in an additional two with a single kidney. The latter suggest that increases in placental cystine aminopeptidase and/or renal metabolism are not the major mechanisms accounting for the augmented MCR, although more data will be needed to establish these speculations. Nonetheless, the marked increment in MCR may explain the previously described decrease in the P_{AVP} response to osmotic stimuli in late gestation. It may also explain the occurrence of certain cases of transient gestational diabetes insipidus, as well as why some women with pre-existing central diabetes insipidus require additional hormone replacement while pregnant (see below).

Mechanisms responsible for the osmoregulatory alterations

Hormonal changes

During pregnancy there are increases in the levels of several hormones that potentially could alter AVP secretion. Data from our laboratory suggest that the fetoplacental unit may be the site of such a compound since pseudo-pregnancy, a state mimicking the hormonal milieu of gestation in the absence of the fetus or placenta, is not accompanied by decrements in P_{osm} (Barron et al, 1983). However, we have been unsuccessful in attempts to alter body tonicity of virgin rats with the administration of placental extracts (Barron and Lindheimer, unpublished observations). Similarly, we have been unable to identify roles for oestrogen, progesterone (Barron et al, 1986), prolactin, endogenous opioids or the renin–angiotensin system in the osmoregulatory alterations of pregnancy. In preliminary experiments, human chorionic gonadotropin appears to lower both basal P_{osm} and the osmotic threshold for AVP release; however, further studies will be needed to confirm these observations and determine if the magnitude of the effect parallels that reported in human pregnancy (Davison and Lindheimer, unpublished observations).

The role of volume and blood pressure

Pregnancy in both humans and rodents is accompanied by substantial increases in blood volume, changes that in theory should suppress AVP secretion. However, it has been suggested that as a consequence of the marked vasodilatation, 'effective circulating volume' is actually *decreased* during pregnancy (Nolten and Ehrlich, 1980; Schrier, 1987), and a recent study of serial haemodynamic and hormonal alterations during pregnancy in the baboon supports such a concept (Phippard et al, 1986). If true, pregnancy would resemble cirrhosis and congestive heart failure, two clinical situations in which extracellular volume is expanded and vasopressin is secreted despite plasma hypotonicity.

We have addressed the above issue in studies using the gravid rat model, hypothesizing that if 'effective' volume were indeed decreased in pregnancy, gravid animals should secrete AVP in an exaggerated manner when subjected to experimental volume depletion. This, however, was not the case; despite a blood volume that at term was nearly twice that of non-gravid animals, both 14-day (midterm) and 21-day (near-term) rats demonstrated exponential rises in P_{AVP} that were virtually identical to those in virgin controls, each group demonstrating a significant increase in plasma levels only when volume depletion exceeded 7% (Figure 5). This meant that AVP levels increased in the gravid rats when circulating volume was still considerably greater than in non-pregnant rats. In other words, the volume-sensing AVP secretory mechanism is reset during pregnancy such that the increased intravascular volume is recognized as normal (Barron et al, 1984b).

In additional investigations we assessed the effect of chronic volume expansion on osmoregulation in gravid rodents. We reasoned that if

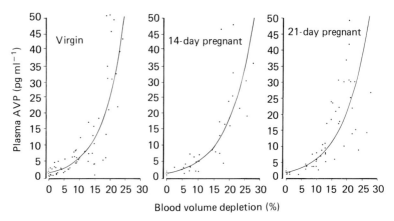

Figure 5. The relationship of P_{AVP} to isosmotic decreases in blood volume in gravid and virgin rats. Experimental animals (● virgin, $n = 64$; 14-day pregnant, $n = 33$; 21-day pregnant, $n = 49$) were injected IP with polyethylene glycol dissolved in isotonic or slightly hypotonic saline, while controls (○) received isotonic saline alone. Each of the regression lines is highly significant ($r = 0.88$–0.92). From Barron et al (1984a) with permission.

reductions in 'effective' blood volume were responsible for alterations in AVP secretion and body tonicity, then experimentally induced volume expansion should increase the basal P_{osm} of gravid rats towards the levels of virgin animals. Beginning on the first day of sperm positivity, pregnant and control rats were treated with standard diet or a high-sodium diet, alone or in combination with daily injections of deoxycorticosterone acetate (DOCA). The volume-expanding regimens led to significant decreases in plasma renin activity and aldosterone levels, indicating that an increase in 'effective' volume had been achieved. Despite this, plasma osmolality and sodium of treated pregnant animals were similar to control pregnant rats: 8–10 mosmol kg^{-1} and 3–5 mmol^{-1}, respectively, below similarly treated virgin groups.

To determine if decrements in blood pressure were responsible for the osmoregulatory changes, gravid rats were treated chronically with norepinephrine and DOCA. Despite significant increases in mean arterial pressure of about 10%, P_{osm} of pregnant animals was unaltered, remaining significantly hypotonic compared to levels in virgin controls. Taken together with the above findings, these observations provide strong support for the hypothesis that factors other than haemodynamic stimuli mediate the alterations in P_{osm} and AVP secretion during pregnancy (Barron et al, 1987).

Additional factors that may influence water handling

Posture

When studied in the supine position, first-trimester and second-trimester gravidas have been observed to excrete a water load normally; however, this ability was impaired in late pregnancy (Janney and Walker, 1932). Hytten and

Klopper (1963) performed similar studies with subjects in the sitting position, and reported enhanced water excretion during early gestation followed by impaired excretory capacity during the third trimester. Others studying the effects of oral water loading in subjects positioned in lateral recumbency observed that water excretion was not decreased during weeks 32–34 of pregnancy when compared to results of postpartum studies (Davison et al, 1981). In addition, several investigators have observed that merely changing from the lateral recumbent to a supine position during late gestation significantly decreases urine flow (Hendricks and Barnes, 1955; Pritchard et al, 1955; Chesley and Sloan, 1964; Lindheimer and Weston, 1969), and quiet standing is progressively more antidiuretic as pregnancy advances (Assali et al, 1959). These results have been attributed to posturally induced haemodynamic alterations caused by the enlarging uterus. Although the mechanism mediating these phenomena remains unknown, alterations in antidiuretic hormone secretion do not appear to be a prerequisite, since posture-induced alterations in water excretion have been observed in a gravida with diabetes insipidus (Whalley et al, 1961). Finally, it should be mentioned that postural effects on water handling are insufficient, by themselves, to account for the decline in P_{osm} during gestation.

Vasopressinase

A fascinating paradox is that although plasma AVP levels are normal in gestation and gravidas have little difficulty concentrating their urine (see below), the blood of pregnant women and non-human primates (but not rodents) contains large quantities of a cystine aminopeptidase (vasopressinase) of presumed placental origin, which in vitro destroys nanogram quantities of AVP per millilitre plasma per minute (Tuppy, 1968; Rosenbloom et al, 1975). The biologic importance of this enzyme, its activity in vivo and its contribution to the augmented metabolic clearance of vasopressin during human pregnancy are unknown. It is essential in investigations involving the measurement of AVP in pregnancy plasma that painstaking attention is paid to the rapid and complete inactivation of vasopressinase at the time blood is removed from gravid subjects (Davison et al, 1984).

Prostaglandins

Plasma and urinary levels of several vasodilatory prostaglandins (e.g. PGE_2, PGI) increase substantially during pregnancy and certain eicosanoids may inhibit the hydro-osmotic action of vasopressin on the renal collecting duct. In this regard, there are conflicting reports as to whether gravid humans (Roth and Slater, 1962; Vorherr and Friedberg, 1964; Torres et al, 1966; Kleeman and Vorherr, 1974; Gallery et al, 1979), rats (Barron et al, 1985) and goats (Sasson et al, 1982) are resistant to the antidiuretic effects of injected aqueous vasopressin. However, even if such resistance were proved, other mechanisms such as enhanced metabolic clearance could explain a relative decrease in urinary concentration following AVP administration during pregnancy. We

Table 2. Urinary concentrating ability in pregnancy.

	Maximum U_{osm} (mosmol kg^{-1})		
Author	Non-pregnant	Pregnant	Comments
Kaitz (1961)	—	935 ± 118 (30)	Dehydrated 24 h
McCartney et al (1964)	—	910 ± 113 (7)	Dehydrated 20 h
Norden and Tuttle (1965)	—	942 ± 207 (34)	Dehydrated 24 h
Reeves and Brumfitt (1968)	—	75% > 850 (33)	Dehydrated 21 h
Williams et al (1969)	1052 ± 92 (20)	930 ± 95 (45)	Dehydrated 24 h
Norden et al (1970)	—	899 ± 133 (75)	Dehydrated 16 h then pitressin injected
Davison et al (1981)	854 ± 107 (6)	725 ± 110 (6)	Dehydrated 17 h
Hutchon et al (1982)	1141 ± 223 (7)	826 ± 223 (8)	Dehydrated 15 h
Hutchon et al (1982)	1109 ± 225 (7)	932 ± 169 (27)	Received desmopressin (dDAVP)
Davison et al (1984)	784 ± 102 (8)	779 ± 121 (8)	Dehydrated 12 h

Figures in parenthesis represent sample size.

are unaware of any studies specifically examining the effect of gestational increases in prostaglandin synthesis on urinary concentrating ability in normal pregnancy.

Urinary concentration and dilution

The marked increment in glomerular filtration rate during pregnancy might be expected to impair maximal urinary concentrating ability due to the large increment in filtered solute per nephron, and there is some evidence to support such a hypothesis. Table 2 summarizes data from nine studies in which urinary concentrating ability of pregnant subjects was studied by measuring urine osmolality after variable periods of dehydration with or without the addition of aqueous arginine vasopressin (Pitressin) or the analogue desmospressin acetate (dDAVP). Although only four reports include non-pregnant controls, the data suggest that maximal urinary concentrating ability is modestly impaired in the gravid women. Nonetheless, it is doubtful that such an observation has any clinical significance, since P_{osm} is equally well defended in pregnant and non-pregnant women when subjected to dehydration (Davison et al, 1981; 1984).

It should be noted that much of the data in Table 2 may not be valid since investigators frequently failed to control for posture. In this regard, it has been noted serendipitously that lateral recumbency interferes with tests of urinary concentration (Davison et al, 1981). In these studies U_{osm} actually decreased in subjects dehydrated for 12 hours when they assumed the lateral decubitus position, but then increased when the test was continued with subjects supine. *Although lateral recumbency is the preferred position for investigation of renal haemodynamics during pregnancy, sitting is the posture of choice when renal concentrating ability is examined.* Authors of the above studies focused on maximal urine concentrating ability, and there are few investigations of the relationship between P_{AVP} and U_{osm} under basal, euhydrated conditions. In one such study, levels of AVP were similar during (1.4 ± 0.6 pg ml^{-1}) and following (1.3 ± 0.6 pg ml^{-1}) pregnancy, and were associated with similar levels of U_{osm} (598 ± 82 mosmol kg^{-1} and 609 ± 101 mosmol kg^{-1}, respectively) suggesting that renal sensitivity to antidiuretic hormone is not significantly altered during gestation (Davison et al, 1981). Such observations have been confirmed in recent studies of steady-state AVP infusions in gravid women (Davison; Barron; Lindheimer; unpublished observations).

The ability to achieve maximal urinary dilution does not appear to be altered during pregnancy; however, the effect of posture remains unclear. Lindheimer and Weston (1969) observed that administration of hypotonic fluid to 12 third-trimester gravidas positioned in lateral recumbency resulted in a U_{osm} of 54 ± 18 mosmol kg^{-1}, a value comparable to that considered normal in non-pregnant individuals. When subjects changed to the supine position, U_{osm} remained the same or decreased in 7 of the 12 subjects. However, in 2 subjects U_{osm} increased to values greater than 120 mosmol kg^{-1}. In contrast, Davison and associates found that minimum U_{osm} following oral water loading was similar during and following pregnancy, and was unaffected by changing from the lateral to the supine position (Davison et al, 1981).

DIABETES INSIPIDUS DURING GESTATION

Because normal pregnancy is accompanied by increased thirst and urinary frequency, physicians are often disinclined to formally evaluate gravidas who complain of increased urination. This may be one reason why diabetes insipidus (DI) complicating gestation is recognized so infrequently. Nonetheless, a number of recent reports suggest that this syndrome might not be as rare as previously believed.

The several diseases that together comprise diabetes insipidus during pregnancy have recently been reviewed in detail (Dürr, 1987). The discussion below focuses on gestation in patients with pre-existing DI and on the syndrome of transient diabetes insipidus of pregnancy.

Pre-existing central diabetes insipidus

Fertility rates, course of gestation, labour, delivery and lactation in women with isolated central DI have not been documented as different from those in the normal population (Hime and Richardson, 1978; Amico, 1985; Dürr, 1987). With regard to the effect of pregnancy on diabetes insipidus Hime and Richardson (1978) analysed reports of 79 gravidas with central DI. Diagnoses were established by modern criteria in only 26 subjects and data relevant to the course of gestation were present in only 22. Of these, disease worsened during pregnancy in 13, remained unchanged in 5 and, surprisingly, improved in 4. In the more recent literature, requirements for replacement therapy, including both AVP and dDAVP, have been described as either increased (Marek et al, 1978; Phelan et al, 1978; Chelvam et al, 1979; Campbell, 1980; Hadi et al, 1985) or unchanged (Sack et al, 1980; Shangold et al, 1983); however, in most instances, the patient's subjective responses rather than objective determinations of urinary volume and concentration have been used to guide dosage requirements. The potential difficulty this poses is described in a recent report of a woman with traumatic central DI successfully treated with dDAVP prior to pregnancy. During the fifth gestational month she complained of increasing thirst and urination, stating that her usual dose of 0.1 ml dDAVP was no longer effective. However, renal responses to this dose of dDAVP during the thirty-sixth week of pregnancy and three months postpartum were marked and virtually identical (Amico, 1985).

There are several potential mechanisms that may cause DI to worsen during gestation. These include enlargement of the pituitary gland or tumours contained therein, hormone destruction by vasopressinase, placental inactivation, increases in renal and/or hepatic metabolism and/or decreased renal responsiveness. However, none of these potential explanations has been established in the reports cited above.

The treatment of choice for central diabetes insipidus complicating pregnancy appears to be dDAVP. This long-acting analogue of AVP has virtually no pressor activity and no maternal or fetal complications have been reported. A theoretic advantage of this preparation over arginine or lysine vasopressin is that unlike the latter two agents, dDAVP is resistant to enzymatic degradation by vasopressinase and hence its metabolic clearance may not increase so markedly during pregnancy. The oral agents available for the therapy of DI – chlorpropamide, clofibrate and the thiazide diuretics – appear to pose greater risks than dDAVP (Briggs et al, 1986) and are not as consistently effective.

Use of dDAVP is of additional value in the gravida with DI who develops pre-eclampsia, since this hypertensive disorder is associated with increased pressor responsiveness to arginine vasopressin, contraindicating the use of Pitressin. It is of note that pre-eclampsia occurs at all in gravidas with DI, and suggests that antidiuretic hormone is not a central component of the pathogenesis of this hypertensive disorder of pregnancy. In the few cases reported, pre-eclampsia has been associated with an improvement in diabetes insipidus (Bloemers, 1961; Gordon and Bradford, 1970; Campbell, 1980; Hadi et al, 1985). Such observations could be the result of decreased glomerular filtration, enhanced sodium reabsorption or decreased metabolic clearance of vasopressin in those pre-eclamptics with liver involvement.

Transient diabetes insipidus of pregnancy

A number of instances of diabetes insipidus appearing *de novo* during pregnancy and resolving postpartum have been described (Blotner and Kunkel, 1942; Carfagno et al, 1953; Feeney et al, 1978; Ferrara et al, 1980; Barron et al, 1984a; Korbett et al, 1985; Baylis et al, 1986; Ford and Lumpkin, 1986; Cammu et al, 1987, Dürr et al, 1987). A recent pathophysiologic classification separates such cases into forms sensitive or resistant to vasopressin (Dürr, 1987).

Vasopressin-responsive DI

It is likely that many of these cases represent mild deficiencies in AVP secretory capacity, brought to clinical attention by one of the mechanisms alluded to earlier. Such a possibility cannot be excluded, since few investigators have established the normality of AVP secretion postpartum via measurement of P_{AVP} responses to osmotic stimulation. In one of the few well-documented cases, Baylis and colleagues described a woman with mild central diabetes insipidus, established by measuring P_{AVP} responses to hypertonic saline infusion postpartum. Prior to conception urine output was less than 2 l per day; however, during each of the two pregnancies volumes more than doubled, necessitating therapy with dDAVP. Following each delivery, thirst, polyuria and polydipsia rapidly resolved (Baylis et al, 1986).

The above circumstance is akin to that observed in heterozygous Brattleboro rats. These animals have a partial defect in hypothalamic AVP synthesis; when they become pregnant, most alter water intake and urine output, and concentrate urine similarly to the normal Long–Evans strain during pregnancy. However, some dams periodically manifest marked increases in water turnover, mimicking that observed in homozygous animals with complete AVP deficiency (Barron et al, 1985). Whether some degree of AVP deficiency is a prerequisite for the development of this form of gestational DI is unknown.

Vasopressin-resistant DI

In 1980 Ferrara and colleagues reported a case, albeit with incomplete details, suggesting a transient form of gestational DI that did not respond to Pitressin (Ferrara et al, 1980). In 1984 we described transient DI unresponsive to large doses of aqueous vasopressin in three gravidas, one of whom had measurable levels of circulating immunoreactive AVP (Barron et al, 1984b). Since excessive endogenous vasopressinase was not excluded as a cause of the syndrome (although one woman did have increased levels), and because the bioactivity of the single measured plasma AVP level could not be verified, we labelled the disorder 'vasopressin-resistant' rather than 'nephrogenic' diabetes insipidus.

Recently, Dürr and colleagues (1987) described a gravida with severe polyuria unresponsive to massive doses of AVP; however, urine volumes fell and U_{osm} rose promptly when dDAVP was administered. Since AVP is rapidly destroyed by vasopressinase while dDAVP is resistant to inactivation, the authors hypothesized that hormone destruction by this enzyme caused the polyuria. This was supported by studies demonstrating excessive quantities of circulating vasopressinase and by the production of marked polyuria and decreased U_{osm} in a bioassay rat injected with the patient's plasma. The woman's urine volume returned to normal by the fortieth postpartum day, at which time plasma vasopressinase activity was minimal. Whether this type of transient DI is due to increased vasopressinase levels *per se* or activation of normally inactive enzyme, remains to be determined.

It is of interest that many of the reported cases of transient DI in pregnancy were associated with abnormal liver and kidney function, which in some instances was accompanied by mildly elevated blood pressure suggesting pre-eclampsia. It is, however, difficult to implicate these developments in the pathogenesis of the syndrome, since the superimposition of pre-eclampsia in gravidas with pre-existing DI typically reduces polyuria. The role of increased prostaglandin synthesis in this disorder was recently investigated by Ford and Lumpkin (1986) who administered indomethacin and sulindac to a single gravida with transient DI; however, no increase in U_{osm} was observed following either drug. Furthermore, there was no urinary response to either AVP or dDAVP, and following a period of water deprivation P_{osm} increased to 292 mosmol kg^{-1} and P_{AVP} was 12 pg ml^{-1}, while U_{osm} was only 275 mosmol kg^{-1}. These data support a diagnosis of transient, true nephrogenic diabetes insipidus, and emphasize the marked heterogeneity of the disorders comprising the syndrome of transient DI of pregnancy.

REFERENCES

Amico JA (1985) Diabetes insipidus and pregnancy. *Frontiers Hormone Research* 13: 266–277.

Assali NS, Dignam WJ & Dasgupta K (1959) Renal function in human pregnancy. II Effects of venous pooling on renal hemodynamics and water, electrolytes and aldosterone excretion during normal pregnancy. *Journal of Laboratory Clinical Medicine* 54: 394–408.

Barron WM & Lindheimer MD (1984) Renal sodium and water handling in pregnancy. *Obstetrics and Gynecology Annual* 13: 35–69.

Barron WM, Stamoutsos BA, Langhofer M & Lindheimer MD (1983) Effect of pseudopregnancy on plasma osmolality and vasopressin. *Clinical Research* 37: 747A.

Barron WM, Stamoutsos BA & Lindheimer MD (1984a) Role of volume in the regulation of vasopressin secretion during pregnancy in the rat. *Journal of Clinical Investigation* 73: 923–932.

Barron WM, Cohen LH, Ulland LA et al (1984b) Transient vasopressin-resistant diabetes insipidus of pregnancy. *New England Journal of Medicine* 310: 442–444.

Barron WM, Dürr JA, Stamoutsos BA & Lindheimer MD (1985) Osmoregulation during pregnancy in homozygous and heterozygous Brattleboro rats. *American Journal of Physiology* 248: 229–237.

Barron WM, Schreiber J & Lindheimer MD (1986) Effect of ovarian sex steroids on osmoregulation and vasopressin secretion in the rat. *American Journal of Physiology* 250: E352–E361.

Barron WM, Dürr J & Lindheimer MD (1987) Do hemodynamic factors mediate the osmoregulatory changes of pregnancy? *Clinical and Experimental Hypertension*, part B 6: 39.

Bayliss PH, Thompson C, Burd J et al (1986) Recurrent pregnancy-induced polyuria due to hypothalamic diabetes insipidus: an investigation into possible mechanisms responsible for polyuria. *Clinical Endocrinology* 24: 459–466.
Bloemers D (1961) Diabetes insipidus and toxaemia of pregnancy. *Journal of Obstetrics and Gynaecology of the British Commonwealth* 68: 322–327.
Blotner H & Kunkel P (1942) Diabetes insipidus and pregnancy. Report of two cases. *New England Journal of Medicine* 227: 287–292.
Briggs GG, Freeman RK & Yaffe SJ (1986) *A Reference Guide to Fetal and Neonatal Risk: Drugs in Pregnancy and Lactation*, 2nd edn. Baltimore: Williams & Wilkins.
Cammu H, Velkeniers B, Charels K et al (1987) Idiopathic acute fatty liver of pregnancy associated with transient diabetes insipidus. Case report. *British Journal of Obstetrics and Gynaecology* 94: 173–178.
Campbell JW (1980) Diabetes insipidus and complicated pregnancy. *Journal of the American Medical Association* 234: 1744–1745.
Carfagno SC, Durant TM & Shuman CR (1953) Diabetes insipidus in pregnancy. *Archives of Internal Medicine* 92: 542–553.
Chelvam P, Puraviappan & Ahmad Z (1979) Clomiphene-induced pregnancy in a patient with diabetes insipidus and hypothyroidism. *Medical Journal of Australia* 2: 316–317.
Chesley LC & Sloan DM (1964) The effect of posture on renal function in late pregnancy. *American Journal of Obstetrics and Gynecology* 89: 754–759.
Davison JM, Vallotton MB & Lindheimer MD (1981) Plasma osmolality and urinary concentration and dilution during and after pregnancy: evidence that lateral recumbency inhibits maximal urinary concentrating ability. *British Journal of Obstetrics and Gynaecology* 88: 472–479.
Davison JM, Gilmore EA, Dürr J, Robertson GL & Lindheimer MD (1984) Altered osmotic thresholds for vasopressin secretion and thirst in human pregnancy. *American Journal of Physiology* 246: F105–F109.
Davison JM, Shiells EA, Philips PR, Barron WM & Lindheimer MD (1987) Metabolic clearance rates (MCR) of vasopressin (AVP) increase markedly in gestation: a possible cause of polyuria in pregnant women. *Clinical Research* 35: 646A.
Dunn FL, Brennan TJ, Nelson AE & Robertson GL (1973) The role of blood osmolality and volume in regulating vasopressin secretion in the rat. *Journal of Clinical Investigation* 52: 3212–3219.
Dürr JA (1987) Diabetes insipidus in pregnancy. *American Journal of Kidney Disease* IX: 276–283.
Dürr JA, Stamoutsos BA & Lindheimer MD (1981) Osmoregulation during pregnancy in the rat. Evidence for resetting of the threshold for vasopressin secretion during gestation. *Journal of Clinical Investigation* 68: 337–346.
Dürr JA, Hoggard JG, Hunt JM & Schrier RW (1987) Diabetes insipidus in pregnancy associated with abnormally high circulating vasopressinase activity. *New England Journal of Medicine* 316: 1070–1074.
Feeney JG, Craig GA & Hancock KW (1978) Pregnancy and Nelson's syndrome. Two case reports. *British Journal of Obstetrics and Gynaecology* 85: 715–718.
Ferrara JM, Malatesta R & Kemmann E (1980) Transient nephrogenic diabetes insipidus during toxemia in pregnancy. *Diagnostic Gynecology and Obstetrics* 2: 227–230.
Ford SM & Lumpkin HL (1986) Transient vasopressin-resistant diabetes insipidus of pregnancy. *Obstetrics and Gynecology* 68: 726–728.
Gallery EDM, Gyory AZ, Lissner D et al (1979) Urinary concentration, white blood cell excretion, acid excretion, and acid base status in normal pregnancy: Alterations in pregnancy-associated hypertension. *American Journal of Obstetrics and Gynecology* 135: 27–36.
Gordon G & Bradford WP (1970) Pregnancy in a patient with diabetes insipidus following induction of ovulation with clomiphene. *Journal of Obstetrics and Gynaecology of the British Commonwealth* 77: 467–469.
Hadi HA, Mashini IS & DeVoe LD (1985) Diabetes insipidus during pregnancy complicated by preeclampsia. A case report. *Journal of Reproductive Medicine* 30: 206–208.
Hendricks CH & Barnes AC (1955) Effect of supine posture on urinary output in pregnancy. *American Journal of Obstetrics and Gynecology* 69: 1225–1232.
Hime MC & Richardson JA (1978) Diabetes insipidus and pregnancy: case report, incidence and

review of literature. *Obstetrics and Gynecology Survey* **33**: 375–379.

Hutchon DJR, Van Zijl JAWM, Campbell-Brown BM et al (1982) Desmopressin as a test of urinary concentrating ability in pregnancy. *Journal of Obstetrics and Gynecology* **2**: 206–209.

Hytten FE (1980) Weight gain in pregnancy. In Hytten F & Chamberlain G (eds) *Clinical Physiology in Obstetrics*, pp. 193–233. Oxford: Blackwell Scientific.

Hytten FE & Klopper AI (1963) Response to a water load in pregnancy. *Journal of Obstetrics and Gynaecology of the British Commonwealth* **70**: 811–816.

Janney JC & Walker EW (1932) Kidney function in pregnancy. I. Water diuresis in normal pregnancy. *Journal of the American Medical Association* **99**: 2078–2083.

Kaitz AL (1961) Urinary concentrating ability in pregnant women with asymptomatic bacteriuria. *Journal of Clinical Investigation* **40**: 1331–1338.

Kleeman CR & Vorherr H (1974) Water metabolism and neurohypophyseal hormones. In Bondy PK & Rosenberg LE (eds) *Duncan's Diseases of Metabolism*, pp 1479–1518. Philadelphia: WB Saunders.

Korbett SM, Corwin HL & Lewis EJ (1985) Transient nephrogenic diabetes insipidus associated with pregnancy. *American Journal of Nephrology* **5**: 442–444.

Lindheimer MD & Weston PV (1969) Effect of hypotonic expansion on sodium, water and urea excretion in late pregnancy: the influence of posture on these results. *Journal of Clinical Investigation* **48**: 947–956.

Lindheimer MD, Barron WM & Davison JM (1985) Water metabolism and vasopressin secretion in pregnancy. In Schrier RW (ed) *Vasopressin*, pp 229–241. New York: Raven Press.

Marek J, Loutocky A, Pacovsky V et al (1978) Ten-year experience with DDAVP in treatment of diabetes insipidus. *Endocrinologie* **72**: 188–194.

McCartney CP, Spargo B, Lorincz A et al (1964) Renal structure and function in pregnancy patients with acute hypertension. Osmolar concentration. *American Journal of Obstetrics and Gynecology* **90**: 579–592.

Nolten WE & Ehrlich EN (1980) Sodium and mineralocorticoids in normal pregnancy. *Kidney International* **18**: 162–172.

Norden CW & Tuttle EP (1965) Impairment of urinary concentrating ability in pregnant women with asymptomatic bacteriuria. In Kass EH (ed.) *Progress in Pyelonephritis*, pp 73–80. Philadelphia: Davis.

Norden CW, Levy PS & Kass EH (1970) Predictive effect of urinary concentrating ability and hemagglutinating antibody titer upon response to antimicrobial therapy in bacteriuria of pregnancy. *Journal of Infectious Disease* **121**: 588–596.

Olsson K, Benlamlih S, Dahlborn K et al (1982) Effects of water deprivation and hyperhydration in pregnant and lactating goats. *Acta Physiologica Scandinavica* **115**: 361–367.

Parboosingh J & Doig A (1973) Renal nyctohemeral excretory patterns of water and solutes in normal human pregnancy. *American Journal of Obstetrics and Gynecology* **116**: 609–615.

Phelan JP, Guay AT & Newman C (1978) Diabetes insipidus in pregnancy: A case review. *American Journal of Obstetrics and Gynecology* **130**: 365–366.

Phippard HF, Horvath JS, Glynn EM et al (1986) Circulatory adaptations to pregnancy – serial studies of haemodynamics, blood volume, renin, and aldosterone in the baboon (*Papio hamadryas*). *Journal of Hypertension* **4**: 773–779.

Pritchard JA, Barnes AC & Bright RH (1955) The effect of the supine position on renal function in the near term pregnant woman. *Journal of Clinical Investigation* **34**: 777–781.

Reeves DS & Brumfitt W (1968) Localization of urinary tract infection. A comparative study of methods. In O'Grady F & Brumfitt W (eds) *Urinary Tract Infection—Proceedings of the First National Symposium*, pp 53–67. Oxford: Oxford University Press.

Robertson GL (1983) Thirst and vasopressin function in normal and disordered states of water balance. *Journal of Laboratory Clinical Medicine* **101**: 351–371.

Robertson GL & Berl T (1986) Pathophysiology of water metabolism. In Brenner BM & Rector FC (eds) *The Kidney*, 3rd edn, pp 385–432. Philadelphia: WB Saunders.

Rosenbloom AA, Sack J & Fisher DA (1975) The circulating vasopressinase of pregnancy: species comparison with radioimmunoassay. *American Journal of Obstetrics and Gynecology* **121**: 316–320.

Roth K & Slater S (1962) Inactivation of vasopressin during pregnancy. *American Journal of Obstetrics and Gynecology* **83**: 1325–1336.

Sack J, Friedman E & Katznelson D (1980) Long-term treatment of diabetes insipidus with a synthetic analog of vasopressin during pregnancy. *Israeli Journal of Medical Sciences* **16:** 406–407.

Schrier RW (1987) Pregnancy—an overfill or underfill state? *American Journal of Kidney Disease* **IX:** 284–289.

Schrier RW, Berl T & Anderson RJ (1979) Osmotic and nonosmotic control of vasopressin release. *American Journal of Physiology* **236:** F321–F332.

Shangold MM, Freeman R, Kumaresan P et al (1983) Plasma oxytocin concentrations in a pregnant woman with total vasopressin deficiency. *Obstetrics and Gynecology* **61:** 662–667.

Torres C, Schewitz LJ & Pollak VE (1966) The effect of small amounts of antidiuretic hormone on sodium and urate excretion in pregnancy. *American Journal of Obstetrics and Gynecology* **94:** 546–558.

Tuppy H (1968) The influence of enzymes on neurohypophysial hormones and similar peptides. In Berde B (ed) *Neurohypophysial Hormones and Similar Polypeptides. Handbook of Experimental Pharmacology*, pp 67–129. New York: Springer-Verlag.

Vorherr H & Friedberg V (1964) The action of antidiuretic hormone in pregnancy. *Klinische Wochenschrift* **42:** 201–204.

Whalley PJ, Roberts AD & Prichard JA (1961) The effects of posture on renal function during pregnancy in a patient with diabetes insipidus. *Journal of Laboratory Clinical Medicine* **58:** 867–870.

Williams GL, Campbell H & Davies KJ (1969) Urinary concentrating ability in women with asymptomatic bacteriuria in pregnancy. *British Medical Journal* **3:** 212–215.

6

Acute renal failure in pregnancy

NATHALIE PERTUISET
JEAN-PIERRE GRUNFELD

Acute renal failure (ARF) has become a very unusual complication of pregnancy. In the 1960s, estimates of the incidence of ARF were 1 case per 1400–5000 gestations (Knapp and Hellman, 1959; Kerr and Elliot, 1967), and pregnancy-related ARF represented as much as 24–40% of all cases of ARF (Kennedy et al, 1973; Chapman and Legrain, 1979). Since 1970 its incidence has decreased markedly in industrialized countries as the result of progress in contraception, liberalized abortion laws and improved obstetric care. Lindheimer et al. (1983) estimate that the current incidence of ARF necessitating dialysis during pregnancy is less than one case per 10 000 in Western countries. Chapman and Legrain (1979) noted that obstetric ARF represented only 4.5% of all their cases of ARF in the last decade. At the National Maternity Hospital, Dublin, from 1961 to 1970, 20 cases of ARF occurred among 57 568 delivered women, whereas from 1971 to 1980 only four cases were observed among 83 713 deliveries (Donohoe, 1983). In less developed countries, however, there had been no decline, and obstetric ARF incidence is still high, for instance in northern India (Chugh et al, 1976). Similarly, at the Mustapha Hospital, Algiers, pregnancy-related ARF represented approximately 20% of all cases of ARF between 1979 and 1983, and this percentage is similar to that found from 1966 to 1978 (A. Merouani and M. Drif, personal communication).

Pregnancy-associated renal failure had at one time a bimodal distribution with peaks at the end of the first and the third trimester (Smith et al, 1965). In early pregnancy, ARF was due mainly to septic abortion, whereas in late pregnancy it had several causes, the major one being eclampsia and uterine bleeding. The initial peak has all but disappeared in industrialized nations, where sterile pregnancy termination is available, but in the last decade a new peak represented by patients with idiopathic postpartum failure is appearing.

The mortality rate in pregnancy-related ARF is low when compared with non-obstetric ARF. Finn (1983) reviewing 25 series published between 1950 and 1979 estimated the average maternal mortality at 16.8%. On the other hand, gravidas with ARF have a high risk of irreversible and/or residual chronic renal failure due to the high incidence of bilateral renal cortical necrosis (BRCN) in this setting. Recent data, however, from the National

Table 1. Comparative statistics over two decades at the National Maternity Hospital, Dublin*.

	1961–1970		1971–1980	
Category	Cases	Incidence	Cases	Incidence
Deliveries	57 568		83 713	
Abruptio placentae	1 091	1 in 53	630	1 in 133
Acute renal failure (ARF)	20	1 in 2900	4	1 in 21 000
Cortical necrosis	6	1 in 10 000	1	1 in 80 000
Complete	4		0	
Incomplete	2		1	
Mortality (ARF)	3		0	

* From McDonald, cited in Donohoe JF (1983).

Maternity Hospital in Dublin showed a decline in the incidence of both abruptio placentae and BRCN during the last decade in pregnant women (Donohoe, 1983). Acute cortical necrosis was observed in only one among 80 000 deliveries between 1971 and 1980 compared with 1 in 10 000 deliveries between 1961 and 1970 (Table 1). In obstetric ARF as a whole, prognosis for survival is poorer for the fetus than for the mother, with a high incidence of abortion and stillbirth.

SEPTIC ABORTION

The dramatic decrease of obstetric ARF in industrialized countries reflects the virtual disappearance of post-abortum ARF. For example, Kleinknecht et al (1980) in a series of 950 patients with ARF observed only one case of post abortum ARF, representing an incidence of 0.06%, and no case has been observed at the Necker Hospital since 1978 (Figure 1). In contrast, ARF due to septic abortion represents a substantial proportion of obstetric ARF in less developed countries. In India, Chugh et al (1976) reported that among 72 patients referred to their dialysis unit for obstetric ARF, 43 cases (59.7%) were related to septic abortion.

Initial symptoms of septic abortion include fever, vomiting, diarrhoea and generalized myalgias, and these appear within 2 days after the attempted abortion. They are rapidly associated with signs of septic shock, jaundice due to intravascular haemolysis, and often anuric renal failure. Skin necrosis of the extremities and other features of disseminated intravascular coagulation (DIC) may be observed in severe cases. Laboratory findings include haemolytic anaemia, thrombocytopenia and clotting abnormalities suggestive of DIC. Bacterial identification may be difficult. In most cases, sepsis is due to gram-negative bacteria. Clostridial infection is now less common, but when present usually leads to severe ARF.

Renal failure is due mainly to acute tubular necrosis. The oliguric or often anuric phase generally persists for 2 or even 3 weeks, then renal function

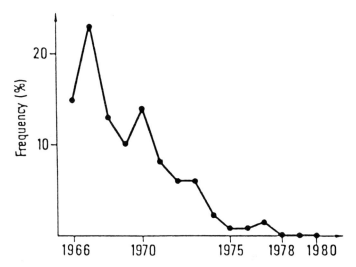

Figure 1. Incidence of ARF after septic abortion among all patients with renal failure referred to the nephrology service at Hôpital Necker from 1966 to 1980.

rapidly returns to normal. However, a high incidence of BRCN has been observed by some authors (Chugh et al, 1983).

The mortality rate in developed countries, once approximately 10%, is certainly much lower now, while in non-industrialized nations such as in northern India, mortality is still quite high (Chugh et al, 1976). Death occurs early in the course of the abortion and is usually due to septic shock rather than to uraemic complications. Initial management should include intensive supportive therapy for shock, immediate use of antibiotics and dialysis. Uterine evacuation may be necessary because of incomplete abortion. In the 1960s, many investigators advocated early abdominal hysterectomy (Bartlett and Yahia, 1969). More recently, Hawkins and colleagues (1975) obtained a favourable outcome, with normal renal function recovery found in 17 out of 19 patients managed with intensive antibiotic therapy, peritoneal dialysis and no surgical procedures. Indeed, modern antibiotic therapy usually eradicates infection from the uterus and prevents bacterial passage into the maternal circulation, but hysterectomy may be indicated in patients with necrotic uterine lesions that accompany abortion induced by chemicals and in rare cases with uncontrolled uterine sepsis.

ACUTE PYELONEPHRITIS

Acute pyelonephritis is one of the most common infectious complications of the pregnant state. In their analysis of 24 000 deliveries, Gilstrap et al (1981) found an incidence of acute pyelonephritis of 2% in pregnant women or women who had recently delivered. Several cases of ARF associated with bacterial pyelonephritis in gravidas without underlying renal disease have

Table 2. Main causes of ARF in 57 pregnant women.

	No. of cases	Mean age (yr)	Nulliparas	Cortical necrosis
Acute pyelonephritis	2	21	2	0
Severe pre-eclampsia or eclampsia	12	28	2	1
Abruptio placentae	13	30	1	7
Prolonged intrauterine fetal death	6	32	1	5
Uterine haemorrhage	4	29	1	2
Postpartum idiopathic ARF	5	24	2	3
Miscellaneous causes (including amniotic fluid, embolism, sepsis, incompatible blood transfusion, etc.)	15		6	1

Adapted from Grünfeld et al (1980).

been reported (Ober et al, 1956; Grünfeld et al, 1980). As in non-gravid patients, gram-negative sepsis and septic shock are the most important pathogenic factors, but acute pyelonephritis per se seems to have a deleterious effect on renal function in gravidas, whereas it does not significantly alter renal function in non-pregnant women. For example, Whalley et al (1975) in an analysis of 130 gravidas with acute pyelonephritis, found a significant decrement of glomerular filtration rate in as many as 20% of the cases. The propensity of pregnant women with acute pyelonephritis to develop renal failure may be related to the increased sensitivity of their renal vasculature to the vasoactive effect of bacterial endotoxins (Whalley et al, 1975). Stasis in the upper urinary tract in pregnancy may also contribute to this more deleterious effect on renal function. Finally, it must be stressed that acute renal impairment may be precipitated or aggravated by the undue use of non-steroidal anti-inflammatory drugs or potentially nephrotoxic antibiotics.

Patients with acute pyelonephritis during pregnancy should be hospitalized to be treated quickly and closely supervised. Early and adequate antibiotic therapy and treatment of shock are the best means to prevent renal failure. Successful use of specific antiendotoxin therapy in the management of septic shock in pregnant women with acute pyelonephritis has been reported (Lachman et al, 1984). Recurrent infections are frequent, and either close surveillance for reinfection or suppressive antimicrobial therapy for the remainder of gestation are recommended. Prevention of acute pyelonephritis during pregnancy is based on identification and eradication of asymptomatic bacteriuria.

RENAL FAILURE DUE TO VOLUME CONTRACTION

Volume contraction is an important mechanism of ARF in pregnancy. In late pregnancy, the most common cause of hypovolaemia is blood loss due to concealed or overt uterine haemorrhage. Ante- and postpartum haemorrhage were noted as the major cause of ARF in 16% of late pregnancy-related ARF by Kennedy et al (1973) and in 7% of our own patients (Table 2). Smith et al

(1965) considered uterine bleeding a precipitating factor in 59% of their obstetric ARF cases, and blood loss was a contributing factor in 79% of obstetric ARF in the study by Chugh et al (1976). Pre-eclamptic women whose intravascular volume is already contracted and who have increased reactivity to vasoconstrictor hormones, or gravidas with abruptio placentae who have severe coagulation disturbances, appear to be particularly susceptible to the detrimental renal effects of blood loss. Hyperemesis gravidarum and particularly late vomiting in pregnancy may also lead to ARF. Volume depletion may also contribute to the development of ARF in gravidas with acute pyelonephritis and in septic abortion. Volume contraction may lead to prerenal ARF, acute tubular necrosis or to bilateral renal cortical necrosis, especially in gravidas with abruptio placentae. Early and adequate blood and fluid replacement is essential for the prevention of renal failure. The attention paid to this preventive measure is probably the main factor involved in the decreased incidence of ARF in pregnancy.

SEVERE PRE-ECLAMPSIA/ECLAMPSIA

Most retrospective studies dealing with ARF in pregnancy list severe pre-eclampsia/eclampsia as an important cause of ARF. For example, evidence of pre-existing hypertension or pre-eclampsia was noted in 62% of gravidas with late pregnancy-related ARF by Smith et al (1965) and in 33% by Kennedy and colleagues (1973). In our own series of cases presenting from 1957 to 1979, severe pre-eclampsia or eclampsia was the apparent cause of ARF in 12 out of 57 pregnant women (Grünfeld et al, 1980). ARF developed preferentially in older gravidas, most often in multiparas. Arteriolar and arterial renal changes consistent with pre-existing nephrosclerosis were documented by autopsy in several of the cases reported by Ober et al (1956). Thus, a substantial number of patients with ARF labelled pre-eclamptic may in fact have been misclassified as they actually had underlying renal vascular disease. In subsequent studies on eclampsia, the incidence of ARF was low, probably because of earlier detection and better management of pre-eclampsia/eclampsia. Pritchard and Pritchard (1975) observed only one case with ARF in 154 eclamptic women, and Lopez-Llera and Linares (1976) found a very low incidence of ARF—1% in 365 cases of eclampsia. However, in the aforementioned Algerian series, eclampsia still represented 56% of the causes of pregnancy-related ARF in the 1979–1983 period (A. Merouani and M. Drif, personal communication).

In severe pre-eclampsia/eclampsia, renal failure is most probably due to acute tubular necrosis. Occasionally, ARF is related to BRCN. The mechanisms of ARF in pre-eclampsia/eclampsia are not clearly identified. It has been suggested that glomerular capillary obstruction resulting from the swelling of glomerular endothelial cells lead to postglomerular ischaemia and acute tubular necrosis or BRCN. However, there is no evidence that glomerular changes are more severe and/or more diffuse in eclamptic women who develop renal failure than in those who do not. Tubular obstruction by intratubular haemoglobin casts may also contribute to ARF, as can occasionally myoglobinuria related to repeated grand mal seizures. Disseminated intravascular dissemination resulting in microangiopathic haemolytic anaemia is rarely involved. Reduced prostacyclin production in the umbilical artery, in amniotic fluid and in plasma from patients with severe pre-eclampsia has been reported and could play a role (De Gaetano et al, 1981). Finally, as noted previously, haemorrhage is a frequent contributing factor of ARF in toxaemic women whose intravascular volume is already contracted and who have an enhanced vascular reactivity. The HELLP syndrome (an acronym for haemolysis, elevated liver enzymes and low platelet count) is a variant of severe pre-eclampsia, which usually resolves following delivery (Weinstein, 1985). ARF develops in approximately 50% of such affected patients but is usually not severe enough to require dialysis. In some cases of pre-eclamptic women with this syndrome, the coagulation problems did not appear to resolve after delivery until plasma exchange was instituted.

ACUTE FATTY LIVER OF PREGNANCY

Acute fatty liver of pregnancy (AFLP) is an uncommon disorder characterized by microvesicular fatty infiltration of the centrilobular hepatocytes, jaundice and rapidly progressive hepatic failure occurring in late pregnancy and often complicated by ARF. This disease was first described by Stander and Cadden in 1934, and then recognized as a distinct entity by Sheehan in 1940. Until 1980, AFLP has been regarded as a rare but often fatal complication of pregnancy. Fewer than 100 cases have been reported (Haemmerli, 1966; Bletry et al, 1979; Davies et al, 1980): the prevalence was approximately 1 per 1 000 000 pregnancies (Haemmerli, 1966) and the published maternal and fetal mortality was 85% (Kaplan, 1985). Since then, many well-documented additional cases have been reported (Burroughs et al, 1982; Hou et al, 1984; Pockros et al, 1984; Kaplan, 1985; Rolfes and Ishak, 1985): estimates of the current incidence is 1 per 13 000 deliveries (Pockros et al, 1984) and maternal and fetal mortality rates are now between 11 and 25% (Pockros et al, 1984). The increased incidence and improved survival has been ascribed to the early recognition of milder cases, better supportive care and prompt delivery once the diagnosis of AFLP has been made. The illness usually begins in the third trimester of pregnancy, most often after the thirty-fifth week. Primagravidas, particularly those carrying twins, have been reported to be the prenatal group most at risk (Koff, 1981; Burroughs et al, 1982). The initial symptoms include nausea, vomiting, fatigue and abdominal pain, and these are rapidly followed by fever, jaundice and hepatic encephalopathy as a result of severe hepatic failure. Various degrees of mental status alteration are observed and may result in part from profound hypoglycaemia. Pre-eclamptic signs are present in 30–50% of the patients (Bletry et al, 1979; Burroughs et al, 1982). Extrahepatic complications such as coagulopathy from DIC, intestinal bleeding from peptic ulceration and pancreatitis may occur later in the course of AFLP.

Hyperbilirubinaemia associated with elevated serum alkaline phosphatase levels are characteristic laboratory findings, but the bilirubin level may be normal early in the course of the disease. Aminotransferase levels are usually only mildly increased. Leucocytosis is common. Thrombocytopenia and microangiopathic haemolytic anaemia may be found (Kaplan, 1985). Serum amylase and blood ammonia levels may be elevated. Severe hypoglycaemia may occur (Hou et al, 1984; Kaplan, 1985; Rolfes and Ishak, 1985). Hyperuricaemia is often observed and has been found before the onset of clinical manifestations in some patients (Pockros et al, 1984).

Renal failure develops in about 60% of cases. In the majority of the patients renal insufficiency is mild and results from prerenal factors. For example, in the study by Burroughs et al (1982), urinary sodium was below 5 mmol/24 h in 7 out of 12 patients who developed renal failure. However, acute tubular necrosis may be observed (Davies et al, 1980; Rolfes and Ishak, 1985). Renal failure is rarely severe enough to require dialysis, and in fatal cases death is due to hepatic failure, bleeding diathesis or pancreatitis rather than to renal failure.

AFLP should be considered a medical emergency and should be suspected in every woman with vomiting and abdominal pain and/or liver dysfunction in the third trimester of pregnancy. Diagnosis is based on the exclusion of other causes of hepatobiliary disease, and on liver biopsy if no other cause is detected and coagulation tests are normal or correctable. When liver biopsy cannot be performed safely, ultrasonography and postpartum computed tomography may be useful procedures for the detection of excess liver fat content (Bydder et al, 1980; Campillo et al, 1986). Acute cholelithiasis may be eliminated by ultrasonography. Intrahepatic cholestasis of pregnancy does not produce liver failure and is characterized by generalized pruritus. Viral hepatitis A and B should be excluded by appropriate serological tests. The main differential diagnosis of AFLP is fulminant hepatitis due to non-A/non-B hepatitis. This disease is usually associated with more marked elevation of serum aminotransferases, and leucocytosis is absent. Liver biopsy with appropriate stains for fat (such as oil red O) would distinguish fulminant hepatitis and AFLP but may be contraindicated because of uncorrectable clotting abnormalities. Finally, hepatic dysfunction is frequently found in pre-eclamptic women, particularly in those with the HELLP syndrome. However, in this disease aminotransferase levels are usually only minimally increased, the bilirubin level is characteristically normal and the liver biopsy is either normal or shows periportal fibrin deposition. In any case, delivery is indicated in severe pre-eclampsia as it is in AFLP.

The characteristic hepatic lesion of AFLP consists of microvacuolar fatty infiltration of hepatocytes with a centrilobular distribution. There is no disturbance of hepatic architecture. Necrosis or inflammatory changes are usually minimal or absent. Pathological data obtained during recovery show progressive clearing of fatty deposits and a return to normal (Burroughs et al, 1982).

The renal pathological findings are variable. Kidney structure may be within normal limits (Cano et al, 1975; Bletry et al, 1979). Fine fatty vacuolization of the tubular cells is frequently observed and may be found in patients with normal renal function (Ober and Lecompte, 1955; Burroughs et al, 1982). Other abnormalities, such as glomerular hypercellularity, focal tubular necrosis and non-specific tubular regenerative changes have also been noted (Recant and Lacy, 1963; Slater and Hague, 1984). Intraglomerular deposition of fibrin has been detected in some patients (Grünfeld et al, 1980; Slater and Hague, 1984).

The aetiology of AFLP is still unclear. It has been suggested that a viral agent, nutritional factors or a urea cycle enzyme deficiency may play a role in this disease. Similarities between AFLP and Reye's syndrome such as the histological appearance and reduced activity of mitochondrial urea cycle enzymes have been pointed out (Weber et al, 1979). However, some differences are worth noting: Reye's syndrome occurs in children and is rarely complicated by ARF; mitochondrial ultrastructure and plasma amino acid abnormalities are different; and accumulation of fat in the hepatocytes is predominantly in the form of triglycerides. Tetracycline administration is known to give a similar clinical syndrome with nearly the same histological features in both non-pregnant women and women at any stage of pregnancy. Since the first report by Kunelis et al (1965) of tetracycline-associated fatty liver of pregnancy, at least 30 cases have been attributed to tetracycline toxicity. However, many cases of AFLP have been reported since the cessation of tetracycline use during pregnancy.

The pathogenesis of ARF is uncertain but ARF appears to be a secondary event. Volume depletion and shock may contribute to ARF in some cases. Disseminated intravascular coagulation has been implicated but histopathological changes consistent with this hypothesis are scanty. Some features resemble those of the so-called 'hepatorenal syndrome' reported in various hepatic disorders.

The treatment of AFLP is non-specific and consists basically of vigorous supportive and corrective measures such as haemodynamic monitoring, adequate treatment of sepsis and hepatic encephalopathy, and correction of hypoglycaemia and clotting defects. Plasma or blood product transfusion may reverse low antithrombin III levels found in cases with disseminated intravascular coagulation (Pockros et al, 1984). Most of the authors advocate immediate delivery either by caesarean section or induction of labour as soon as the diagnosis is ascertained (Kaplan, 1985). There have been no recurrences of AFLP in 13 surviving mothers who have had subsequent pregnancies (Burroughs et al, 1982).

IDIOPATHIC POSTPARTUM RENAL FAILURE

The idiopathic postpartum renal failure is a syndrome of acute, rapidly progressive renal failure occurring shortly after an uneventful pregnancy. This rare and often lethal syndrome was noted as 'malignant nephrosclerosis in women postpartum' in 1967 by Sheer and Jones and first described as a specific entity by Robson et al in 1968 as 'irreversible postpartum renal failure'. Since then, 'postpartum intravascular coagulation with acute renal failure' (Rosenmann et al, 1969), 'postpartum renal failure with microangiopathic haemolytic anaemia' (Luke et al, 1970), 'the postpartum haemolytic uraemic syndrome' (Eisinger, 1972) and 'idiopathic postpartum renal failure' (Sun et al, 1975) have been reported in the literature. This syndrome affect previously healthy women and occurs 1 day to several weeks after an apparently normal pregnancy and delivery. The patients usually present with an influenza-like illness, followed by a rapidly progressive oliguric or often anuric renal failure. Blood pressure is either normal or slightly elevated at the onset, but severe or malignant hypertension develops as the disease progresses. Symptoms of congestive heart disease and grand mal seizures are common features. Severe microangiopathic haemolytic anaemia (with anisocytosis, numerous schizocytes, high reticulocyte count and a low serum haptoglobin level) and thrombocytopenia are found in approximately 75% of the cases, which can thus be termed 'postpartum haemolytic and uraemic syndrome' (HUS). Elevated serum levels of fibrinogen degradation products are frequently noted, but abnormalities of blood coagulation that are compatible with DIC are rarely observed. Hypocomplementemia has been noted in a few patients. Diagnosis of idiopathic postpartum renal failure may be established after the exclusion of other common causes of postpartum ARF such as abruptio placentae, postpartum haemorrhage, amniotic fluid emboli and puerperal sepsis. It should be kept in mind that renal failure, microangiopathic haemolytic anaemia and thrombocytopenia may be associated in pregnant women in various entities, for example:

1. Severe pre-eclampsia
2. So-called HELLP syndrome
3. AFLP
4. Thrombotic thrombocytopenic purpura
5. Prepartum haemolytic–uraemic syndrome

Distinction between idiopathic postpartum renal failure and some of these disorders may be difficult since they may persist in the postpartum period. Although there is clinically a broad overlap between these conditions, correct identification is necessary since specific investigations or therapy are needed in some. Finally, oral contraceptives may provoke HUS, whose manifestations are close to those observed in idiopathic postpartum ARF. Hauglustaine et al (1981), in a review of 52 patients with haemolytic uraemic postpartum syndrome, noted that five of these patients were receiving oral contraception at the onset of the disease. It is unknown whether these latter cases should be attributed to current oral contraception or to recent pregnancy.

Prognosis of postpartum ARF is poor. In a review of 49 patients with postpartum ARF by Segonds et al (1979), death occurred in 61%, complete recovery of renal function occurred in only 9.5% and 12% of the patients had terminal renal failure requiring maintenance haemodialysis. Improvement of renal function usually occurs early in the course of postpartum ARF, but may be delayed for as long as $1\frac{1}{2}$ years after the onset of renal failure (Segonds et al, 1979). Recurrent postpartum HUS has been reported (Gomperts et al, 1978). Renal transplantation may be successful, although recurrence of the lesion of HUS in kidney allografts has been occasionally observed.

Renal biopsy is useful for the diagnosis of idiopathic postpartum ARF when there is no clinical evidence of HUS. In patients with clinically unequivocal HUS, renal biopsy must be discussed only with regard to its value in the therapeutic decision because of the high incidence of post biopsy bleeding (Sun et al, 1975; Grünfeld et al, 1980). Renal histopathological changes (Sun et al, 1975; Schoolwerth et al, 1976; Segonds et al, 1979; Hayslett, 1985) involve glomeruli, afferent arterioles and intralobular arteries. Glomerular capillaries and arteriolar changes may be characteristic of thrombotic microangiopathy and similar to those found in HUS in children. Glomerular lesions are characterized by a thickening of the capillary walls due to endothelial swelling and subendothelial deposition of a pale, granular, fibrin-like material leading to capillary obstruction. Other findings include capillary thrombi and occasionally proliferative changes. Intimal swelling, subintimal deposits and fibrinoid necrosis with thrombosis in the lumen are found in the arterioles. In other patients, however, renal changes most closely resemble those found in malignant nephrosclerosis or scleroderma. The glomerular lesions are of ischaemic type with retracted tufts and wrinkled membranes, and vascular changes involve intralobular arteries. Immuno-fluorescent studies usually show fibrin and complement component three (C3) in the mesangium, capillary walls and arterioles (Morel-Maroger et al, 1979; Segonds et al, 1979). The two types of glomerular lesions may represent successive stages of the disease and may co-exist on the same biopsy specimen. The ischaemic type of lesion, however, is often prominent in idiopathic postpartum renal failure as it is in non-obstetric HUS in adults. Morel-Maroger et al (1979) have shown that severe arterial involvement carries a poor prognosis, whereas glomerular changes have less prognostic value.

Various hypotheses and tentative classifications have been put forward concerning idiopathic postpartum ARF and HUS (Hayslett, 1985). These syndromes have been regarded as clinical counterparts of the generalized Shwartzman reaction. Moreover Conger et al (1981) have demonstrated that a single dose of endotoxin induces the Shwartzman reaction in rats during the postpartum period, whereas a second injection is required in virgin animals. The lack of evidence for consumptive coagulopathy or benefit from antico-agulation is against the Shwartzman hypothesis. It has been suggested that the endothelial damage constitutes the key lesion in HUS. This mechanism may be involved in many cases, including the post-infectious form. In recent studies, infection with *Escherichia coli* producing a vero-cell cytotoxin (verotoxin) has been found in several cases of HUS (Karmali et al, 1983). It has been hypothesized that endotoxin might trigger the endothelial damage. A role of verotoxin-producing *E. coli* has also been emphasized in a woman with reversible postpartum HUS (Steele et al, 1984). Others have suggested that deposition of platelet thrombi in the microvasculature is the primary event. Platelet aggregation may result from endothelial damage induced by bacterial endotoxins, from a deficient synthesis of prostacyclin (PGI_2) or from a lack of plasma factor regulating endothelial PGI_2 production (Remuzzi and Rossi 1985). Additional pathogenic mechanisms have been proposed in HUS. As noted previously, oral contraceptive-induced HUS closely resembling idio-pathic postpartum ARF has been described and a role for hormonal changes has been suggested (Hayslett, 1985). Genetic and environmental factors have been implicated in a few kindreds, as they have in thrombotic thrombocytope-nic purpura, idiopathic HUS and post-pill HUS (Grottum et al, 1975). Of interest is a recent report of two HLA-identical sisters, one of whom developed postpartum HUS and the other post-pill HUS (Modesto et al, 1984). A pathogenic role for immunological factors has also been proposed, as transient hypocomplementenia has been reported in some patients. There is, as yet, no convincing evidence of an immune complex-like disease in idiopathic postpartum renal failure (Segonds et al, 1979; Neame, 1980).

The heterogeneous nature of HUS should be recognized. Classification based on pathophysiological findings may be helpful for the choice of therapy (Drummond, 1985). Conservative management by peritoneal dialysis or haemodialysis and antihypertensive agents is crucial. Angiotensin-converting enzyme inhibitors have abolished the need for bilateral nephrectomy in refractory hypertension. The usefulness of anticoagulation type therapy is disputed. A beneficial effect of heparin on mortality has been noted in uncontrolled trials (Segonds et al, 1979). However, no evidence of heparin effectiveness was found in a controlled trial in children with HUS (Hayslett, 1985). Most authors advocate the use of heparin therapy in the early stage of the disease (Sun et al, 1975; Morel-Maroger et al, 1979). The beneficial effect of fibrinolytic therapy on renal function has not yet been demonstrated. It should be stressed that severe haemorrhagic complications have been frequently reported in patients treated by heparin or fibrinolytic agents. Improvement of renal function has been ascribed to antithrombin III infusion in women with postpartum HUS (Brandt et al, 1981). Fresh frozen plasma infusion, PGI_2 infusion, plasma exchange and antiplatelet therapy are 'currently in vogue' and improvement has been ascribed to their use in uncontrolled studies (Drummond, 1985).

BILATERAL RENAL CORTICAL NECROSIS

Obstetric complications represent the most common causes of acute BRCN. In the recent series reported by Chugh et al (1983) in India, 71% of 49 cases of BRCN were of obstetric origin. Bilateral cortical necrosis may develop early in pregnancy after septic abortion. However, it is more likely to be associated with obstetric complications occurring during the third trimester of the postpartum period. For example, in our own series BRCN was diagnosed in 21% of the cases of postpartum ARF but in only 1.5% of post-abortion ARF, which is similar to the incidence of BRCN in the non-gravid population (Kleinknecht et al, 1973). Similarly, in the report of Smith et al (1965) none of the 52 women with post-abortum ARF had BRCN.

Abruptio placentae with either concealed or overt haemorrhage is the most frequent presenting event. In our series, BRCN was present in 45% of ARF-complicated abruptio placentae (Kleinknecht et al, 1973). Other obstetric complications associated with coagulation abnormalities such as prolonged intrauterine death, puerperal sepsis, postpartum haemorrhage or amniotic fluid embolism are much less frequent causes of BRCN.

Typically, renal cortical necrosis occurs primarily in multiparas aged 30 years or older. The diagnosis should be suspected in gravidas when ARF develops early in the trimester of pregnancy, especially between weeks 26 and 30 (Kleinknecht et al, 1973). An association with pre-eclampsia is disputed. In

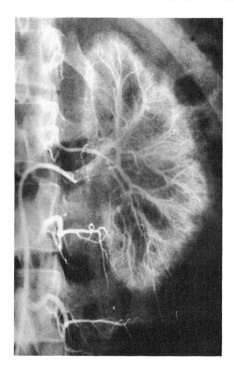

Figure 2. Selective left renal arteriogram in total cortical necrosis. Cortical nephrogram is completely absent. The outer edge of the cortex is poorly outlined and is separated from the inner layer by a clear, non-vascularized area. From Kleinknecht et al (1973), with permission.

contrast with earlier literature the incidence of pre-eclampsia associated to BRCN appears to be low in most recently published series. For example, Sheehan and Lynch (1973) noted that BRCN was present in only 2% of gravidas with eclampsia. In the recent study by Chugh et al (1983), pre-eclampsia was present in only 4 out of 35 patients with obstetric renal cortical necrosis. Furthermore, Kleinknecht et al (1973) noted that the incidence of pre-eclampsia was lower in gravidas with BRCN than in pregnant women with acute tubular necrosis.

BRCN is suggested clinically by the presence of anuria or severe oliguria of long duration (lasting 15–20 days or longer) (Kleinknecht et al, 1973; Chugh et al, 1983). The definite diagnosis rests on histological examination of renal biopsy and/or selective renal angiography (Kleinknecht et al, 1973). Both methods may also provide information on the extent of the lesion and therefore have a prognostic value. Diffuse renal cortical necrosis is characterized by complete cortical destruction with only a thin rim of preserved subcapsular and juxtamedullary tissue. With light microscopy most glomeruli are necrotic and the cortical nephrogram is absent on the arteriogram (Figure 2). In patchy necrosis, which is supposed to be of better prognosis, a lower percentage of glomeruli are destroyed and the cortical nephrogram appears

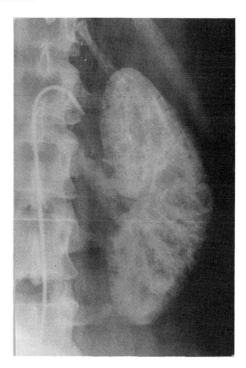

Figure 3. Selective left renal arteriogram in partial cortical necrosis. The cortical nephrogram shows a mottled, non-homogeneous appearance with alternating clear necrotic areas and dense, striped, vascularized regions. From Kleinknecht et al (1973), with permission.

heterogeneous, with a striated aspect (Figure 3). In this latter type of renal necrosis the diagnosis may be missed by the biopsy because of the 'patchy' nature of the lesion. A selective arteriography may be of great value in that case. Computed tomography may provide a non-invasive technique for differentiating cortical necrosis from acute tubular necrosis (Papo et al, 1985). Cortical calcifications may be seen on X-rays after a few weeks.

The prognosis for survival of BRCN is still poor, especially in diffuse renal cortical necrosis. Chugh et al (1983) noted a maternal mortality as high as 32%. In series from developed countries, where supportive therapy with haemodialysis can be provided over a long period, the mortality is only 36% (Grünfeld et al, 1980). In most patients who survive the acute phase of ARF, residual renal function resumes. Creatinine clearance may therefore increase slowly over a period of 1–3 years and dialysis be discontinued. Nevertheless, in a significant number of patients a subsequent deterioration in renal function may occur in the following months or years. Glomerular haemodynamic changes in the surviving nephrons have been incriminated as a possible cause of subsequent renal deterioration (Brenner et al, 1983). Transplantation has been performed in patients with terminal renal failure, but a high incidence of hyperacute graft rejection has been reported by Gelfand et al (1974).

BRCN is being currently considered as the clinical counterpart of the experimental Sanarelli–Shwartzman reaction. In pregnant animals, a generalized Shwartzman reaction may be induced by a single dose of endotoxin (Conger et al, 1981). The severe clotting disorders observed in certain obstetric complications such as abruptio placentae or amniotic fluid embolism may contribute to the pathophysiology of BRCN. However, features of DIC are not particularly frequent in gravidas with BRCN compared to women with acute tubular necrosis. The initial event in the genesis of cortical necrosis is probably endothelium damage due to a local effect on endotoxin, and thromb formation in situ therefore ensue (Raij et al, 1977).

MISCELLANEOUS CAUSES OF ACUTE RENAL FAILURE

Occasionally, obstructive ARF may occur in gravidas with polyhydramnios (Quigley and Cruickshank, 1977), incarcerated gravide uterus, or even in women with uncomplicated gestation (Bennett and Adler, 1982).

Amniotic fluid embolism, which occurs primarily in multiparas after prolonged labour, may also induce ARF. Pregnant women with underlying renal disease are more prone to develop acute tubular necrosis even in the absence of chronic renal insufficiency, especially when increased blood pressure or superimposed pre-eclampsia is present (Lindheimer et al, 1983).

Finally, ARF in gravidas may be caused by coincidental factors such as acute glomerulonephritis, drug nephrotoxicity, incompatible blood transfusions or bacterial endocarditis. Goodpasture's syndrome in a pregnant woman has been recently reported (Nilssen et al, 1986). We are aware of one rare instance where non-caseating granulomas were identified and the gravida then undergoing dialysis responded to steroids with a return of renal function and successfully completed the gestation (Warren et al, 1988). Parenthetically the kidney was the only organ involved in this patient' sarcoidosis. In effect sudden renal failure during pregnancy with non-apparent cause is an indication for prepartum biopsy. These pregnancy-unrelated cases of ARF represent only about 5% of all obstetric ARF.

MANAGEMENT OF ACUTE RENAL FAILURE IN PREGNANCY

Management of ARF in gravidas is the same as that in non-pregnant patients. The vital importance of blood replacement and even 'overtransfusion' in those women with frequent and severe uterine haemorrhage must be recalled. Dialysis should be undertaken early in order to maintain urea nitrogen at around 30 mg/dl. Both peritoneal dialysis and haemodialysis may be used in gravidas with ARF (Kelleher and Berl, 1981). The advantages of these two techniques are disputed (see Chapter 14). Smith et al (1965) considered peritoneal dialysis to be the best method and stressed that 'neither pelvic peritonitis nor enlarged uterus are contraindications'. The catheter must be inserted under direct vision through a small incision and high in the abdomen. Nevertheless, haemodialysis has been used with success in several patient

(Grünfeld et al, 1980). Preservation of a good uteroplacental perfusion requires a careful monitoring of fluid balance during dialysis. Close attention to the possibility of haemorrhagic complications due to heparinization is necessary. Fetal survival in gravidas undergoing haemodialysis has been reported (Cole et al, 1980; Hou, Chapter 10).

SUMMARY

Acute renal failure has become a very rare complication of pregnancy. This results from the virtual disappearance of septic abortion ARF and from the improvement of prenatal care, including the prevention of volume contraction which is mainly due to uterine haemorrhage, early diagnosis, and treatment of other classic maternal complications such as pre-eclampsia and acute pyelonephritis. The incidence of BRCN has also been declining during the last decade. Acute fatty liver, a potentially fatal disease, is often complicated by ARF. Early recognition of this disorder with prompt termination of pregnancy and intensive supportive therapy can reduce fetal and maternal mortality rate. The syndrome of idiopathic postpartum renal failure is also associated with a high morbidity and mortality. Beyond supportive treatment including haemo- or peritoneal dialysis, the use of potent antihypertensive drugs to control blood pressure and blood transfusion if necessary, specific therapy as plasma infusion, plasma exchange and antiplatelet drugs may be of value. Both peritoneal dialysis and haemodialysis may be used in gravidas with ARF. Early 'prophylactic' dialysis should be applied to pregnant women. Careful monitoring of fluid balance and anticoagulation is necessary during dialysis.

REFERENCES

Bartlett RH & Yahia C (1969) Management of septic chemical abortion with renal failure: report of five consecutive cases with five survivors. New England Journal of Medicine 281: 747–753.

Bennett AH & Adler S (1982) Bilateral ureteral obstruction causing anuria secondary to pregnancy. Urology 20: 631–633.

Bletry O, Roche-Sicot J, Rueff B & Degott C (1979) Steatose hepatique aigue gravidique. Nouveau Presse Médecale 8: 1835–1838.

Brandt P, Jespersen J & Gregersen G (1981) Postpartum haemolytic–uraemic syndrome treatment with antithrombin-III. Nephron 27: 15–18.

Brenner BM, Meyer TW & Hostetter TH (1983). Hemodynamically mediated glomerular injury and the progressive nature of kidney disease. Kidney International 23: 647–655.

Burroughs AK, Seong NGH, Dojcinov DM, Sheuer PJ & Sherlock SVP (1982) Idiopathic acute fatty liver of pregnancy in 12 patients. Quarterly Journal of Medicine 204: 481–497.

Bydder GM, Kreel L, Chapman RWG, Harry D & Scherlock S (1980) Accuracy of computed tomography in diagnosis of fatty liver. British Medical Journal 281: 1042.

Campillo B, Bernau J & Witz MO (1986) Ultrasonography in acute fatty liver of pregnancy. Annals of Internal Medicine 105: 383–384.

Cano RI, Delman MR, Pitchumoni CS, Lev R & Rosenthal WS (1975) Acute fatty liver of pregnancy: complicated by intravascular coagulation. Journal of the American Medical Association 231: 159–161.

Chapman A & Legrain M. Acute tubular necrosis and interstitial nephritis. In Hamburger J et al (eds) *Nephrology*, pp 383–410. New York: John Wiley.

Chugh KS, Singhal PC, Sharma BK et al (1976) Acute renal failure of obstetric origin. *Obstetrics and Gynecology* **48:** 642–646.

Chugh KS, Singhal PC, Kher VK et al (1983) Spectrum of acute cortical necrosis in Indian patients. *American Journal of Medical Science* **286:** 10–20.

Cole EH, Bear RA & Steinberg W (1980) Acute renal failure at 24 weeks of pregnancy: a case report. *Canadian Medical Association Journal* **112:** 1161–1162.

Conger JD, Falk SA & Guggenheim SJ. (1981) Glomerular dynamics and morphologic changes in the generalized Shwartzman reaction in postpartum rats. *Journal of Clinical Investigation* **67:** 1334–1346.

Davies MH, Wilkinson SP, Hanid MA et al (1980) Acute liver disease with encephalopathy and renal failure in late pregnancy and the early puerperium: a study of fourteen patients. *British Journal of Obstetrics and Gynaecology* **87:** 1005–1014.

De Gaetano G, Livio M, Donati MB & Remuzzi G (1981) Platelet and vascular prostaglandins in uraemia, thrombotic microangiopathy and preeclampsia. *Philosophical Transactions Royal Society London (B)* **294:** 339–342.

Donohoe JF (1983) Acute bilateral cortical necrosis. In Brenner BM & Lazarus JM (eds) *Acute Renal Failure*, pp 252–268. Philadelphia: WB Saunders.

Drummond KN (1985) Hemolytic uremic syndrome. Then and now. *New England Journal of Medicine* **312:** 116–118.

Eisinger AJ (1972) The postpartum hemolytic uremic syndrome. *Journal of Obstetrics and Gynaecology of the British Commonwealth* **79:** 139–143.

Finn WF (1983) Recovery from acute renal failure. In Brenner BM & Lazarus JM (eds) *Acute Renal Failure*, pp 252–268. Philadelphia: WB Saunders.

Gelfand MC, Friedman EA, Knepshield JH & Karpatkin S (1974) Detection of antiplatelet antibody in patients with renal cortical necrosis. *Kidney International* **6:** 426–430.

Gilstrap LC, Cunningham FG & Whalley PJ (1981) Acute pyelonephritis during pregnancy: an anterospective study. *Obstetrics and Gynecology* **57:** 409–413.

Gomperts ED, Sessel L, Du Plessis V & Hersch C (1978) Recurrent postpartum haemolytic uraemic syndrome. *Lancet* **i:** 48.

Grottum KA, Flatmark A, Myhre E et al (1975) Immunological hereditary nephropathy. *Acta Medica Scandinavica (Supplement)* **197:** 571.

Grünfeld JP, Ganeval D & Bournerias F. (1980) Acute renal failure in pregnancy. *Kidney International* **18:** 179–191.

Haemmerli VP (1966) Jaundice during pregnancy with special emphasis on recurrent jaundice during pregnancy and its differential diagnosis. *Acta Medica Scandinavica (Supplement)* **444:** 1–111.

Hauglustaine D, Vandamne B, Vanrenterghem Y & Michielsen P (1981) Recurrent hemolytic uremic syndrome during oral contraception. *Clinical Nephrology* **15:** 147–153.

Hawkins DF, Sevitt LH, Fairbrother PF & Tothill AU (1975) Management of septic chemical abortion with renal failure: use of a conservative regimen. **292:** 722–725.

Hayslett JP (1985) Current concepts: postpartum renal failure. *New England Journal of Medicine* **312:** 1556–1559.

Hou SH, Levin S, Ahola S et al (1984) Acute fatty liver of pregnancy survival with early cesarean section. *Digestive Diseases and Sciences* **29:** 449–452.

Kaplan ML (1985) Acute fatty liver of pregnancy. *New England Journal of Medicine* **313:** 367–370.

Karmali MA, Petric M, Steele BT & Limb C (1983) Sporadic cases of haemolytic–uraemic syndrome associated with faecal cytotoxin and cytotoxin-producing Escherichia coli in stools. *Lancet* **i:** 619–620.

Kelleher S & Berl T (1981) Acute renal failure in pregnancy. *Seminars in Nephrology* **1:** 61–68.

Kennedy AC, Burton JA, Luke RG et al (1973) Factors affecting the prognosis in acute renal failure. *Quarterly Journal of Medicine* **42:** 73–86.

Kerr DNS & Elliot W (1967) Renal disease in pregnancy. *Practitioner* **190:** 459–467.

Kleinknecht D, Grunfeld JP, Cia Gomez P, Moreau JF & Garcia-Torres R (1973) Diagnostic procedures and long-term prognosis in bilateral renal cortical necrosis. *Kidney International* **4:** 390–400.

Kleinknecht D, Bochereau G & Chauveau P (1980) Y a-t-il encore des accidents graves de l'avortement provoqué? *Nouvelle Presse Medicale* **9:** 460.

Knapp RC & Hellman LH (1959) Acute renal failure in pregnancy. *American Journal of Obstetrics and Gynecology* **78:** 570–577.

Koff RS (1981) Case records of Massachusetts General Hospital. *New England Journal of Medicine* **304:** 216–224.

Kunelis CT, Peters JL & Edmonson HA (1965) Fatty liver of pregnancy and its relationship to tetracycline therapy. *American Journal of Medicine* **38:** 359–377.

Lachman E, Pitsoe S & Gaffin SL (1984) Anti-lipopolysacharride immunotherapy in management of shock of obstetric and gynaecological origin. *Lancet* **i:** 981–983.

Lindheimer MD, Katz AI, Ganeval D & Grünfeld JP (1983) Acute renal failure in pregnancy. In Brenner BM & Lazarus JM (eds) *Acute Renal Failure*, pp 510–526. Philadelphia: WB Saunders.

Lopez-Llera M & Linares GR (1976) Factors that influence maternal mortality in eclampsia. In Lindheimer MD et al (eds) *Hypertension in Pregnancy*, p. 41. New York: John Wiley.

Luke RG, Siegel RR, Talbert W & Holland N (1970) Heparin treatment for postpartum renal failure with microangiopathic hemolytic anemia. *Lancet* **ii:** 750–752.

Modesto A, Durand D, Orfila C & Suc JM (1984) Syndrome hemolytique uremique chez deux germains HLA identiques. *Nephrologie* **5:** 47–48.

Morel-Maroger L, Kanfer A, Solez K, Sraer JD & Richet G (1979) Prognostic importance of vascular lesions in acute renal failure with microangiopathic hemolytic anemia (hemolytic-uremic syndrome): clinicopathologic study in 20 adults. *Kidney International* **15:** 548–558.

Neame PB (1980) Immunologic and other factors in thrombotic thrombocytopenic purpura (TTP). *Seminars in Thrombosis and Homeostasis* **6:** 416–429.

Nilssen DE, Talseth T & Brodwall (1986) The many faces of Goodpasture's syndrome. *Acta Medica Scandinavica* **220:** 489–491.

Ober WB & Lecompte PM (1955) Acute fatty metamorphosis of the liver associated with pregnancy. *American Journal of Medicine* **19:** 743–758.

Ober WE, Reid DE, Romney SL & Merill JP (1956) Renal lesions and acute renal failure in pregnancy. *American Journal of Medicine* **21:** 781–810.

Papo J, Peer G, Aviram A & Paizer R (1985) Acute renal cortical necrosis as revealed by computerized tomography. *Israeli Journal of Medical Science* **21:** 862.

Pockros PJ, Peters RL & Reynolds TB (1984) Idiopathic fatty liver of pregnancy: findings in ten cases. *Medicine* (Baltimore) **63:** 1–11.

Pritchard JA & Pritchard SA (1975) Standardized treatment of 154 consecutive cases of eclampsia. *American Journal of Obstetrics and Gynecology* **123:** 543–549.

Quigley MM & Cruikshank DP (1977) Polyhydramnios and acute renal failure. *Journal of Reproductive Medicine* **19:** 92.

Raij L, Keane WF & Michael AF (1977) Unilateral Shwartzman reaction: cortical necrosis in one kidney following in vivo perfusion with endotoxin. *Kidney International* **12:** 91–95.

Recant L & Lacy P (1963) Fulminating liver disease in a pregnant woman at term. *American Journal of Medicine* **35:** 231–240.

Remuzzi G & Rossi EC (1985) The hemolytic uremic syndrome. *International Journal of Artificial Organs* **8:** 171–173.

Robson JS, Martin AM, Ruckley VA & MacDonald MK (1968) Irreversible postpartum renal failure: a new syndrome. *Quarterly Journal of Medicine* **37:** 423–435.

Rolfes DB & Ishak KG (1985) Acute fatty liver of pregnancy: a clinicopathologic study of 35 cases. *Hepatology* **5:** 1149–1158.

Rosenmann E, Kanter A, Bacani RA, Pirani CL & Pollak VE (1969) Fatal late postpartum intravascular coagulation with acute renal failure. *American Journal of Medical Science* **257:** 259–273.

Schoolwerth AC, Sandler RS, Klahr S & Kissane JM (1976) Nephrosclerosis postpartum and in women taking oral contraceptives. *Archives of Internal Medicine* **136:** 178–185.

Segonds A, Louradour N, Suc JM & Orfila C (1979) Postpartum hemolytic uremic syndrome: a study of 3 cases with a review of the literature. *Clinical Nephrology* **12:** 229–242.

Sheehan HL & Lynch JB (1973) Pathology of toxaemia of pregnancy. Edinburgh: Churchill Livingstone, p. 287.

Sheehan H (1940) The pathology of acute yellow atrophy and delayed chloroform poisoning. *Journal of Obstetrics and Gynaecology of the British Commonwealth* **47:** 49–62.

Sheer RL & Jones DB (1967) Malignant nephrosclerosis in women postpartum: a note on microangiopathic hemolytic anemia. *Journal of the American Medical Association* **201:** 106–110.

Slater DN & Hague WM (1984) Renal morphological changes in idiopathic acute fatty liver of pregnancy. *Histopathology* **8:** 567–581.

Smith K, Browne JCM, Schackman R & Wrong OM (1965) Acute renal failure of obstetric origin: an analysis of 70 patients. *Lancet* **ii:** 351–354.

Stander HJ & Cadden JF (1934) Blood chemistry in preeclampsia and eclampsia. *American Journal of Obstetrics and Gynecology* **28:** 856–871.

Steele BT, Goldie J & Alexopolou I (1984) Postpartum haemolytic uraemic syndrome and verotoxin-producing Escherichia coli. *Lancet* **i:** 511.

Sun NCJ, Johnson WJ, Sung DTW & Woods JE (1975) Idiopathic postpartum renal failure: review and case report of a successful renal transplantation. *Mayo Clinic Proceedings* **50:** 395–401.

Warren GV, Sprague SM & Corwen HL (1988) Sarcoidosis presenting as acute renal failure in pregnancy. *American Journal of Kidney Disease* (in press).

Weber FL, Snodgrass PJ, Powell DE et al (1979) Abnormalities of urea cycle enzyme activities and hepatic ultrastructure in acute fatty liver of pregnancy. *Journal of Laboratory and Clinical Medicine* **94:** 27–41.

Weinstein L (1985) *Philosophical Transactions of the Royal Society of London.* Preeclampsia/eclampsia with hemolysis, elevated liver enzymes, and thrombocytopenia. *Obstetrics and Gynecology* **66:** 657–660.

Whalley PJ, Cunningham FG & Martin F (1975) Transient renal dysfunction associated with acute pyelonephritis of pregnancy. *Obstetrics and Gynecology* **46:** 174–177.

7

Urinary tract infections complicating pregnancy

F. GARY CUNNINGHAM

Urinary tract infections in non-pregnant women are common, and if uncomplicated they are usually innocuous. Although most women with antepartum urinary infections are asymptomatic, covert bacteriuria when superimposed upon pregnancy-induced dilatation of the urinary tract (part of which is obstructive in origin), may lead to cystitis or pyelonephritis. Thus, during pregnancy acute pyelonephritis is common and may cause considerable morbidity. Because of these serious sequelae, routine screening to detect and eradicate asymptomatic bacteriuria is recommended by most American and British investigators.

ASYMPTOMATIC BACTERIURIA

Asymptomatic or covert bacteriuria indicates persistent, actively multiplying bacteria within the urinary tract without symptoms of infection. By convention, bacteriuria is considered 'significant' if these organisms are quantified to be at least 100 000 colonies per ml in freshly voided urine collected by the midstream clean-catch technique. More recently, Stamm and colleagues (1982) reported evidence that lower colony counts may represent active infection. This has also been our experience with pregnant women at Parkland Memorial Hospital; acute pyelonephritis commonly follows untreated bacteriuria with urine colony counts of 20 000 to 50 000 per ml.

While the exact mechanisms are unclear, in some women perineal bacteria gain urethral access, and then go on to colonize the bladder or kidneys. This is an exciting area of research, and much has been learned of some mechanisms by which normal gut bacteria became 'pathogenic' for their unimpaired hosts. Most bacteria have *adhesins*, which allow attachment to uroepithelial cells, and these are usually characterized as *fimbriae*, an example of which is shown in Figure 1. These structures, also called *pili*, are attracted to uroepithelial receptors dictated by their glycoprotein/glycolipid constituency. In at least some *Escherichia coli*, P-fimbriation is a marker of virulence. For example,

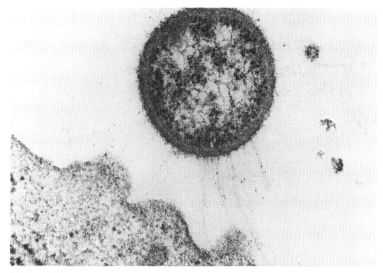

Figure 1. Transmission electron microscopy shows fimbriated *E. coli* adhering to transitional cell (original × 180 000). From Roberts (1986) reprinted with permission of *Infections in Surgery*.

while only 10% to 15% of strains that cause urinary infections have P-fimbriae, nearly all cases of non-obstructive pyelonephritis are caused by P-fimbriated *E. coli* (Väisänen et al, 1981; Svanborg Eden et al, 1982).

Prevalence

The prevalence of asymptomatic bacteriuria during pregnancy ranges from 2% to 7% and is largely dependent upon socioeconomic factors, with infections being five times more common in indigent women. Moreover, this risk is doubled in the woman with sickle cell trait (Pritchard et al, 1973), and it is appreciably increased in diabetes.

Significance

Pregnant women who develop symptomatic urinary infections mostly do so as a result of covert bacteriuria that antedates gestation (Whalley, 1967). Nearly 30% of women with early pregnancy bacteriuria go on to develop acute pyelonephritis if not treated, and it has been convincingly shown that eradication of silent infection usually circumvents this. Thus, it seems reasonable to recommend routine screening to detect bacteriuria, at least in high-risk obstetrical populations. This may not be cost-effective if the prevalence is low (Campbell-Brown et al, 1987).

A small number of women, perhaps 1%, acquire bacteriuria during pregnancy, and again, 25% to 30% of these will develop pyelonephritis (Whalley, 1967). It is apparent that routine, one-time early screening does not prevent all symptomatic infections: in fact, at Parkland Hospital, women who

Table 1. Comparison of adverse pregnancy outcomes in 248 women with renal or bladder bacteriuria.*

| | Bacteriuric women (%) | | Non-bacteriuric controls (%) |
Pregnancy complications	Renal ($N=114$)	Bladder ($N=134$)	($N=248$)
Haematocrit less than 30	2.6	3.7	2.1
Hypertension	12	15	14
Low-birthweight infants	10	13	13
Growth-retarded infants	8	8	8
Preterm delivery	4	8	5

* Modified after Gilstrap et al (1981b).

had sterile screening cultures constituted about a third of cases admitted for antepartum pyelonephritis. Because of the small yield (1%), it is difficult to make a convincing argument for a second screening culture later in pregnancy.

While the import of asymptomatic bacteriuria in the genesis of bladder and kidney infections is unquestioned, for decades there has been considerable debate regarding its potential morbidity for other pregnancy outcomes (Whalley, 1967; Editorial, 1985). In his earliest studies, which he summarized in 1978, Kass reported that untreated bacteriuria was associated with a four-fold increased incidence of low-birthweight infants when compared to treated women (Kass, 1978). Kincaid-Smith and Bullen (1965) reported similar findings, except they observed that treatment did not substantively alter adverse perinatal outcome. Subsequently other studies, including one from our institution (Gilstrap et al, 1981a), have offered proof that asymptomatic bacteriuria is not a prominent factor in the genesis of low-birthweight or preterm infants.

Anaemia and pregnancy-induced hypertension have also been associated with covert bacteriuria. Using invasive methods, it was shown that bacteriuria was of bladder or kidney origin in approximately equal proportions (Fairley et al, 1966). The assumption followed that adverse perinatal outcomes might be more frequent in women with chronic renal infections, and a new vista for study was opened. This was expanded when Thomas and her colleagues developed the technique for identifying antibody-coated bacteria, using fluorescein-tagged antiglobulin (Thomas et al, 1974). We applied these methods in a large group of pregnant women with asymptomatic infections, and confirmed the distribution of bladder (54%) and renal (46%) bacteriuria (Gilstrap et al, 1981a). Our purpose was to compare prospectively pregnancies in these women to non-bacteriuric controls, to determine if covert infection caused an adverse outcome. Intuitively at least, it seemed logical that pre-eclampsia and anaemia might be increased with renal bacteriuria. However, in this case-controlled study, as shown in Table 1, we were unable to document these associations.

Treatment

Bacteria most frequently isolated are normal commensurals of bowel flora. *E. coli* is predominant (80%), and *Klebsiella, Proteus,* and *Enterobacter* species constitute most of the remainder. A small number of infections are caused by staphylococci and by group B and enterococcal streptococci. Initial selection of an antimicrobial is empirical, and a number of drugs, including nitrofurantoin, one of the sulphonamides, ampicillin or cephalosporins have all been used in pregnant populations and appear to be safe and effective. The simplest regimen with which we have experience is nitrofurantoin, 100 mg given orally at bedtime for 10 days. This has proved to be as effective as ampicillin, sulphonamide or cephalexin given 4 times daily for 21 days. The success of this daily bedtime dose is probably because the drug remains in the urinary collecting system for longer periods.

Treatment for covert bacteriuria has evolved from long-term courses that ranged from 6 weeks to continuous therapy until delivery, to shorter courses of 10 days to 3 weeks. More recently, single-dose therapy has been advocated by some (Harris et al, 1981; Bailey, 1985). Bailey and colleagues examined the comparative efficacy of either single-dose or 5-day treatment with trimethoprim or trimethoprim–sulphamethoxazole, and all regimens tested were equally successful in eradicating bacteriuria (Bailey et al, 1983, 1986).

Regardless of the regimen chosen or the duration of therapy (except for continuous therapy), approximately 30% of women will develop recurrent bacteriuria during the same pregnancy. These patterns of recurrent infection are interesting. It would seem, again intuitively, that renal bacteriuria would be more difficult to eradicate, and in earlier localization studies it was shown that recurrent renal infection was more likely to be a relapse, defined as infection with the same organism (which presumably was not eradicated). When we localized bacteriuria by using the antibody-coated bacteria test, we found that recurrent infection following 10-day therapy was more likely to be renal in origin (Leveno et al, 1981). Conversely, while bladder bacteriuria was usually easily eradicated with short-term therapy, reinfection—the same or different organism isolated after an intervening sterile culture—was the most common mode of recurrence.

Since we showed that a longer course of therapy (21 days) was more effective in eradicating renal bacteriuria, it is tempting to suggest an alternative regimen of initial empirical treatment: single-dose ampicillin or amoxycillin followed by 21-day therapy (nitrofurantoin, 100 mg at bedtime) for those women with recurrence. In this scheme, most recurrences would be relapses, and most of these would be renal infections.

For success of any scheme for detection and treatment of bacteriuria, continued surveillance of women who have recurrent infection is important, since 25% to 30% of these will develop acute pyelonephritis. For women with persistent bacteriuria despite two or three courses of therapy, we have found that nitrofurantoin, 100 mg at bedtime given for the remainder of pregnancy, usually prevents symptomatic infection.

CYSTITIS

Acute bacterial cystitis complicates 1–2% of pregnancies (Harris and Gilstrap, 1981; Editorial, 1985). Interestingly, Harris and Gilstrap (1981) reported that cystitis seldom follows asymptomatic bacteriuria, but rather arises *de novo*. They showed that surveillance programmes to eradicate covert bacteriuria, while dramatically decreasing the incidence of pyelonephritis, had no such salutary effect on cystitis. Finally, in most cases of cystitis, the bacteria recovered were not antibody-coated, leading the investigators to conclude that cystitis is a different entity from chronic covert bacteriuria and pyelonephritis.

Treatment

Women with symptomatic bacterial cystitis respond rapidly to any of the several antimicrobial regimens described for covert bacteriuria. For example, Harris and Gilstrap (1981) reported a 97% cure rate using a 10-day course of ampicillin. Since most of these infections appear to be localized to the bladder, single-dose antimicrobial therapy seems reasonable; however, appropriate studies have not yet been conducted during pregnancy. Moreover, since we observed that 40% of women with acute antepartum pyelonephritis have concomitant lower urinary tract symptoms (Gilstrap et al, 1981a), early pyelonephritis must be confidently excluded before giving 1-dose therapy.

ACUTE PYELONEPHRITIS

Nearly 1% of all pregnancies are complicated by acute pyelonephritis, and thus it is the most common serious bacterial infection of pregnancy (Editorial, 1985). The population incidence varies, and depends on the prevalence of covert bacteriuria and whether it is treated. At Parkland Hospital, nearly 80% of women attend antenatal clinics where routine bacteriuria screening is performed and treatment is given for the 8% that are infected. Prior to our introduction of routine screening, nearly 3% of pregnancies were complicated by pyelonephritis, which now complicates only 1% of our annual 15 000 pregnancies. Before treatment programmes were initiated, the majority (around 70%) of women with pyelonephritis had preceding covert bacteriuria, and a third of these cases apparently followed bacteriuria newly acquired during gestation. This situation is now reversed, and as expected, infections following early pregnancy bacteriuria have substantially decreased.

Like covert infections, the pathogenesis of acute pyelonephritis seems to depend upon the virulence or invasiveness of the perineal bacteria that ultimately colonize urine and cause ascending infection. As discussed earlier, virulence has been attributed to bacterial P-fimbriae which attach to specific receptors on uroepithelial membranes (Svanborg Eden et al, 1982). These receptors are globoseries glycolipids which are antigens of the P blood group system. As schematically depicted in Figure 2, bacterial pili bind to α-D-

Bacterium

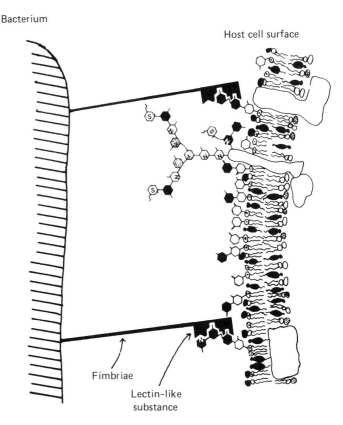

Host cell surface

Fimbriae

Lectin–like
substance

Figure 2. Schematic representation of P-fimbriae and uroepithelial cell receptors. From Svanbor
Eden (1982) with permission.

galactopyranosyl-$(1 \rightarrow 4)$-β-D-galactopyranoside disaccharides. Interestingly
these adhesins are more commonly identified in bacteria causing non
obstructive pyelonephritis than in those associated with infection and chronic
obstruction (reflux). Their prevalence has not been evaluated in uncompli
cated pyelonephritis in pregnant women.

Diagnosis

Acute pyelonephritis is usually diagnosed easily by clinical findings and
microscopic bacteriuria subsequently verified by culture. In our report
describing 656 pregnant women with pyelonephritis, 82% presented with back
pain and chills (Gilstrap et al, 1981a); 40% also had lower urinary tract
symptoms that usually included dysuria and frequency. Physical findings
include fever and tenderness to fist percussion at the costovertebral angle.

Bacteriuria is confirmed by quantitative culture, and *E. coli* remains the
most common isolate. In our previous experiences (Gilstrap et al, 1981a), *E*

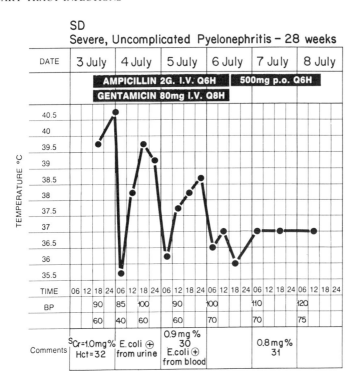

Figure 3. Vital signs graphic chart from a 25-year-old primigravida with acute antepartum pyelonephritis at 34 weeks gestation.

coli was isolated from 72% of 656 women, and Faro and colleagues (1984) reported this organism in 60% of their patients. In a survey of nearly 100 pregnant women recently admitted for pyelonephritis, we identified *E. coli* in 81%, *Klebsiella pneumoniae* and *Enterobacter* each in 6% and *Proteus mirabilis* in 2% (S. Cox and G. Cunningham, unpublished observations).

Almost all symptoms and findings in these women can ultimately be attributed to endotoxaemia, and as described below, so can the serious complications of acute pyelonephritis. The most obvious is thermoregulatory instability characterized by high spiking fever, with sublingual temperatures fluctuating from as low as 34 °C to as high as 42 °C (Figure 3). This reaction is mediated in the anterior hypothalamus by endotoxin-stimulated interleukin-1, previously termed endogenous pyrogen (Dinarello, 1984).

Treatment

Hospitalization is recommended since these women are quite ill and, indeed, 15% to 20% have bacteraemia. Moreover, they are usually dehydrated and unable to tolerate oral medication because of nausea and vomiting. Finally,

Table 2. Management of the pregnant woman with acute pyelonephritis.

1. Hospitalization
2. Urine and blood cultures
3. Complete blood count, serum creatinine and electrolytes
4. Frequent vital sign monitoring, including urinary output
5. Intravenous hydration to establish a minimum urinary output of 30 ml per hour (indwelling bladder catheter if necessary)
6. Intravenous antimicrobials (see text)
7. Chest x-ray if dyspnoea or tachypnoea
8. Repeat haematology and chemistry studies in 48 hours
9. Oral antimicrobials begun when afebrile
10. Discharge after afebrile 24 hours, continue antimicrobials 10 to 21 days
11. Urine culture 1 to 2 weeks after antimicrobials completed

serious complications of acute pyelonephritis are common in pregnancy and careful monitoring is necessary.

A general outline of the management approach that we use at Parkland Hospital is shown in Table 2. A modicum of laboratory evaluation done at admission includes cultures of urine and blood, serum electrolytes and creatinine concentration, and a complete blood count. For the woman with uncomplicated pyelonephritis, further laboratory work is seldom necessary.

During at least the first few days of therapy, these women must be monitored carefully for evidence of bacterial shock, as well as other serious complications. Close observation with frequent determination of vital signs, including urinary output, is integral to their care. Initial treatment is directed at restoration of the contracted blood volume, and this is accomplished by intravenous crystalloid, either normal saline or lactated Ringer's solution, given rapidly over the first few hours to ensure urinary output of 30 to 50 ml h^{-1}. In a small number of women, usually those in whom endotoxaemia is severe, this simple measure does not result in appreciable urinary output, and further measures are described below.

The choice of antimicrobial therapy is empirical; however, if the woman has had a previous urinary infection during the pregnancy, then in vitro sensitivities are reviewed to select specific therapy. For more than two decades ampicillin has been used successfully for treatment, and for the woman with uncomplicated pyelonephritis, we recommend 2 g given intravenously by 'piggyback' infusion every 6 hours until she is afebrile. Oral ampicillin, 500 mg 4 times daily, is then substituted, and this is continued after discharge for a total treatment course of 10 days. This regimen is safe and effective, as demonstrated by Cunningham and colleagues at Charity Hospital in New Orleans, where 85% of women so treated became afebrile within 48 hours (Cunningham et al, 1973).

In the past several years, many uropathogens that cause community-acquired pyelonephritis have become resistant to ampicillin as determined by in vitro studies. For example, at Parkland Hospital, only 33% of E. coli, 2% of K. pneumoniae, and no Enterobacter cloacae isolated from pregnant women admitted for pyelonephritis in 1986 were sensitive to ampicillin (S. Cox and G. Cunningham, unpublished observations). However, concentrations against which bacteria are tested are almost minuscule when compared to renal parenchymal and urinary concentrations achieved with ampicillin in doses recommended, and this may explain our experiences in which there is usually clinical cure despite in vitro resistance. On the other hand, Duff (1984) reported a clinical failure rate of 27% in 131 women given ampicillin initially, and it seems reasonable to prescribe antimicrobials to which bacteria are more sensitive. Surprisingly, there are few clinical studies in which the efficacy of other regimens has been evaluated systematically.

Concern for in vitro resistance frequently prompts the addition of an aminoglycoside, usually gentamicin, to the ampicillin regimen. Gentamicin is an excellent choice for treatment of severely ill women; however, we are concerned that nearly 20% of these women have significant renal dysfunction (Whalley et al, 1975). Thus, synergistic nephrotoxicity from endotoxin and aminoglycoside, as well as the potential for ototoxicity in both mother and fetus, is a worrisome aspect of such therapy. Serial monitoring of serum creatinine is mandatory, and some recommend measurements of peak and trough aminoglycoside concentrations, with appropriate alternations in dosage (Duff, 1984).

Current microbial sensitivity profiles indicate that any of a number of cephalosporins is a reasonable alternative. We have now had considerable experience with intravenous cephalothin, 2 g given intravenously by 'piggy-back' infusion every 6 hours, for which the salutary clinical response was equivalent to ampicillin (Cunningham et al, 1973). Duff (1984) recommends cefazolin, 1 to 2 g given intravenously every 8 hours. Faro and colleagues (1984) reported a 96% clinical cure rate in 23 women given cefuroxime, 750 mg intravenously every 8 hours for 5 days. Unfortunately, in vitro antimicrobial resistance is now reported with cephalothin. While there is no published experience with other cephalosporins, it seems reasonable that most would be equally satisfactory.

The 'extended-spectrum' penicillins are ideally suitable for these ill women. The spectrum of these drugs against most uropathogens is excellent, and they have the inherent safety of the penicillin group. We now have experience with two ureidopenicillins, piperacillin and mezlocillin, both of which have excellent in vitro microbiocidal spectra. We recently treated more than 100 women with mezlocillin, 3 g given intravenously every 4 hours, and the cure rate exceeded 95%. We also treated 50 women with piperacillin, 4 g given intravenously every 8 h and the cure rate was 90% (S. Cox and G. Cunningham, unpublished observations).

In the majority of cases, with appropriate intravenous hydration and antimicrobial treatment, rapid clinical improvement is forthcoming. From earlier experiences (Cunningham et al, 1973), we showed that 85% of such women given ampicillin, cephalothin or chloramphenicol were afebrile after 48 hours, and we recently confirmed this. Failure to improve clinically within the first 72 hours suggests complications that frequently are associated with underlying obstruction such as urolithiasis or anatomic anomalies.

In some very ill women preterm labour ensues, and indeed, 10% of the 487 women whom we admitted for antepartum pyelonephritis were in labour

(Gilstrap et al, 1981a). Although Duff (1984), as well as others, recommends tocolysis in this situation, we have never used this. Most of these women are quite ill, and beta-mimetics actually simulate endotoxin-induced cardiovascular effects.

COMPLICATIONS OF PYELONEPHRITIS

Acute pyelonephritis during pregnancy can be devastating, and perhaps as many as a fourth of women with severe infections have evidence for multisystem derangement. Although complications such as pyonephrosis and perinephric cellulitis or abscesses occur more frequently when obstruction is present, it is not a requisite for severe sequelae. In general, these complications tend to be multiple, and are more common in the woman who clinically appears very ill, or 'toxic'.

Urinary calculi

In the absence of a prompt clinical response, there should be a search for obstructive urinary tract lesions. In most cases, these are from urinary calculi, the removal of which usually prompts rapid resolution of infection. In some cases passage of a double-J ureteral stent may relieve the obstruction (Krieger, 1986). For the woman who remains substantively febrile after 72 hours of appropriate therapy, a plain abdominal radiograph is indicated, since nearly 90% of renal stones are radiopaque. Possible benefits far outweigh any minimal fetal risk from radiation. If negative, then we recommend intravenous pyelography modified by the number of radiographs taken after contrast injection. The 'one-shot pyelogram', in which a singe radiograph is obtained 30 minutes after contrast injection, usually allows adequate collecting-system imaging to detect stones or structural anomalies. Occasionally, a second or even a third radiograph may be indicated. Unilateral non-visualization may suggest an end-stage obstructed kidney with pyonephrosis as a cause of continuing sepsis. In these cases, calculi frequently co-exist, and removal of the infected kidney may be life-saving.

While some prefer renal sonography to detect underlying lesions, the issue is not settled (Benson et al, 1986). Pyelocalyceal dilatation, urinary calculi and possibly intrarenal or perinephric abscesses may be visualized. Our experiences with sonar have not always been successful, and a negative examination should not terminate the work-up in a woman with continuing urosepsis. Although results are promising, we have insufficient experience with 'limited' computerized axial tomography. Finally, magnetic resonance may be used to characterize these lesions; although probably safe, it is not widely available.

Perinephric cellulitis and abscess

In a very small number of women, more commonly those who present after several days of symptoms or those with calculi, infection spreads beyond the renal capsule causing perinephric cellulitis. In its earliest stages there is a phlegmon, and with intensive antimicrobial therapy clinical resolution ensues within several more days. Rarely, there is perinephric space suppuration, and surgical drainage may be life-saving. These infections are quite serious and emphasize the need for continuing investigation when the typical prompt response is not forthcoming.

Other uncommon lesions have been described in these 'non-responders'. *Emphysematous pyelonephritis* is characterized by a particularly virulent infection with gas-producing Enterobacteriaceae which results in a gangrenous kidney. Mortality is high and nephrectomy is mandatory (Ahlering et al, 1985). Typical radiographic findings and a nephrectomy specimen are shown in Figure 4.

Acute segmental pyelonephritis, also called lobar nephronia, has been described using computed axial tomography, and probably represents a segmental intrarenal phlegmon (Costas, 1972). It usually resolves with continued antimicrobial therapy; however, some recommend serial ultrasound examinations should a renal abscess develop that would be amenable to percutaneous drainage.

Septicaemic shock

Although bacteraemia is demonstrated in 15 to 20% of women with severe pyelonephritis, the septic shock syndrome is uncommon. Continuing hypotension and diminished perfusion following endotoxaemia must be differentiated from hypotension caused by hypovolaemia, fever, anorexia, nausea and vomiting. While many of these women have further evidence for endotoxaemia, only a few have continuing hypotension after appropriate fluid resuscitation. Those women that do usually appear seriously ill, and frequently have multisystem involvement. Even then, in most of these cardiac output and tissue perfusion is restored after intravenous fluid resuscitation, although blood pressure may remain low as a result of diminished systemic vascular resistance. Occasionally we have infused dopamine at 5 μg kg^{-1} min^{-1} to maintain systolic pressure at 90 mmHg. The classic septic shock syndrome is characterized by overt capillary endothelial damage and severely diminished vascular resistance with low cardiac output that responds poorly to intravenous fluids and vasopressors. These women need intensive observation and care is usually facilitated by pulmonary artery catheterization.

Most of the complications described are probably variants of the septic shock syndrome, and arise as the result of endotoxaemia. Whether pregnant women are more susceptible to these aberrations is unknown; however, it is inferential that they are.

Renal dysfunction

In a prospective study of 220 women with antepartum pyelonephritis, we found that nearly a fourth had seriously diminished glomerular filtration rates (Whalley et al, 1975). Fortunately (as shown in Figure 5) such renal dysfunction is transient, and is usually reversible within several days although it sometimes persists for weeks. There is good evidence that this is mediated by endotoxin lipopolysaccharide (Richman et al, 1980). Management includes

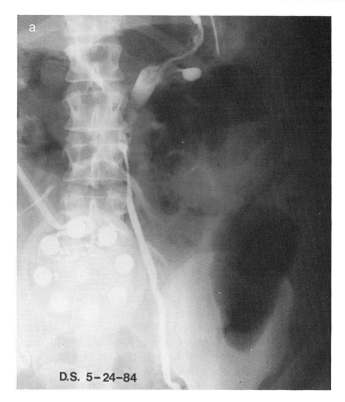

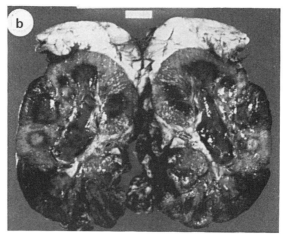

Figure 4. Emphysematous pyelonephritis. (a) Plain abdominal radiograph in a 20-year-old nullipara at 24 weeks' gestation. The area of the left kidney is occupied by a large gas collection. At surgical exploration, 600 ml of purulent material was removed, along with the gangrenous kidney. (b) Photograph of nephrectomy specimen. From Ahlering (1985) Emphysematous pyelonephritis: a 5-year experience with 13 patients. *Journal of Urology* **134:** 1086–1088. With permission from Williams & Wilkins.

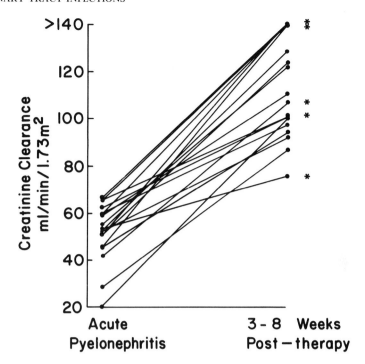

Figure 5. Glomerular filtration as determined by endogenous creatinine clearance in 18 pregnant women with acute pyelonephritis. These women had moderate to severe renal dysfunction which approached normal by 3 to 8 weeks after therapy. From Whalley et al (1975) *Obstetrics and Gynecology* **46:** 174–180.

close observation with serial creatinine determination, and treatment with intravenous fluids and antimicrobials without substantial nephrotoxicity (or with appropriate dosage reduction of those that are nephrotoxic). In Figure 6, the hospital course of such a woman is summarized. We have managed only one woman in whom dialysis was necessary, and her course was further complicated by purpura fulminans and continuing sepsis from skin sloughage.

Haematological dysfunction

Haematological aberrations are common, but seldom of clinical importance. For example, thrombocytopaenia and minimally elevated fibrin–fibrinogen split products in serum are frequently identified. In the rare case, endotoxin activates intravascular coagulation, and treatment for such consumptive coagulopathy is directed toward eliminating the infection. Unless operative intervention is planned, reversal of the coagulopathy follows such treatment and blood component replacement is unnecessary.

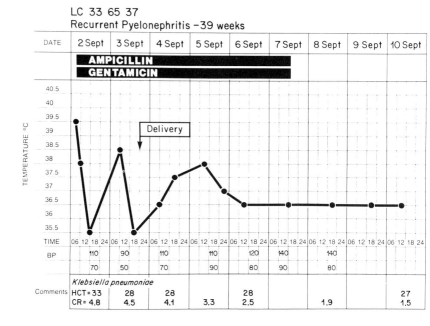

Figure 6. Recurrent pyelonephritis at 39 weeks gestation further complicated by severely diminished renal function for which gentamicin dosage was appropriately reduced. By discharge on day 9, renal dysfunction had improved considerably, although it was still significantly impaired.

There is now abundant evidence that endotoxaemia causes haemolysis, and anaemia is common with antepartum pyelonephritis (Brumfitt, 1975; Gilstrap et al, 1981b). Erythrocyte transfusions are seldom indicated in otherwise uncomplicated infection; however, we have found them necessary in nearly half of women with pulmonary injury described below. More commonly, worrisome anaemia develops after pyelonephritis, and it is not unusual for the haematocrit to reach 25 volumes per cent. The woman whose course is shown in Figure 6 is typical for this complication, and unless there is underlying chronic renal disease, restoration of the haemoglobin mass is usually prompt if there is adequate iron.

Pulmonary injury

Approximately 1 in 50 women with severe antepartum pyelonephritis develop evidence for respiratory insufficiency (Cunningham et al, 1987). Endotoxin alters alveolar–capillary membrane permeability with subsequent pulmonary oedema (Asbaugh et al, 1967; Rinaldo and Rogers, 1982). Fortunately, in most women, clinical manifestations are transient and respond promptly to increased inspired oxygen concentration. However, the respiratory distress syndrome may be life-threatening, and careful attention should be given to the respiratory rate and other evidence for arteriovenous oxygen shunting. Most

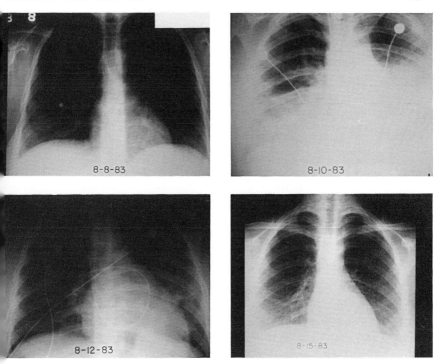

Figure 7. This 18-year-old multipara at 20 weeks gestation had a normal radiograph upon admission 8 August. Respiratory distress 20 hours later was accompanied by a left-sided pulmonary infiltrate which became bilateral by 10 August. She had normal cardiovascular function determined by pulmonary artery catheterization. The X-ray was normal by 12 August. From Cunningham et al (1987) with permission.

women with pulmonary injury have clinical manifestations within 48 hours of admission, and tachypnoea must be promptly investigated by chest radiograph and arterial blood gas analysis. Prompt recognition and appropriate respiratory therapy, which occasionally includes intubation and mechanical ventilation, prevents severe hypoxaemia that may cause fetal death or preterm labour. The clinical case of a woman with severe pulmonary involvement is shown in Figure 7.

Pulmonary injury frequently coexists with other complications already discussed. For example (as shown in Table 3), women with pulmonary capillary injury commonly have associated haematological aberrations and renal dysfunction. These syndromes are more common in women with proven bacteraemia, and it has also been our experience that infections caused by *K. pneumoniae* are usually more severe. It is unclear whether prompt treatment with antimicrobials directed against this organism will prevent these complications. Unfortunately, we have been unable to enumerate risk factors that identify prospectively a woman at risk for these complications. As illustrated in Table 3, these women tend to be more seriously ill; however, most factors that indicate severity of illness are recognized only in retrospect.

Table 3. Selected factors for women with pyelonephritis and pulmonary injury compared with similarly infected women without respiratory distress.*

Factor	Respiratory distress	No distress	Comparison
Symptoms (mean)	2.6 days	2.5 days	NS
Maximal temperature (mean)	39.7 °C	39.1 °C	$P=0.002$
Renal dysfunction	57%	20%	$P=0.018$
Haematocrit (mean)	30.1	32.3	$P=0.012$
Platelet count/mm^3:			
Lowest (mean)	153 000	242 000	$P=0.02$
Less than 100 000	40%	0	$P=0.003$
Bacteraemia	43%	22%	$P=0.16$
Klebsiella or *Proteus*	40%	13%	$P=0.05$
Days febrile (mean)	3.2	1.9	$P=0.004$
Preterm delivery	21%	4%	$P=0.10$

* Modified from Cunningham et al (1987).

SUMMARY

Urinary infections, with a spectrum from covert bacteriuria to severe pyelonephritis, commonly complicate pregnancy. Serious infections follow untreated silent bacteriuria in a fourth of cases, and routine screening can be justified in high-risk populations, particularly those from lower socioeconomic strata. Despite an initial salutary response to a number of antimicrobial regimens, covert bacteriuria recurs in one-third of treated women whose risk of pyelonephritis remains at 25%. Acute cystitis may be unrelated to these other infections and responds readily to a number of regimens; however, single-dose therapy is not recommended since early pyelonephritis can be mistaken for uncomplicated cystitis.

Pyelonephritis is the most common severe bacterial infection complicating pregnancy. These women are frequently quite ill, and hospitalization is recommended. Since 85% to 90% respond within 48 hours to intravenous fluids and antimicrobials, continued fever and evidence of sepsis after two or three days should prompt a search for underlying obstruction. Perhaps 20% of women with severe pyelonephritis develop complications that include septic shock syndrome or its presumed variants. These latter include renal dysfunction, haemolysis and thrombocytopaenia, and pulmonary capillary injury. In most of these women, continued fluid and antimicrobial therapy result in a salutary outcome, but there is occasional maternal mortality.

REFERENCES

Ahlering TE, Boyd SD, Hamilton CL et al (1985) Emphysematous pyelonephritis: a 5-year experience with 13 patients. *Journal of Urology* **134:** 1086–1088.

Asbaugh DG, Bigelow DB, Petty TL & Levine BE (1967) Acute respiratory distress in adults. *Lancet* **ii:** 319–323.

Bailey RR, Bishop V & Peddie BA (1983) Comparison of single dose with a 5-day course of co-trimoxazole for asymptomatic (covert) bacteriuria of pregnancy. *Australian and New Zealand Journal of Obstetrics and Gynaecology* **23:** 139–141.

Bailey RR (1985) Single-dose therapy for uncomplicated urinary tract infections. *New Zealand Medical Journal* **98:** 327–329.

Bailey RR, Peddie BA & Bishop V (1986) Comparison of single dose with a five-day course of trimethoprim for asymptomatic (covert) bacteriuria of pregnancy. *New Zealand Medical Journal* **99:** 501–503.

Benson M, Li Puma JP & Resnick MI (1986) The role of imaging studies in urinary tract infection. *Urologic Clinics of North America* **13:** 605–625.

Brumfitt W (1975) The effects of bacteriuria in pregnancy on maternal and fetal health. *Kidney International* (Supplement) **8:** 113–120.

Campbell-Brown M, McFadyen IR, Seal DV & Stephenson ML (1987) Is screening for bacteriuria in pregnancy worth while? *British Medical Journal* **294:** 1579–1582.

Costas S, Ripey JJ & Van Blerk PJP (1972) Segmental acute pyelonephritis. A precursor to renal carbuncle or abscess? *British Journal of Urology* **44,** 399.

Cunningham FG, Morris GB & Mickal A (1973) Acute pyelonephritis of pregnancy: a clinical review. *Obstetrics and Gynecology* **42:** 112–116.

Cunningham FG, Lucas MJ & Hankins GDV (1987) Pulmonary injury complicating antepartum pyelonephritis. *American Journal of Obstetrics and Gynecology* **156:** 797–807.

Dinarello CA (1984) Interleukin-1 and the pathogenesis of the acute-phase response. *New England Journal of Medicine* **311:** 1413–1418.

Duff P (1984) Pyelonephritis in pregnancy. *Clinical Obstetrics and Gynecology* **27:** 17–31.

Editorial (1985) Urinary tract infection during pregnancy. *Lancet* **ii:** 190–192.

Fairley KF, Bond AG & Adey FD (1966) The site of infection in pregnancy bacteriuria. *Lancet* **i:** 939–943.

Faro S, Pastorek JG, Plauche WC et al (1984) Short-course parenteral antibiotic therapy for pyelonephritis in pregnancy. *Southern Medical Journal* **77:** 455–457.

Gilstrap LC, Cunningham FG & Whalley PJ (1981a) Acute pyelonephritis in pregnancy: an anterospective study. *Obstetrics and Gynecology* **57:** 409–413.

Gilstrap LC, Leveno KJ, Cunningham FG et al (1981b) Renal infection and pregnancy outcome. *American Journal of Obstetrics and Gynecology* **141:** 709–716.

Harris RE & Gilstrap LC (1981) Cystitis during pregnancy: a distinct clinical entity. *Obstetrics and Gynecology* **57:** 578–580.

Harris RE, Gilstrap LC & Pretty A (1981b) Single-dose antimicrobial therapy for asymptomatic bacteriuria during pregnancy. *Obstetrics and Gynecology* **59:** 546–549.

Kass EH (1978) Horatio at the orifice: the significance of bacteriuria. *Journal of Infectious Disease* **138:** 546–557.

Kincaid-Smith P & Bullen M (1965) Bacteriuria in pregnancy. *Lancet* **i:** 395–401.

Krieger JN (1986) Complications and treatment of urinary tract infections in pregnancy. *Urologic Clinics of North America* **13:** 685.

Leveno KJ, Harris RE, Gilstrap LC et al (1981) Bladder versus renal bacteriuria during pregnancy: recurrence after treatment. *American Journal of Obstetrics and Gynecology* **139:** 403.

Pritchard JA, Scott DE, Whalley PJ et al (1973) The effects of maternal sickle hemoglobinopathies and sickle cell trait on reproductive performance. *American Journal of Obstetrics and Gynecology* **117:** 662–670.

Richman AV, Gerber LI & Baks JU (1980) Peritubular capillaries. A major target site of endotoxin-induced vascular injury. *Laboratory Investigation* **43:** 327–334.

Rinaldo JE & Rogers RM (1982) Adult respiratory-distress syndrome: changing concepts of lung injury and repair. *New England Journal of Medicine* **306:** 900–909.

Roberts JA (1986) Pathophysiology of pyelonephritis. *Infections in Surgery* November: 633–638.

Stamm WE, Counts GW, Running KR et al (1982) Diagnosis of coliform infection in acutely dysuric women. *New England Journal of Medicine* **307:** 463.

Svanborg Eden C, Hagberg L, Leffler H & Lonberg H (1982) Recent progress in the understanding of the role of bacterial adhesion in the pathogenesis of urinary tract infection. *Infection* **10:** 327–332.

Thomas V, Shelokov A & Forland M (1974) Antibody-coated bacteria in the urine and the site of urinary tract infections. *New England Journal of Medicine* **290:** 588–592.

Väisänen V, Elo J, Tallgren LG et al (1981) Mannose-resistant haemagglutination and P antigen recognition are characteristic of *Escherichia coli* causing primary pyelonephritis. *Lancet* **ii:** 1366–1369.

Whalley PJ (1967) Bacteriuria of pregnancy. *American Journal of Obstetrics and Gynecology* **97:** 723–738.

Whalley PJ, Cunningham FG & Martin FG (1975) Transient renal dysfunction associated with acute pyelonephritis of pregnancy. *Obstetrics and Gynecology* **46:** 174–180.

8

Nephrolithiasis and gestation

PATSY MAIKRANZ
FREDRIC L. COE
JOAN H. PARKS
MARSHALL D. LINDHEIMER

Although nephrolithiasis is uncommon during pregnancy, it is associated with an increased incidence of maternal urinary tract infections (Coe et al, 1978), and kidney stone passage can precipitate premature labour (Drago et al, 1982). Detection and management of kidney stones are more complicated than in the non-gravid state because most of the diagnostic and therapeutic interventions commonly employed in stone disease can potentially affect the developing fetus. This review focuses on the incidence, aetiology, diagnosis, natural history and management of kidney stones during pregnancy, and discusses mechanisms that may be responsible for this complication of pregnancy.

INCIDENCE

The incidence of stone disease during pregnancy is reported to range between 0.03% and 0.53% (Coe et al, 1978; Miller and Kakkis, 1982; Horowitz and Schmidt, 1985). The true incidence of kidney stones in pregnancy is not clearly established because most of the literature is selective: patients are identified because their stones become symptomatic. A non-selective survey by our group in 1978 revealed no increased incidence of kidney stones either developing of recurring during gestation.

Geography may influence the occurrence of stones as mountainous and hot areas of the world (Figure 1) have the highest incidence of nephrolithiasis (Drach, 1978). In the western hemisphere, calcium nephrolithiasis occurs most frequently in industrialized countries (Lemann et al, 1979), perhaps because of increased dietary intake of protein in these countries. Increased dietary intake of protein leads to increased acid production and increased urinary calcium and uric acid excretions (Robertson et al, 1979), thus increasing the substrates available for stone formation. Given these geographic variations it is difficult to compare one's findings to those in the literature, which come from diverse locations.

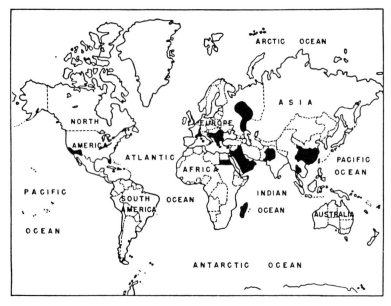

Figure 1. The occurrence of kidney stones worldwide. From Drach (1978) with permission.

AETIOLOGY

Certain anatomical and physiological changes which occur during gestation may facilitate stone formation. Calyces, ureters and renal pelves dilate during the first trimester and remain so until delivery. Concomitant with these anatomical changes, ureteral peristaltic activity decreases (Waltzer, 1981). These anatomical changes have been ascribed to either hormonal or mechanical factors, but a combination of these factors seems the most likely explanation. Decreased ureteral peristalsis occurring in the dilated collecting system can lead to urinary stasis and infection that promotes growth of pre-existing stones and allows new stones to form.

The glomerular filtration rate (GFR) increases by up to 25–50% early in normal pregnancy (Lindheimer and Katz, 1986). The filtered loads of calcium, sodium and uric acid increase along with the increase in GFR. For either uric acid stones to form or crystalluria to develop, the urine must be severely oversaturated from dehydration, hyperuricosuric or very acidic (Favus and Coe, 1986). Urine is slightly alkaline during gestation (Lim et al, 1976; Maikranz et al, 1987b) and this may provide some protection against uric acid stone formation.

Our own studies of urinary solutes during pregnancy confirm those of others (Pedersen et al, 1984) and show that urinary calcium excretion may increase by one- to two-fold during gestation. Urinary supersaturation, an expression of concentration and solubility with respect to calcium salts, also markedly increases during gestation (Kristensen et al, 1985; Maikranz et al, 1987a). Although increased supersaturation should promote stones during

Table 1. Types of stones formed and their frequency of occurrence.

Stone composition	Number of women	Percentage
Calcium oxalate	244	58
Calcium phosphate	12	3
Calcium + uric acid	24	5.5
Uric acid	9	2
Cystine	8	2
Struvite	76	18
Unknown	49	11.5
	422	

Taken from Coe FL, Parks JH (1988) Nephrolithiasis and treatment **Yearbook** (in press).

pregnancy, women who form stones form no more when they are pregnant than when they are not. Perhaps they are protected by increased urinary excretion of both magnesium and citrate, known inhibitors of calcium kidney stones. An acidic glycoprotein called nephrocalcin is normally present in urine and inhibits calcium oxalate stone formation (Nakagawa et al, 1985). Nephrocalcin excretion increases markedly during normal pregnancy (Wabner et al, 1987). Thus the hypercalciuric and very supersaturated urine of normal gravidas may be balanced by increased inhibitory factors, especially nephrocalcin.

One mechanism for gestational hypercalciuria may be that circulating levels of 1,25-dihydroxyvitamin D (calcitriol) increase during gestation (Kumar et al, 1979). Calcitriol increases intestinal calcium absorption (Coburn et al, 1973) and can cause hypercalciuria in humans (Kaplan et al, 1977; Brickman et al 1974). Hypercalciuria from calcitriol is not due to increased filtered load of calcium but rather to reduced renal calcium reabsorption, because calcitriol reduces serum levels of parathyroid hormone (PTH) (Chertow et al, 1975; Slatopolsky et al, 1984; Norris et al, 1985). PTH normally stimulates tubular calcium reabsorption at the level of the distal convoluted tubule and the connecting segment (Shareghi and Stoner, 1978) and also in the thick ascending limb of the loop of Henle (Bourdeau and Burg, 1980). PTH secretion is suppressed by both increased serum calcium (Sherwood et al, 1968; Brown, 1982) and by calcitriol itself (Chertow et al, 1975). Several groups have investigated PTH levels during pregnancy and, unfortunately, have reported widely varying values; some authors have attributed the variations to differences in the assay methods (Pedersen et al, 1984). Gestational hypercalciuria may merely represent an overadaptation—gastrointestinal calcium absorption in excess of what the fetus uses to create its skeleton; mechanisms responsible for gestational calcitriol excess are unknown.

Struvite kidney stones only form when the urinary tract is infected with

Table 2. Presentation of nephrolithiasis in pregnancy.

Symptoms	Signs
Fever	Pyrexia
Nausea	Pyuria
Emesis	Crystalluria
Flank pain	Haematuria
Abdominal pain	Costovertebral angle tenderness
Dysuria	
Urgency	

Modified from Maikranz et al (1987b), with permission.

organisms that possess urease, for example *Proteus* species. These infection stones can form around a nidus of calcium, uric acid or cystine, or may consist only of magnesium ammonium phosphate (struvite) admixed with calcium carbonate—an inevitable calcium precipitate in alkaline urine. Women who produce pure struvite stones present with infection rather than stone passage, are usually not hypercalciuric, and have a high frequency of urological surgery and contralateral stone formation (Kristensen et al, 1987, in press). Although struvite stones can form in completely normal collecting systems, the anatomical changes of the urinary tract during pregnancy may predispose to struvite stone formation. Very little has been written about struvite stones in pregnancy.

Types and relative percentages of kidney stones occurring in non-gravid women studied at our institution are given in Table 1. Most of the available review papers on nephrolithiasis during gestation that provide case details have incomplete information on kidney stone analysis, but from the sparse data available it appears that the relative percentages of the occurrence of kidney stones are about the same as in our non-gravid women.

DIAGNOSIS

It has been observed (Folger, 1955) that the most common non-obstetric cause of abdominal pain requiring hospitalization during pregnancy is renal colic. In the more recent series of patients reported by Jones et al (1978), Lattanzi et al (1980), Drago et al (1982) and Perreault et al (1982), the most common presenting symptom of stones during gestation was pain. Other common presenting symptoms are the same as those in non-gravid stone formers (Table 2).

A good history and physical examination remain the foundation of the approach to the pregnant patient with suspected nephrolithiasis. Specific areas to be included are: age at onset of stone disease, family members with stone disease, diet and medications, prior urinary tract infections, results of previous abdominal radiographs, and other medical disorders or prior surgeries (Smith, 1978). Laboratory evaluation of the patient with kidney stones can often be influenced by the history. Currently, even routine testing is expensive, and given the importance of cost containment in medical care, it is of value to individualize the diagnostic approach to each patient.

Ultrasonography is ideal for stones in pregnancy because it does not expose the fetus to ionizing radiation. In a prospective comparison study with excretory urograms in non-gravidas, renal ultrasound provided 74% specificity and 98% sensitivity (Ellenbogen et al, 1978). Because most symptomatic stones in pregnancy are located in the ureters (Horowitz and Schmidt, 1985), ultrasonography may be a less sensitive test in this situation. In addition, the physiological dilatation of the collecting system which accompanies gestation makes identification of obstruction from kidney stones more difficult than in non-gravidas.

The risk of congenital anomalies is increased from 1 to 3% when large doses of radiation (5–15) rad are delivered to the maternal pelvis (Swartz and Reichling, 1978). The effect of lesser amounts of radiation exposure is unknown. Standard excretory urograms usually deliver less than 1.5 radiation absorbed doses to the fetus. To decrease fetal radiation exposure, one should film only the involved side, shield the maternal pelvis and limit the number of films obtained. Current indications for an excretory urogram during gestation include: (1) symptoms of calculi unresponsive to conservative therapy (2) a decline in renal function in association with symptoms of kidney stones (3) severely symptomatic pyelonephritis refractory to antibiotics, especially in a gravida with a past history of nephrolithiasis (Maikranz et al, 1987b). In any case it is important to remember that radiological studies necessary for maternal health care delivery should not be withheld for fear of fetal radiation exposure, especially after mid-trimester. In 1987, information on the use of magnetic resonance imaging to detect stones in gravidas is unavailable, but this technique has merit on theoretical grounds.

Spontaneous passage of a symptomatic kidney stone provides relief for the patient and often confirms the diagnosis for the physician. Eighty-three stones were identified during 74 pregnancies in the series of patients reported by Coe (1978), Jones et al (1978), Lattanzi et al (1980), Drago et al (1982) and Perreault et al (1982); of these, 62 (74%) were passed spontaneously and those remaining required interventions either during pregnancy or in the puerperium. The percentage of women requiring intervention was greater in the series of Horowitz and Schmidt (1985) compared to other reports. Progressive ureteral dilatation may account for the high rate of spontaneous passage in gestation.

Stones occurring during gestation are more frequently diagnosed in the second and third trimesters (Lattanzi and Cook, 1980) and in multiparas (Jones et al, 1978). The higher incidence in multiparas may reflect the fact that stone disease increases with age in both sexes (Drach et al, 1978); the increased rate of occurrence later in gestation may be due to the passage of previously asymptomatic stones through the dilated ureter to the level of the pelvic brim. The ureters resume their normal calibre at this level, and trap stones that obstruct urine flow and cause symptoms.

Symptomatic stones occur with equal frequency on both sides during

Table 3. The passage of kidney stones.

Source	n*	Stones passed spontaneously	Non-operative† procedures	Operative procedures	Other‡
Coe (1970)	20(15)	20	0	0	0
Drago et al (1982)	12 (9)	9	1	2	0
Horowitz and Schmidt (1985)	17(17)	5	10	2	0
Jones et al (1978)	21(20)	12	2(1§)	5(4§)	2
Lattanzi and Cook (1980)	11(11)	7	2	0	2
Perreault et al (1982)	19(19)	14	0	4(1§)	1

Modified from Maikranz et al (1987b), with permission.
*the number of stones reported, with the number of pregnancies in parentheses.
†cystoscopy, percutaneous nephrostomy and basket extraction.
‡patients either lost to follow-up or without clinical evidence of stone passage.
§the number of procedures done postpartum.

pregnancy, even though the right ureter is usually more dilated than the left. This equality is presumably because both sides of the collecting system do dilate during normal pregnancy. The location of newly formed or migrating stones may be influenced by pre-existing anatomical abnormalities.

NATURAL HISTORY

A review of the literature on kidney stones in pregnancy reveals that conservative management alone results in spontaneous passage of at least 50% of symptomatic stones. Although operative and non-operative interventions may be necessary during pregnancy in up to 30% of patients (Table 3), in the remaining gravidas procedures can often be avoided until after delivery. If a stone cannot be left to pass by itself, the best alternative is cystoscopy to either remove the stone or relieve the obstruction by passing a stent catheter (Jones et al, 1978; Loughlin and Bailey, 1986). If cystoscopy is unsuccessful or surgically undesirable, either a percutaneous nephrostomy or an open procedure must usually be performed (Horowitz and Schmidt, 1985). None of the surgical interventions listed in Table 3 caused fetal demise or maternal complications. All procedures, both operative and non-operative, should be delayed until the postpartum period when possible. Specific indications for interventions during pregnancy include (1) persistent infection proximal to an obstructing stone, (2) intractable pain, (3) renal colic precipitating premature labour that is refractory to drug therapy, (4) worsening renal function with a persistent obstruction, and (5) obstruction of a solitary kidney (Maikranz et al, 1987b).

The most common non-obstetric complication of kidney stones during gestation is urinary tract infection, reportedly occurring in up to 10–20% of gravidas with stone disease (Coe et al, 1978). Oral antibiotic therapy usually eradicates lower tract infection. More serious infections, pyelonephritis and calculus pyelonephritis require hospitalization and parenteral antibiotic therapy, and perhaps intervention to remove an obstructing stone.

Table 4. Postpartum evaluation of stone disease.

Serum levels
  Calcium
  Phosphorus
  Uric acid
  Creatinine

Spot urine
  Urinalysis
  Culture
  Fasting pH

Urine chemistries (24-h collection)
  Creatinine
  Uric acid
  Calcium
  Phosphorus
  Oxalate
  Citrate

Stone analysis (if stone is available)

Radiology
  Flat plate of abdomen
  Excretory urogram (not always indicated)

Modified from Smith (1979), with permission.

Premature labour from renal colic is the most common obstetric complication of kidney stones (Drago et al, 1982). β_2-Agonist therapy usually arrests premature labour, and the risk of premature labour ceases completely with stone passage or removal. Armon (1977) reported a patient with a large vesicular stone that impeded labour and necessitated caesarean section for delivery. In 1980, Honore reported results of a retrospective study of stone disease and pregnancy in which he concluded that a past history of stone disease predisposed gravidas to spontaneous abortion. He theorized that abnormalities in calcium homeostasis may cause some abnormal hormone secretion by the corpus luteum or placenta, have teratogenic effects on the zygote, or cause myometrial hyperirritability which accounted for the increased number of spontaneous abortions he identified in this group of women.

Gravid stone formers or stone-forming women who are contemplating pregnancy frequently seek counselling prior to conception or early in gestation about how pregnancy will affect their stone disease and vice versa. Data from our retrospective study of 1978, as well as our continuing clinical experience, suggest that pregnancy has no adverse effects on stone disease. Neither the severity nor the activity of stone disease appears to change during gestation. The incidence of urinary tract infections is increased in gravidas with pre-existing stone disease, and questionably the incidence of spontaneous abortions is increased in this group. The latter observation needs more careful investigation before a true cause and effect can be established.

MANAGEMENT

Conservative therapy, that is hydration, bed rest and administration of analgesics, should be the initial approach to gravidas with symptomatic stones. This approach alone should result in spontaneous passage of at least 50% of symptomatic stones during gestation (Jones et al, 1978). When possible, stones should be saved and crystallography performed, as very valuable information regarding long-term postpartum therapy can be gained from stone analysis. Metabolic evaluation of stone disease should be delayed until at least 3 months after parturition and lactation, as changes in the metabolism of calcium, urate and other urinary ions during these periods produce urine chemistry values that are irrelevant to the patients' stone disease. A practical initial postpartum evaluation of stone disease is outlined in Table 4. An attempt to delay non-operative and operative urological interventions until after delivery is the most prudent approach, but this is not always possible. These interventions have become less hazardous in the last two decades with advances in fetal and maternal health care.

Medications commonly prescribed for patients with stone disease have many unacceptable side-effects during pregnancy. Thiazides enhance distal renal tubular reabsorption of calcium, thereby reducing urinary excretion of calcium (Lemann et al, 1979); these drugs are commonly used to treat hypercalciuric states (Coe, 1977; Yendt and Cohanim, 1978). This class of drugs has few side-effects but has been reported to cause fetal thrombocytopenia (Rodriguez et al, 1964), hypoglycaemia (Gray, 1968) and hyponatraemia (Gray, 1968). Unfortunately, this group of drugs may also impair the normal volume expansion of pregnancy thought to be important for optimum fetal development. Instead of using thiazides to treat hypercalciuric disorders during pregnancy, patients should be instructed to increase their fluid intake and avoid excessive ingestion of calcium until after parturition, when thiazides can safely be administered. Urine output needs to be at least $2-2\frac{1}{2}$ l/day to keep the urine appropriately dilute. Depending on the severity of the stone disease, a lower calcium diet may also be of value. Most prenatal vitamins contain only 100–200 milligrams of calcium and may be continued with mild stone disease; however, for severe calcium stone disease a non-calcium-containing vitamin may be preferable.

Xanthine oxidase inhibitors, used in the treatment of uric acid stone disease, halt purine metabolism at the level of hypoxanthine and thus decrease both serum and urinary uric acid. Effects on the human fetus are unestablished, but no adverse effects on fetal animals have been noted. Still, this class of drugs should also probably be avoided during gestation. Therapeutic measures to treat uric acid stones in pregnancy include increasing urine volume, modestly limiting purines in the diet and alkalinizing the urine to at least pH 6.0 using any oral alkali preparation in a dose of 0.5–2.0 mmol/kg/day in four divided doses.

Cystine stones are often treated with D-penicillamine. Part of its therapeutic action occurs by forming the disulphide of cysteine and penicillamine, which is more soluble than cysteine (cysteine-cysteine) and is thus more readily excreted. Penicillamine has been reported to be teratogenic in rats. Solomon et al (1977) have described fetal abnormalities in infants of mothers who took the drug during pregnancy. Because of the possibility of teratogenic effects, Gregory and Mansell (1983) discontinued the drug between the sixth and twentieth weeks of gestation in the 22 patients with cystinuria that they took care of during pregnancy. They reported no fetal anomalies related to maternal penicillamine ingestion. Alternate ways to treat cystinuria in gravidas is mainly by increasing urine volume and alkalinizing the urine.

When preparing this review we were unable to find any reports of experience with extracorporeal shockwave lithotripsy in either animal or human gravidas. Lithotripsy cannot be recommended for the treatment of nephrolithiasis in pregnancy until its safety during gestation is firmly established.

NEW FRONTIERS

Our work continues on mineral metabolism in gestation as well as on the acidic glycoproteins known to inhibit calcium oxalate stone formation. Our preliminary data suggest that the excretion of these inhibitors increases during the first trimester of normal pregnancy and remains elevated throughout gestation. Postpartum, the levels fall rapidly to values normal for non-gravid, non-stone-forming women. This observation is important because the hypercalciuria of pregnancy also develops during the first trimester, persisting until after delivery. This work (Wabner et al, 1987), together with previous work on kidney stones and the inhibitor proteins (Nakagawa et al, 1985), has ed us to hypothesize that these glycoproteins may play a biological role in preventing kidney stone formation during gestational hypercalciuria. Ongoing clinical work in this area on both normal and stone-forming gravidas is needed to firmly establish this concept.

SUMMARY

Although both anatomical and physiological changes in pregnancy may predispose to kidney stone formation, it still remains an uncommon occurrence. Correct diagnosis is often difficult. Ultrasound has become the primary diagnostic tool, and a limited study excretory urogram is only necessary for complicated cases. Nephrolithiasis during pregnancy occurs more frequently during the later stages of gestation in multiparas, and without a difference in laterality. Conservative management with bed rest, hydration and analgesia can result in spontaneous passage of the majority of stones in gravidas. Past experience indicates that cystoscopy and/or surgery can usually be done safely when absolutely necessary. Pre-existing stone disease can increase the incidence of maternal urinary tract infections by 10–20%. The most common obstetric complication of stones during gestation is the precipitation of premature labour by renal colic. Unfortunately, most drugs used to treat stone disease are contraindicated in gestation. Experimental evidence suggests that known inhibitors of stone formation are present in gestation, and may help to explain why the incidence of stones is not increased in this particularly hypercalciuric state.

Acknowledgements

This study was supported by grant AM33949 from the National Institutes of Health.

REFERENCES

Armon PJ (1977) Obstructed labour due to a vesical calculus. *British Medical Journal* ii: 498.

Bourdeau JE & Burg MB (1980) Effect of parathyroid hormone on calcium transport across the cortical thick ascending limb of Henle's loop. *American Journal of Physiology* 239: F121–126.

Brickman AS, Coburn JW, Norman AW et al (1974) Short-term effects of 1.25-dihydroxychole-calciferol on disordered calcium metabolism of renal failure. *American Journal of Medicine* 57: 28–33.

Brown EM (1982) Parathyroid hormone secretion in vivo and in vitro. Regulation by calcium and other secretagogues. *Mineral Electrolyte Metabolism* 8: 130–150.

Chertow BS, Baylink DJ, Wergedal JF et al (1975) Decrease in immunoreactive parathyroid hormone in rats and in parathyroid hormone secretion in vitro by 1,25-dihydroxycholecalciferol. *Journal of Clinical Investigation* 56: 668–678.

Coburn JW, Hartenbower DL & Massry SG (1973) Intestinal absorption of calcium and the effect of renal insufficiency. *Kidney International* 4: 96–104.

Coe FL (1977) Treated and untreated recurrent calcium nephrolithiasis in patients with idiopathic hypercalciuria, hyperuricosuria, or no metabolic disorder. *Annals of Internal Medicine* 87: 404–410.

Coe FL, Parks JH & Lindheimer MD (1978) Nephrolithiasis during pregnancy. *New England Journal of Medicine* 298 (6): 324–326.

Drach GW (1978) Urinary lithiasis. In Harrison JH et al (eds) *Campbell's Urology*, Chap. 22, pp 779–878. Philadelphia: WB Saunders.

Drago JR, Rohner TJ Jr & Chez RA (1982) Management of urinary calculi in pregnancy. *Urology* 20 (6): 578–581.

Ellenbogen PH, Scheible FW, Talner LB et al (1978) Sensitivity of gray scale ultrasound in detecting urinary tract obstruction. *American Journal of Roentgenology* 130: 731–733.

Favus MJ & Coe FL (1986) Disorders of stone formation. In Brenner B & Rector F (eds) *The Kidney*, Chap. 32, pp 1403–1442. Philadelphia: WB Saunders.

Folger GK (1955) Pain and pregnancy. *Obstetrics and Gynecology* 5: 513–518.

Gray MJ (1968) Use and abuse of thiazides in pregnancy. *Clinics in Obstetrics and Gynecology* 11 568–578.

Gregory MC & Mansell MA (1983) Pregnancy and cystinuria. *Lancet* 19: 1958–1960.

Honore LH (1980) The increased incidence of renal stones in women with spontaneous abortion a retrospective study. *American Journal of Obstetrics and Gynecology* 137 (1): 145–146.

Horowitz E & Schmidt JD (1985) Renal calculi in pregnancy. *Clinical Obstetrics and Gynecology* 28 (2): 324–338.

Jones WA, Correa RJ Jr & Ansell JS (1978) Urolithiasis associated with pregnancy. *Journal of Urology* 122: 333–335.

Kaplan RA, Haussler MR, Deftos LJ et al (1977) The role of 1,25-dihydroxyvitamin D in the mediation of the intestinal hyperabsorption of calcium in primary hyperparathyroidism and absorptive hypercalciuria. *Journal of Clinical Investigation* 59: 756–760.

Kristensen C, Abraham PA, Davis M et al (1985) Hypercalciuria and risk factors for calcium nephrolithiasis during pregnancy. *Kidney International* 327: 144 (abstract).

Kristensen C, Parks JH, Lindheimer M et al (1987) Reduced glomerular filtration rate and hypercalciuria in primary struvite nephrolithiasis. *Kidney International* **32:** 749–753.

Kumar R, Cohen WR, Silva P et al (1979) Elevated 1,25-dihydroxyvitamin D plasma levels in normal human pregnancy and lactation. *Journal of Clinical Investigation* **63:** 342–344.

Lattanzi DR & Cook WA (1980) Urinary calculi in pregnancy. *Obstetrics and Gynecology* **56** (4): 462–466.

Lemann J Jr, Adams ND & Gray RW (1979) Urinary calcium excretion in human beings. *New England Journal of Medicine* **301** (10): 535–541.

Lim VS, Katz AI & Lindheimer MD (1976) Acid-base regulation in pregnancy. *American Journal of Physiology* **231** (6): 1764–1770.

Lindheimer MD & Katz AI (1986). The kidney in pregnancy. In Brenner B & Rector F (eds) *The Kidney*, Chap. 28, pp 1253–1296. Philadelphia: WB Saunders.

Loughlin KR & Bailey RB (1986) Internal ureteral stents for conservative management of ureteral calculi during pregnancy. *New England Journal of Medicine* **315:** 1647–1649.

Maikranz P, Parks JP, Coe FL et al (1987a) Urinary calcium oxalate and calcium carbonate supersaturations increase in pregnancy. *Kidney International* **31:** 209 (abstract).

Maikranz P, Coe FL, Parks JP & Lindheimer MD (1987b) Nephrolithiasis in pregnancy. *American Journal of Kidney Disease* **9:** 354–358.

Miller RD & Kakkis J (1982) Prognosis, management and outcome of obstructive renal disease in pregnancy. *Journal of Reproductive Medicine* **28:** 199–201.

Nakagawa Y, Abram V, Parks JH et al (1985) Urine glycoprotein crystal growth inhibitors. *Journal of Clinical Investigation* **76:** 1455–1462.

Norris KC Kraut JA, Andress DL et al (1985) Intravenous calcitriol for severe secondary hyperparathyroidism in dialysis patients. *Kidney International* **27:** 168 (abstract).

Pederson EB, Johannesen P, Kristensen S et al (1984) Calcium, parathyroid hormone and calcitonin in normal pregnancy and preeclampsia. *Gynecologic and Obstetric Investigation* **18:** 156–164.

Perreault JP, Paquin JM, Faucher R et al (1982) Urinary calculi in pregnancy. *Canadian Journal of Surgery* **25** (4): 453–454.

Robertson WG, Peacock M & Hodgkinson A (1979) Dietary changes and the incidence of urinary calculi in the U.K. between 1958 and 1976. *Journal of Chronic Diseases* **32:** 469–476.

Rodriguez SU, Leiken SL & Hiller MC (1964) Neonatal thrombocytopenia associated with antepartum administration of thiazide drugs. *New England Journal of Medicine* **270:** 881–884.

Shareghi GR & Stoner LC (1978) Calcium transport across segments of the rabbit distal nephron in vitro. *American Journal of Physiology* **235:** F367–375.

Sherwood LM, Mayer GP, Ramberg CF et al (1968) Regulation of parathyroid hormone secretion: proportional control by calcium, lack of effect of phosphate. *Endocrinology* **83:** 1043–1051.

Slatopolsky E, Weerts C, Thielan J et al (1984) Marked suppression of secondary hyperparathyroidism by intravenous administration of 1,25-dihydroxycholeciferol in uremic patients. *Journal of Clinical Investigation* **4:** 2136–2143.

Smith L (1978) Calcium-containing renal stones. *Kidney International* **13:** 383–389.

Solomon L, Abrams G, Dinner M et al (1977) Neonatal abnormalities associated with D-penicillamine treatment during pregnancy. *New England Journal of Medicine* **296:** 54–55.

Swartz HM & Reichling BA (1978) Hazards of radiation exposure for pregnant women. *Journal of the American Medical Association* **239** (18): 1907–1909.

Wabner C, Sirivongs D, Maikranz P et al (1987) Evidence for increased excretion in pregnancy of nephrocalcin, a urinary inhibitor of crystal growth. *Kidney International* **31:** 359 (abstract).

Waltzer WC (1981) The urinary tract in pregnancy. *Journal of Urology* **125:** 271–276.

Wendt ER & Cohanim M (1978) Prevention of calcium stones with thiazides. *Kidney International* **13:** 397–409.

9

Gestation in women with kidney disease: prognosis and management

MARSHALL D. LINDHEIMER
ADRIAN I. KATZ

This chapter reviews the obstetric outcome and long-term prognosis of gravidas with renal disease, and highlights prevailing controversies in this field of reproductive medicine. Two entities discussed in detail elsewhere in this book, diabetic nephropathy and reflux nephropathy, are mentioned only briefly here.

THE INTERACTION OF GESTATION AND RENAL DISEASE

The combination of pregnancy and underlying renal parenchymal disease was once considered quite worrisome, and many such gestations were interrupted on the basis of selective or poorly documented literature. In the last decade, however, a number of studies have been published which, although largely retrospective, include several hundred patients whose renal disease has been diagnosed by renal biopsy (Katz et al, 1980; Surian et al, 1984; Jungers et al, 1986; Abe et al, 1986; Barcelo et al, 1986). Critical review of these reports suggests the following general conclusions:

1. Women with underlying renal disease but with preserved or only mildly decreased renal function and normal blood pressure at conception will do well, and pregnancy will not affect adversely the course of their disease. (This statement has to be tempered somewhat for certain nephropathies that appear more sensitive to intercurrent gestation, such as lupus nephropathy and membranoproliferative glomerulonephritis, and does not apply to scleroderma and periarteritis, in which pregnancy is contraindicated.) Authorities disagree as to whether or not gestation adversely influences the natural history of IgA nephropathy, focal glomerulosclerosis and reflux nephropathy (Surian et al, 1984; Kincaid-Smith and Fairley, 1987).

2. Prognosis is more guarded if renal function is moderately impaired (serum creatinine ≥ 1.5 mg dl^{-1}) or if hypertension is present before conception; a substantial proportion (about one-third) of such patients will experience

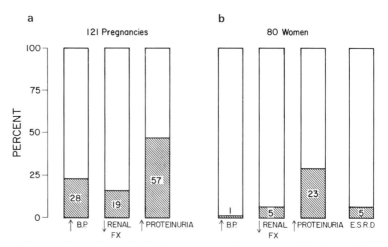

Figure 1. Course of renal disease; (a) during pregnancy and puerperium; (b) at the end of follow-up. Based on data from Katz et al (1980).

renal function deterioration during pregnancy, and accelerated progression of the underlying disease after delivery (Imbasciati et al, 1984; Hou et al, 1985).

3. Women with severe renal dysfunction (serum creatinine ≥ 3 mg dl^{-1}) are usually infertile. On the rare occasion when they do conceive the likelihood of a successful outcome is low, and the gestation is attended by high maternal morbidity—two compelling reasons to discourage pregnancy in such patients.

Pregnancy when renal function is preserved

In 1980 we published a combined prospective and retrospective study that evaluated the immediate and long-term effects on antecedent kidney disease of 121 gestations in 89 women whose diagnosis had been established by renal biopsy (Katz et al, 1980). All these gravidas had normal, or at most slightly impaired, renal function (serum creatinine ≤ 1.4 mg dl^{-1}) before conception, and only 20% had hypertension, usually of a mild degree. Chronic focal and diffuse glomerulonephritis and chronic interstitial nephritis were the most common diagnoses, accounting for two-thirds of all cases. Women with lupus nephritis were not included, as their data were reported separately in another collaborative investigation (Hayslett and Lynn, 1980).

Figure 1 summarizes the effects of pregnancy on blood pressure, renal function and proteinura during 121 gestations, as well as the remote follow-up of these parameters in 80 of the women. It is evident on examining this figure that the immediate and long-term gestational effects on the kidney were quite different, as the incidence of high blood pressure, functional decline and proteinuria were considerably higher during pregnancy and the immediate puerperium than at the end of the follow-up period. Although significant hypertension was a problem in 23% of the pregnancies, it developed *de novo* in only half of them, and was usually associated with a glomerular lesion. Renal function declined in 16%, most often in women with diffuse glomerulonephritis, but in most cases the decrement was only mild to moderate and reversed post partum. More important, many gravidas experienced the expected increments in creatinine clearance (as evidenced by declines in serum creatinine levels), as well as in true glomerular filtration rate (GFR) measured by the inulin clearance, which increased in 26 women studied prospectively. In contrast, abnormal proteinuria was both common and severe, exceeding 3 g per day in 39 of 57 proteinuric women, and leading frequently to nephrotic oedema. Heavy proteinuria was associated with nearly all the glomerular diseases, and as expected was uncommon in patients with chronic interstitial nephritis. Interestingly, these instances of nephrotic-range proteinuria appeared for the first time during gestation in a substantial number of women. However, they were usually well tolerated and had little, if any, influence on the subsequent course of the renal disease.

Table 1 summarizes the gestational outcome in this series. There were 5 stillbirths and 6 neonatal deaths, giving a success rate of 91% for these 123 fetuses. Such data are quite encouraging, especially when one considers that these infants were born in the 1960s and 1970s. It is probably safe to assume that perinatal mortality would be halved today given the advances in perinatal medicine of the last decade. The incidence of preterm deliveries (20%) was high, reflecting in part medical decision, as many of these pregnancies were induced medically or terminated by caesarean section because of concern for maternal well-being. Finally, 24% of the infants were considered small for gestational age, also a high statistic. However, the 76% that were of adequate size defied the anecdotal dictum that most women with renal disease deliver growth-retarded infants.

At the end of follow-up (3 months to 23 years, mean 62 months), the prevalence and severity of hypertension or renal function abnormalities were considerably lower than those observed during pregnancy (Figure 1). Glomerular filtration rate had declined slightly (highest creatinine now 1.7 mg dl^{-1}) in 5 women, and an additional 5 had progressed to end-stage renal disease. In 4 of the latter women kidney failure occurred 2 to 8 years after the index pregnancy and thus bore no temporal relationship to it. In addition, all 5 women had diseases with ominous prognoses (amyloidosis, focal glomerulosclerosis, polycystic kidney disease and diffuse or crescentic glomerulonephritis). Finally, proteinuria was not only less frequent than during pregnancy, but also milder, excretion in the nephrotic range being observed in only 5 cases.

Our main conclusion in the 1980 report was that renal disease may become clinically apparent or worsen during gestation, but its natural course is probably not affected by gestation. We emphasized that this conclusion applied to gravidas whose kidney function was preserved prior to conception, and that more information was required before the prognosis of gravidas with renal insufficiency could be evaluated. Finally, we noted that the incidence of fetal or neonatal deaths, although moderately higher than in healthy gravidas at our institution, did not warrant discouraging women with renal disease from becoming pregnant.

Table 1. Outcome of pregnancy in relation to type of disease.

Biopsy diagnosis	Patients	Pregnancies	Perinatal deaths*	Preterm deliveries	Small-for-dates babies	Birthweight of live infants†			
						<1500 g	<2000 g	<2500 g	>2500 g
Diffuse glomerulonephritis	26	33	5	13	9	6	3	6	13
Focal glomerulonephritis	12	26	3	1	6	0	1	7	18
Membranoproliferative glomerulonephritis	4	4	0	0	1	0	0	1	3
Membranous nephropathy	7	10	0	1	1	0	0	2	5
Lipoid nephrosis	3	6	0	1	4	0	0	4	2
Focal glomerulosclerosis	1	1	0	0	0	0	0	0	1
Interstitial nephritis (pyelonephritis)	21	26	2	4	2	0	1	4	20
Arteriolar nephrosclerosis	8	8	0	3	3	2	2	0	4
Others‡	7	7	1	1	1	1	0	1	4
Totals	89	119§	11	24	27	9	7	25	70
Per cent			9	20	24	8	6	23	63

* Five stillbirths and six neonatal deaths.
† Birthweights available for only 111 of 116 live infants.
‡ Includes sickle cell nephropathy (2 cases) and polycystic disease, IgA nephropathy, diabetic glomerulosclerosis, renal amyloidosis, bilateral renal artery stenosis (1 case of each).
§ Two sets of twins. Two late second trimester abortions included in earlier analyses have been excluded.
Modified from Katz et al (1980).

Table 2. Immediate and long-term effects of pregnancy in women with chronic renal disease.

	No. of women/ no. of pregnancies	Course during pregnancy or postpartum							Time (yr)	Status at the end of follow-up		
		Hypertension	Increased proteinuria	Decreased kidney function	Preterm deliveries	Small-for-date babies	Still-births	Neonatal deaths		Hypertension	Increased proteinuria	Decreased kidney function
Katz et al (1980)	89/119	28 (23%)	57 (47%)	19 (16%)	24 (20%)	27 (24%)	5 (4%)	6 (5%)	5.3	1 (1%)	23 (29%)	5 (6%)
Surian et al (1984)	86/123	24 (20%)	—	10 (8%)	17 (14%)	7 (6%)	12 (10%)	5 (4%)	1	11 (9%)	—	4 (3%)
Barcelo et al (1986)*	48/66	13 (20%)	10 (15%)	2 (3.3%)	7 (11%)	3 (5%)	2 (3%)	1 (2%)	5	17 (37%)	11 (24%)	8 (18%)
Jungers et al (1986)†	122/240	80 (33%)	81 (33%)	17 (7%)	41 (17%)	22 (12%)	7 (4%)	6 (3%)	6.7	41 (34%)	34 (38%)	7 (6%)

* In 5 women in this series plasma creatinine was 1.3–1.9 mg dl⁻¹ before pregnancy. Data at end of follow-up are not significantly different from control group with similar renal diseases who had not been pregnant.

† Seven women in this series had non-pregnant plasma creatinine levels > 1.4 mg dl⁻¹. Only included are data from patients with primary chronic glomerulonephritis. This series includes 60 abortions (therapeutic and spontaneous), whereas the other series listed here do not.

Several studies dealing with this subject have appeared since 1980 and are summarized in Table 2. These reports, which now comprise over 400 gestations, tend to confirm ours both in respect to the natural history of the renal disease and to the fetal outcome. Furthermore, when problems such as functional deterioration or a major fetal complication did arise, it was usually in women with antecedent hypertension, while normotensive gravidas with minimal renal dysfunction did best. Surian et al (1984), however, cautioned that women with membranoproliferative glomerulonephritis have a propensity to experience renal functional deterioration, and that patients with IgA nephropathy tend to develop persistent hypertension during and after pregnancy.

A contrasting view that attributes to pregnancy an adverse influence on the natural history of renal disease and a poorer gestational outcome in such women has been published periodically, and was reviewed most recently by Becker et al (1985) and by Kincaid-Smith and Fairley (1987). The diseases most affected by pregnancy, according to these authors, appear to be IgA nephropathy, focal glomerulosclerosis, and reflux nephropathy. The controversy regarding reflux nephropathy is detailed by Jungers et al in Chapter 11; IgA nephropathy and focal glomerulosclerosis are discussed below.

IgA nephropathy

Kincaid-Smith and Fairley (1987) reviewed 102 gestations in 65 patients with IgA nephropathy and observed that proteinuria occurred or worsened in 77%, while renal function declined in 22%; this decline persisted postpartum in 2 women. Hypertension was a major feature in these pregnancies, occurring in 63% and persisting postpartum in 16. Fetal loss was 27%, possibly related in part to early termination of the pregnancies. This same group (Becker et al, 1985) previously reported that renal lesions seen at biopsy were apt to be more severe in women with IgA nephropathy who had been pregnant compared to those who had not.

Contrasting with the above is the experience of Jungers et al (1987), who failed to detect any adverse effects of pregnancy on the natural history of IgA nephropathy (Figure 2). These investigators, like Surian et al (1984), noted a tendency to aggravated hypertension during pregnancy in some of the patients, but believed this to be merely a predictive sign of high blood pressure that will develop later as part of the natural history of the disease. Fetal loss of 15% (10 of 66 pregnancies) included 5 instances where the women evidenced pre-existing chronic hypertension. Thus, patients normotensive at conception did well in this series. Fetal outcome in the series reported by Abe et al (1985) and Barcelo et al (1986) was also quite satisfactory, as 91% (48 of 53) of the gestations succeeded.

Focal glomerulosclerosis (FGS)

Kincaid-Smith and Fairley (1987) reviewed 28 gestations in 15 women with FGS. Hypertension, often severe, developed during 71% of these pregnancies, and persisted postpartum in 18%. Proteinuria worsened in 93%, while renal

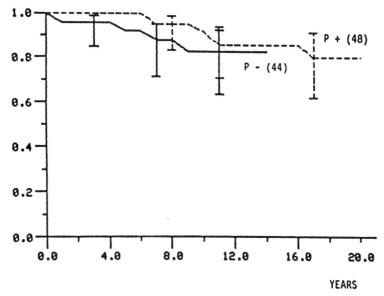

Figure 2. Effect of pregnancy on IgA nephropathy. The fraction of patients free of chronic renal failure is plotted as a function of time (p+, 48 patients who had been pregnant once or more; p−, 44 patients who had never been pregnant). From Jungers et al (1987) with permission.

function declined in 31% of gestations, and in 4 women the decrement persisted after delivery. Fetal loss was 29%, again in part due to early deliveries. In contrast to these data there were no instances of rapid functional decline during any of the 25 gestations in 19 women with FGS reported by Surian et al (1984), but fetal loss in this series (26%) was high. Jungers et al (1987), however, recorded only one spontaneous abortion and a single fetal loss in 9 gestations. The combined number of patients from these three reports is small, and the contested issues may require collaborative prospective studies to resolve.

Collagen disease

The outlook for gravidas with lupus nephropathy but preserved renal function is considerably more complex than in women with the conditions discussed above. Clearly, exacerbations of the systemic disease or its first appearance do occur both during pregnancy and postpartum. Although the effects of gestation on lupus nephropathy (LN) are more difficult to evaluate, a consensus seems nonetheless to be emerging. Hayslett and Lynn (1980) analysed via a retrospective mail survey 65 pregnancies in 47 patients, 36 of whom had a tissue diagnosis of LN. The authors concluded that the course of LN during pregnancy and postpartum correlated better with the activity of the systemic disease in the six months preceding conception than with the type of renal lesion. In another study Fine and colleagues described 52 gestations in which the women had either undetectable or only mild functional abnormalities. No measurable deterioration of renal function could be found in 40 of the 52 pregnancies, while during 7 others a mild but reversible decline was observed. However, in the remaining 5 GFR worsened and remained depressed during the first year of follow-up (Fine et al, 1981). Most recently, Bobrie et al (1987) reviewed the literature as well as their own experience with 72 gestations in patients with lupus nephropathy prior to conception. Their observations agree in general with those of Hayslett and Lynn. A dissenting view, albeit based on a small series (26 gestations in 19 patients with biopsy-proven disease), was reported by Imbasciati et al (1984), who failed to observe any relationship between disease activity prior to conception and the course of renal disease. Three women experienced moderate worsening of renal function during gestation, which persisted in one. More alarming, however, was the occurrence of acute renal failure after delivery in 4 gravidas. The apparent uniqueness of this latter series raises the question whether the authors had been consulted on a selected group of patients.

Fetal outcome in women with systemic lupus erythematosus (SLE) is poorer than with most other renal diseases with preserved glomerular filtration (Hayslett and Reece, 1985). This is due to a higher rate of spontaneous abortion as well as fetal complications secondary to placental transmission of several maternal serum factors such as the lupus anticoagulant and the soluble tissue ribonucleoprotein, anti-Ro(SS-A). Even so, when the disease was in remission and kidney function preserved at conception, approximately 85% of the gestations succeeded (Hayslett and Reece, 1985).

Whereas the prognosis of gravidas with SLE is debated, it is benign enough to allow conception in women who so desire. In contrast, the outcome of pregnancy in patients with renal involvement due to polyarteritis nodosa or scleroderma is considered sufficiently poor to preclude conception or to recommend termination in women already pregnant (reviewed in Lindheimer and Katz, 1986). Both diseases have been associated with hypertensive crises, accelerated loss of renal function and maternal deaths. Thus, although successful gestations have been described, the danger to the mother appears too great to permit even 'trials' of gestation.

Moderate and severe renal insufficiency

The term 'moderate' insufficiency categorizes women who have lost one-third or more of their renal function (serum creatinine ≥ 1.5 mg dl^{-1}) but have not yet reached the advanced stages of renal failure, where successful gestation is unusual (see below). There seems to be less controversy regarding the effects of pregnancy on the renal disease of these women, but there are also considerably fewer data on which conclusions were drawn. It should be remembered that as renal function declines a greater portion of excreted creatinine is due to tubular secretion, the amount of which may vary depending on the lesion. Thus, attempts to judge the amount of residual glomerular filtration from creatinine levels or its clearance are less reliable than when renal function is well preserved. With these reservations in mind, the consensus is that whereas gestation can be uneventful in many women with only moderate renal insufficiency, a substantial proportion will experience a significant deterioration of function during pregnancy, which often is irreversible and hastens the downhill course of their disease. Bear (1976) and Kincaid-Smith et al (1967) noted that approximately half of their patients with moderate renal insufficiency (5 of 11 in one series, 4 of 8 in the other) experienced substantial functional deterioration during gestation, often associated with poorly controlled, moderate to severe hypertension. More recently, Hou et al (1985) and Imbasciati et al (1986) reviewed 39 pregnancies in 37 patients with creatinine levels exceeding 1.4 and 1.6 mg dl^{-1}, respectively. Although over 85% of these gestations succeeded, 24 of the 39 pregnancies were complicated by severe hypertension, and one-fourth of the patients experienced acceleration of their renal disease.

The majority of women with advanced renal failure (defined as creatinine levels above 3 mg dl^{-1}) have amenorrhoea or anovulatory menstrual cycles (see Chapter 14). Data on such patients are limited, and therefore it is difficult to evaluate whether pregnancy has a detrimental effect on their disease. This issue is of limited practical importance, however, because of the already advanced stage of pre-existing renal dysfunction. Anecdotal and personal experience suggest that gestation will aggravate an already difficult management problem, including hectic hypertension and severe fluid retention, with little chance of successful fetal outcome. One should be aware, however, that even women undergoing dialytic therapy occasionally conceive, a topic reviewed elsewhere in this book.

The nephrotic syndrome

As noted in Figure 1 on p. 922 and in the text, proteinuria increases during gestation in over half the women with underlying renal disease, frequently to nephrotic levels. Not surprisingly, this heavy proteinuria is associated with glomerular rather than tubulointerstitial diseases. It is important not to confuse 'physiological' changes of pregnancy with an exacerbation of the patient's disease. For instance, increases in urinary protein may be a consequence of the increments in renal haemodynamics that accompany pregnancy, or may perhaps be due to a rise in renal vein pressure (as the abdominal contents enlarge), or both. Furthermore, serum albumin usually decreases by 0.5 to 1 g dl^{-1} in normal gestation, and when this occurs in patients with renal disease oedema may form (or worsen if already present). Accordingly, an entity termed 'cyclic nephrotic syndrome of pregnancy' may only reflect those instances in which quiescent renal disease becomes more apparent during gestation. Other alterations of normal pregnancy simulating progression of nephrotic syndrome are increments in the plasma levels of cholesterol and other circulating lipids.

The maternal prognosis and fetal outcome in women with the nephrotic syndrome appear good if renal function is preserved and hypertension absent. One dissenting view, however, is that of Jungers et al (1986), who claim that florid nephrosis in early gestation was associated with poor fetal outcome in their series. Lipoid nephrosis in remission is not likely to exacerbate during gestation (Makker and Heyman, 1972).

Some authors suggest that hypoalbuminaemia and the associated decrease in intravascular volume result in small-for-date infants, but most of the women we have observed have adequate-for-date newborns (Katz et al, 1980). Suggestions that children of normotensive mothers with severe proteinuria during gestation manifest impaired neurological or mental development require further study (management of nephrotic syndrome in pregnancy is discussed below).

Renal biopsy in pregnancy

Closed renal biopsy, introduced in the 1950s, is a major reason for the progress in our understanding of kidney pathology and the natural history of many specific disorders. Biopsy techniques were also applied to pregnant populations (Dieckmann et al, 1957), especially in women with pre-eclampsia. Renal biopsies were in general performed for the same diagnostic indications as for non-pregnant subjects, but the primary use of this procedure in pregnant women was to differentiate the various causes of hypertension during the latter half of pregnancy. It was believed at that time that demonstrating the characteristic lesion of pre-eclampsia would be an indication to terminate the pregnancy, while observation of another lesion might lead to specific therapeutic interventions aimed at ensuring continuation of the pregnancy to a point where fetal survival would be improved.

In 1965, Schewitz et al published an oft-quoted report entitled 'Bleeding after renal biopsy in pregnancy'. This group had initially (from 1954 to 1959) noted few adverse reactions and had considered the procedure safe. However, in their next 77 biopsy attempts 16.7% of the women experienced gross haematuria, 4.4% perirenal haematomas, and there was one maternal death— a very worrisome statistic indeed. Some time ago we analysed the experience at our own institution and that reported in the literature (Lindheimer et al, 1975; Lindheimer and Katz, 1977) and concluded the following. In series where major complications were reported, many of the biopsies had been performed antepartum, and in some of them tissue was obtained via the anterior (transperitoneal) route during caesarean section. Women had frequently been biopsied while still hypertensive, and much of this experience predated recognition of the coagulation abnormalities that may accompany pre-eclampsia. At Chicago Lying-in Hospital, McCartney (1964) observed gross haematuria in only 3.5% of 400 women who underwent a kidney biopsy during pregnancy or puerperium. Our subsequent experience at the same institution was similar. The experience of most other centres (cited by Lindheimer et al, 1975, and Lindheimer and Katz, 1977) was comparable to that of McCartney; that is, complications after renal biopsy appeared to be no different from those in non-pregnant patients.

Packham and Fairley (1987) have recently reported on 111 biopsies in pregnant women, all preterm, confirming and extending the impression that risks of the procedure resemble those in the non-pregnant population. In fact, their incidence of transient gross haematuria, 0.9% (all patients undergoing biopsy have microscopic haematuria unless one has missed the kidney!) was considerably lower than in non-pregnant patients, where it is 3–5%. Such excellent statistics no doubt reflect the experience and technical skills of the authors, one of whom (KF) has been performing renal biopsy for over twenty years. Statistics are probably also improved by refinement of the prebiopsy evaluation, which includes verifying that the patient has not ingested drugs that interfere with clotting (i.e. aspirin) for at least 7–10 days prior to the procedure, as well as the usual tests to exclude bleeding diatheses.

Given the above data, it is fair to say that pregnancy adds little or no risk to the procedure. However, because complications do occur, it is important to define indications for kidney biopsy in pregnant women. Packham and Fairley (1987) suggest that closed (percutaneous) needle biopsies ought to be performed quite often, because they believe certain glomerular disorders to be adversely influenced by pregnancy, and that this effect might be blunted by specific therapy, such as antiplatelet agents. We disagree with such broad indications, and conclude that renal biopsy should be performed infrequently during gestation (Lindheimer and Davison, 1987). It is worth remembering that even in non-pregnant populations reasons for renal biopsy are not clearly defined, and experts categorize indications as 'most useful', 'possibly useful' and of 'little or no use' (Cutler and Striker, 1985). The following summarizes our current recommendations, revised from those suggested ten years ago (Lindheimer et al, 1975; Lindheimer and Katz, 1977).

We recommended biopsy when there is sudden deterioration of renal function prior to 32 weeks' gestation and no obvious cause is apparent. This is because certain forms of rapidly progressive glomerulonephritis may respond to aggressive treatment with steroid 'pulses', chemotherapy and perhaps plasma exchange, when diagnosed early. We are also aware of a rare instance of sudden renal failure in which non-caseating granulomas were identified and the gravida, then undergoing dialysis, responded to steroids with a return of renal function and successfully completed the pregnancy (Warren et al, in press).

Another situation in which biopsy is recommended is symptomatic nephrotic syndrome occurring before 32 weeks' gestation. While some might consider a therapeutic trial of steroids in such cases, we prefer to determine beforehand whether the lesion is likely to respond to steroids, because pregnancy is itself a hypercoagulable state prone to worsening by such treatment. On the other hand, proteinuria alone in a normotensive woman with well-preserved renal function, who has neither marked hypoalbuminaemia nor intolerable oedema, would lead us to examine the patient at more frequent intervals and defer the biopsy to the postpartum period. This is because the consensus among most investigators (Katz et al, 1980; Surian et al, 1984; Abe et al, 1985; Barcelo et al, 1986; Jungers et al, 1986) is that prognosis is determined primarily by the level of renal function and the presence or absence of hypertension. We take a similar position in the management of pregnancies with asymptomatic microscopic haematuria alone, when neither stone nor tumour is suggested by ultrasonography.

One 'grey area' is a presentation characterized by 'active urinary sediment' (red and white blood cells and casts) with proteinuria and borderline renal function, in a patient who had not been evaluated in the past. One could argue that diagnosis of a collagen disorder such as scleroderma or periarteritis would be grounds for termination of the pregnancy, or that classification of the type of lesion in a woman with systemic lupus erythematosus would determine the type and intensity of therapy. The first two diseases are only infrequently diagnosed by renal biopsy, and a normotensive woman with stable renal function and neither systemic involvement nor laboratory evidence of these collagen disorders is watched closely without intervening. Biopsy may be indicated, however, in the latter condition, i.e. in selected patients with SLE and lupus nephropathy of uncertain histopathology.

In summary, renal biopsy in pregnancy does not entail increased risks. There are indications for its use, such as sudden renal insufficiency or massive nephrotic syndrome of unknown origin occurring prior to the final two months of pregnancy. Such occurrences are fortunately unusual. On the other hand, the antenatal progress of normotensive women with mild or moderate proteinuria and/or asymptomatic microscopic haematuria but well-preserved renal function should be monitored frequently, and a more extensive evaluation of their disease deferred to the postpartum period.

PATIENT MANAGEMENT

When counselling patients with renal disorders about the advisability of conception or whether to continue a gestation already in progress, neither answers nor decisions come simply! Patient expectation is high, and the desire for motherhood so strong as to tempt the sympathetic physician to take unwarranted risks. Furthermore, patients may conceive against advice, or refuse termination for religious or emotional reasons, in which case the doctors must be ready to manage a difficult gestation and be prepared for serious complications.

We recommend that pregnancy should not be undertaken if serum creatinine exceeds 1.5 mg dl^{-1}. Some would allow gestation in women with preconception levels up to 2 mg dl^{-1}, especially in women with a single kidney, transplant recipients with stable function (preferably for two years) and individuals with primary interstitial disease. In all instances diastolic blood pressure prior to conception should be 90 mmHg or less. The adverse influence of hypertension on fetal outcome is best documented in the studies of Surian et al (1984) (Table 3) and Jungers et al (1986), which demonstrate the change in prognosis even when renal function is well preserved. Hypertension present in the first trimester and 'uncontrolled' was associated with 100% fetal loss in the series of Jungers et al (1986).

Guidelines

All pregnant women with renal disease are best managed at a tertiary care centre under the coordinated care of a fetal–maternal specialist and a nephrologist. The initial laboratory tests should include a data base, which helps in the early detection of renal functional loss as well as of superimposed pre-eclampsia. Thus, besides the usual prenatal screening tests, the following renal parameters should be sought.

Table 3. Chronic renal disease and pregnancy: effect of level of blood pressure on pregnancy complications in 123 pregnancies in 86 women.

	Renal deterioration	Small-for-date babies	Preterm delivery
Normotension	3.0%	2.3%	11.4%
Hypertension*	15.0%	15.6%	20.0%

*BP consistently ≥ 140/90 mmHg.
Based on Surian et al (1984) with permission.

1. Serum creatinine and its timed clearance.
2. Serum urea nitrogen, albumin and cholesterol concentrations.
3. Electrolytes, urine analysis and screening bacterial culture; 24-hour protein excretion.
4. Uric acid levels, oxaloacetic and pyruvate transaminases, lactic dehydrogenase, prothrombin time, partial thromboblastin time and platelet count (superimposed pre-eclampsia screening tests) should also be determined.

We suggest biweekly prenatal visits until gestational week 32, after which the patient should be seen weekly. Renal parameters should be tested every 4–6 weeks, unless more frequent evaluations become necessary. Fetal assessment, in particular electronic monitoring, is best started early (e.g. 30–32 weeks), especially in nephrotic patients with hypoalbuminaemia.

Try to avoid diuretics, especially in nephrotic gravidas, as these women are already oligaemic and further intravascular volume depletion may impair uteroplacental perfusion. Furthermore, since blood pressure normally declines during pregnancy, saliuretic therapy could conceivably precipitate circulatory collapse or thromboembolic episodes. This recommendation, however, is relative, because we have observed occasional patients whose kidneys were retaining salt so avidly that diuretics had to be cautiously used.

Table 4. Pregnancy and renal disease: functional renal status and prospects.

	Category		
Prospects	Mild	Moderate	Severe
Pregnancy complications	22%	41%	84%
Successful obstetric outcome	95%	90%	47%
Long-term sequelae	< 5%	25%	53%

Based on literature survey of 1162 pregnancies in 804 women in reports published between 1973 and 1987. These data do not include collagen diseases.

Table 5. Chronic renal disease and pregnancy.

Renal disease	Effects
Chronic glomerulonephritis and focal glomerular sclerosis (FGS)	Increased incidence of high blood pressure late in gestation, but usually no adverse effect if renal function preserved and hypertension absent prior to gestation. Some disagree, believing that coagulation changes in pregnancy exacerbate disease, especially IgA nephropathy, membranoproliferative glomerulonephritis and FGS.
Systemic lupus erythematosus	Controversial: prognosis most favourable if disease in remission 6 or more months prior to conception. Many authorities increase steroid dosage in the immediate puerperium.
Periarteritis nodosa and scleroderma	Fetal prognosis is poor. Associated with maternal deaths. Reactivation of quiescent scleroderma can occur during pregnancy and postpartum. Therapeutic abortion should be considered.
Diabetic nephropathy	No adverse effect on the renal lesion. Increased frequency of infections, oedema and/or pre-eclampsia.
Chronic pyelonephritis (infectious tubulointerstitial disease)	Bacteriuria in pregnancy may lead to exacerbation.
Polycystic disease	Functional impairment and hypertension usually minimal in child-bearing years, and are not affected by pregnancy.
Urolithiasis	Ureteral dilatation and stasis do not seem to affect natural history, but infections can be more frequent. Stents have been successfully placed during gestation.
Permanent urinary diversion	Depending on original reason for surgery, there may be other malformations of the urogenital tract. Urinary tract infection common during pregnancy, and renal function may undergo reversible decrease. No significant obstructive problem but caesarean section might be necessary for abnormal presentation.
After nephrectomy, solitary and pelvic kidneys	Pregnancy well tolerated. Might be associated with other malformations of the urogenital tract. Dystocia rarely occurs with a pelvic kidney.

Some authorities recommend the use of prophylactic anticoagulation (i.e. miniheparin) in nephrotic gravidas, but there are no data to prove the efficacy of such treatment.

Dietary counselling

High-protein diets were advocated in the past for patients with nephrotic proteinuria, especially during gestation when anabolic requirements increase. In 1987, nephrologists are treating most patients with renal disease (with or without nephrotic syndrome) with protein-restricted diets. The theoretical reasons for this are as follows. Increased glomerular filtration accelerates the progression of renal disease because the combination of hyperfiltration and increased intraglomerular capillary pressure in residual (intact) nephrons of patients (or of individuals with a single kidney following uninephrectomy) causes glomerulosclerosis and leads to progressive loss of glomerular filtration rate (GFR). Protein restriction protects the kidney by preventing glomerular hyperfiltration and decreasing intraglomerular capillary pressure and, paradoxically, may increase plasma albumin in severely nephrotic patients, due to decreased urinary protein loss and perhaps to decrements in the albumin catabolic rate (Kaysen et al, 1986).

Should protein be restricted in gravidas with renal dysfunction, a suggestion already published in the literature (Ferris, 1986)? We caution against this view, and recommend that such therapeutic regimens be avoided in pregnancy until more is known regarding fetal outcome and especially brain development, first from studies in animal models and then in carefully conducted clinical trials. (Also, see Chapter 2, which presents preliminary evidence that protein loading does not affect adversely pregnant rats that were uninephrectomized or had experimental glomerular disease.)

Course of gestation

Glomerular filtration rate and blood pressure are the two parameters that decide the course of the gestation. Evidence of renal functional deterioration or the appearance (or rapid worsening) of hypertension is best evaluated in hospital, and failure to reverse these events is grounds for termination of the gestation. Since plasma creatinine determinations may be quite variable in some laboratories, decisions should not be made until the direction and rate of change are very clear from repeat tests. It is important to remember that a decrement in creatinine clearance of 15–20% may occur normally near term, and that increased proteinuria in the absence of hypertension need not cause alarm, therefore such changes do not suggest a need for hospitalization.

Gravidas with pre-existing renal disease or essential hypertension are more susceptible than control populations to superimposed pre-eclampsia, which frequently occurs in midpregnancy or early in the third trimester. Superimposed pre-eclampsia, however, may be difficult to differentiate from aggravation of the underlying disease, especially in women with glomerular disease who are prone to hypertension and proteinuria. In this context it is of interest that in our study (Katz et al, 1980) there were 13 women diagnosed on clinical grounds to have superimposed pre-eclampsia, but postpartum biopsy revealed glomerular capillary endotheliosis in only 7. In any event, when these situations occur the patient should be hospitalized and treated as if she has superimposed pre-eclampsia, a prudent policy considering the potentially explosive and dangerous nature of this disorder (Lindheimer and Katz, 1986).

SUMMARY

Physicians may be called upon to guide patients with renal disease on the advisability of conceiving or maintaining a gestation, or to manage pregnancies permitted to continue. The prevailing view is that the degree of functional impairment and the presence or absence of hypertension prior to conception determine both pregnancy outcome and the effect of gestation on the natural history of the kidney disorder (Table 4). Normotensive women with minimal dysfunction have a 90% chance of success and there is little evidence that gestation will adversely affect the disease. Presence of hypertension increases the complications rate substantially, and prognosis is also poorer in women with moderate renal dysfunction. Most gestations in the latter group succeed, but at considerable maternal risk: over 20% of these women experience renal functional deterioration, and 30–40% of them have major problems with hypertension. Thus we tend not to recommend pregnancy in patients with moderate renal insufficiency, and definitely discourage gestation when GFR is severely impaired.

There are a number of diseases in which pregnancy should not be undertaken, including scleroderma and periarteritis. Some authors believe that women with membranoproliferative glomerulonephritis also do poorly, and opinions differ on the effects of gestation on IgA nephropathy, focal glomerulosclerosis, and reflux nephropathy. Table 5 summarizes our view concerning pregnancy in a number of specific renal disorders.

Finally, in addition to the controversies noted above, there are other unresolved problems requiring further study. For instance, protein restriction should be avoided until the effect of this therapeutic manoeuvre on fetal development is evaluated. Also needed are conclusive studies on whether or not the physiological hyperfiltration of human pregnancy affects adversely pre-existing renal disease.

Acknowledgements

We thank Mrs Penny Papadatos for her secretarial assistance. Some of the work cited was supported by grants from the National Institutes of Health (HD5572, AM13601 and RR55), the American Heart Association, and the Mother's Aid Foundation of Chicago Lying-In Hospital

REFERENCES

Abe S, Amagasaki Y, Konishi K, Kato E, Sakagachi H & Iyori S (1985) The influence of antecedent renal disease on pregnancy. *American Journal of Obstetrics and Gynecology* **153** 508–514.

Barcelo P, Lopez-Lillo J, Cabero L & Del Rio G (1986) Successful pregnancy in primary glomerular disease. *Kidney International* **30**: 914–919.

Bear RA (1976) Pregnancy in patients with renal disease: a study of 44 cases. *Obstetrics and Gynecology* **48**: 13–18.

Becker GJ, Fairley KF & Whitworth JA (1985) Pregnancy exacerbates glomerular disease. *American Journal of Kidney Diseases* **6**: 266–272.

Bobrie G, Liote F, Houillier P, Grünfeld JP & Jungers P (1987) Pregnancy in lupus nephritis and related disorders. *American Journal of Kidney Diseases* **9**: 339–343.

Cutler RE & Striker GE (1983) Renal biopsy. In Massry SG & Glassock RJ (eds) *Textbook of Nephrology*, pp 10.14–10.17. Baltimore: Williams & Wilkins.

Dieckmann WM, Potter EL & McCartney CP (1957) Renal biopsies from patients with toxemia of pregnancy. *American Journal of Obstetrics and Gynecology* **73**: 1–16.

Ferris T (1986) Pregnancy and chronic renal diseases. *The Kidney* **19**: 1–4.

Fine LG, Barnett EV, Danovitch GM et al (1981) Systemic lupus erythematosus in pregnancy. *Annals of Internal Medicine* **94**: 667–677.

Hayslett JP & Lynn RI (1980) Effect of pregnancy in patients with lupus nephropathy. *Kidney International* **18**: 207–220.

Hayslett JP & Reece EA (1985) Systemic lupus erythematosus in pregnancy. *Clinics in Perinatology* **12**: 539–550.

Hou SH, Grossman SD & Madias NE (1985) Pregnancy in women with renal disease and moderate renal insufficiency. *American Journal of Medicine* **78**: 185–194.

Imbasciati E, Surian M, Bottino S et al (1984) Lupus nephropathy and pregnancy. A study of 26 pregnancies in patients with systemic lupus erythematosus and nephritis. *Nephron* **36**: 46–51.

Imbasciati E, Pardi G, Capetta P et al (1986) Pregnancy in women with chronic renal failure. *American Journal of Nephrology* **6**: 193–198.

Jungers P, Forget D, Henry-Amar M et al (1986) Chronic kidney disease and pregnancy. *Advances in Nephrology* **15**: 103–141.

Jungers P, Forget D, Houillier P, Henry-Amar M & Grünfeld JP (1987) Pregnancy in IgA nephropathy, reflux nephropathy, and focal glomerular sclerosis. *American Journal of Kidney Diseases* **9**: 334–338.

Katz AI, Davison JM, Hayslett JP, Singson E & Lindheimer MD (1980) Pregnancy in women with kidney disease. *Kidney International* **18**: 192–206.

Kaysen GA, Gambertoglio J, Jimenez I, Jones H & Hutchison FN (1986) Effect of dietary protein intake on albumin homeostasis in nephrotic patients. *Kidney International* **29**: 572–577.

Kincaid-Smith P & Fairley KF (1987) Renal disease in pregnancy. Three controversial areas: Mesangial IgA nephropathy, focal glomerulosclerosis (focal and segmental hyalinosis and sclerosis), and reflux nephropathy. *American Journal of Kidney Diseases* **9**: 328–333.

Kincaid-Smith P, Fairley KF & Bullen M (1967) Kidney disease and pregnancy. *Medical Journal of Australia* **2**: 1155–1159.

Lindheimer MD & Davison JM (1987) Renal biopsy in pregnancy. To b— or not to b—. *British Journal of Obstetrics and Gynaecology* **94**: 932–934.

Lindheimer MD & Katz AI (1977) *Kidney Function and Disease in Pregnancy*, pp 149–150. Philadelphia: Lea & Febiger.

Lindheimer MD & Katz AI (1986) The kidney in pregnancy. In Brenner BM & Rector FC (eds) *The Kidney*, 3rd edn, pp 1235–1295. Philadelphia: WB Saunders.

Lindheimer MD, Spargo BH & Katz AI (1975) Renal biopsy in pregnancy-induced hypertension. *Journal of Reproductive Medicine* **15**: 189–94.

Makker SP & Heymann W (1972) Pregnancy in patients who have had the idiopathic nephrotic syndrome in childhood. *Journal of Pediatrics* **81**: 1140–1144.

McCartney CP (1964) Pathological anatomy of acute hypertension of pregnancy. *Circulation* **30** (Suppl 2): 37–42.

Packham D & Fairley KF (1987) Renal biopsy: indications and complications in pregnancy. *British Journal of Obstetrics and Gynaecology* (in press).

Schewitz LJ, Friedman EA & Pollak VE (1965) Bleeding after renal biopsy in pregnancy. *Obstetrics and Gynecology* **26**: 295–304.

Surian M, Imbasciati E, Cosci P et al (1984) Glomerular disease and pregnancy. A study of 123 pregnancies in patients with primary and secondary glomerular diseases. *Nephron* **36**: 101–105.

Warren GV, Sprague SM & Corwin HC (1987) Sarcoidosis presenting as acute renal failure in pregnancy. *American Journal of Kidney Diseases* (in press).

10

Managing diabetic patients with nephropathy and other vascular complications

JOHN P. HAYSLETT
E. ALBERT REECE

Although the term 'diabetes' is used to characterize the condition of glucose intolerance, it is recognized that there are numerous causes of this metabolic derangement, involving both hereditary and environmental factors. In clinical practice diabetes is a heterogeneous condition, varying from minor degrees of carbohydrate intolerance to severe forms with major vascular complications. Diabetes is relatively common among pregnant women; it is estimated that 1 in 200 pregnancies is complicated by overt diabetes, while an additional 5 in 200 pregnancies are associated with gestational diabetes. The association of pregnancy and diabetes raises special concerns regarding the pregnancy performance and outcome because of a high incidence of diabetes-related maternal complications, a higher than normal incidence of perinatal deaths, and alterations in fetal growth and development.

The occurrence of diabetic nephropathy presents additional problems for the gravida and her fetus, including complications related to proteinuria, and often renal insufficiency. This subset of women also has a high incidence of hypertension, a factor that may reduce the overall pregnancy performance and outcome. Recent experience has shown, however, that advances in perinatal and neonatal care have eliminated maternal mortality and reduced the perinatal death rate to levels that approach those observed in diabetics without renal disease. This chapter analyses the maternal and fetal risks in gravidas with diabetic nephropathy, outlines the major metabolic complications in the diabetic pregnancy and discusses the course of diabetic pregnancies in general. Lastly, we outline our approach towards the perinatal management of diabetic women.

Numerous attempts have been made to classify diabetes in pregnant women to anticipate maternal and fetal complications, and to evaluate different management regimens. The most widely used is the Priscilla White classification (White, 1949), shown in Table 1, which is based on the assumption that there is a proportionality between age at onset, duration of disease and vascular complications, and the likelihood of complications during pregnancy. This classification does not specifically include gestational diabetes, defined as the onset or recognition of carbohydrate intolerance during

Table 1. White classification of diabetes mellitus during pregnancy.

Class	Onset	Duration	Therapy
A	Any age	During pregnancy	None needed
B	Age > 20 *and*	< 10 years	Insulin
C	Age 10–20 *or*	10–20 years	Insulin
D	Age < 10 *or* benign background retinopathy *or*	> 20 years	Insulin
F	Any nephropathy	Any length	Insulin
R	Any proliferative retinopathy	Any length	Insulin

From White (1949).

pregnancy and disappearance of carbohydrate intolerance post partum. Theoretically, gestational diabetes can be class A, B or C, depending on the severity of carbohydrate intolerance, the requirement for insulin therapy and the age of the patient.

A more recent attempt to classify diabetic patients during pregnancy is shown in Table 2, proposed by the National Diabetes Data Control Group of the National Institutes of Health (1979). This classification recognizes the major metabolic alterations among patients with diabetes, and is useful in understanding the specific nutritional and hormone replacement requirements of patients with the diabetic syndrome

METABOLIC ALTERATIONS DURING PREGNANCY

A description of clinically important metabolic alterations in the pregnant diabetic necessitates an understanding of alterations in maternal metabolism during normal pregnancy. During gestation, the maternal endocrine–metabolic environment changes rapidly to accommodate the rapidly growing fetus, as recently reviewed by Hollingsworth (1983). The placenta develops *de novo* as an endocrine gland to modulate the delivery of maternal fuels to the fetus. As shown in Tables 3 and 4, maternal carbohydrate metabolism during the first trimester is modified by a rise in serum levels of oestrogen and progesterone. Pancreatic beta-cell hyperplasia occurs and results in an increase in the release of insulin. Hyperinsulinaemia leads to an increase in peripheral glucose utilization, a decline in fasting plasma glucose levels, increased tissue storage of glycogen and decreased hepatic glucose production. These changes presumably occur to ensure ample nutrients for rapid cellular multiplication in the fetus. During late pregnancy, maternal fuel adjustments include a sparing of glucose with decreased maternal levels of glucose and amino acids, a shift to an increased production of fatty acids and ketones, and pancreatic islet cell hyperplasia with an increased insulin response to glucose.

Figure 1 demonstrates the central role of the placenta in the transfer of maternal fuels to the fetus (adapted from Hollingsworth, 1983). Glucose crosses the placenta by carrier-mediated facilitated diffusion, while amino

Table 2. Classification of diabetes mellitus during pregnancy.

New nomenclature	Old names	Clinical characteristics
Type I Insulin-dependent diabetes mellitus (IDDM)	Juvenile diabetes (JD) Juvenile-onset diabetes (JOD) Ketosis-prone diabetes Brittle diabetes	Ketosis prone. Insulin-deficient due to islet cell loss. Often associated with specific HLA types, with pre-disposition to viral insulitis auto-immune (islet cell antibody) phenomena. Occurs at any age, common in youth.
Type II Non-insulin-dependent diabetes mellitus (NIDDM) Non-obese Obese	Adult-onset diabetes (AOD) Maturity-onset diabetes (MOD) Ketosis-resistant diabetes Stable diabetes Maturity-onset diabetes of youth (MODY)	Ketosis resistant. More frequent in adults but occurs at any age. May be seen in family aggregates as an auto-somal dominant genetic trait. May require insulin for hyperglycaemia during stress. Invariably requires insulin during pregnancy.
Gestational diabetes (GDM)	Gestational diabetes	This classification is retained for women whose diabetes begins (or is recognized) during pregnancy. They have an above-normal risk of peri-natal complications. Glucose intolerance may be transitory, but it frequently recurs. Diagnosis requires at least two abnormal values on a 3-hour oral glucose tolerance test (100 g glucose). Plasma glucose　　mg dl^{-1} 　Fasting　　　　105 　1 h　　　　　190 　2 h　　　　　160 　3 h　　　　　145

From National Diabetes Data Control Group (1979).

Table 3. Carbohydrate metabolism in early pregnancy (to 20 weeks' gestation).

Hormonal change	Effect	Metabolic change
↑ Oestrogen and ↑ progesterone ↓ β-Cell hyperplasia and ↑ insulin secretion	↑ Tissue glycogen storage ↓ Hepatic glucose production ↑ Peripheral glucose utilization ↓ Fasting plasma glucose	Anabolic ↑ Due to sex steroids + Hyperinsulinaemia

From Hollingsworth (1983).

Table 4. Carbohydrate metabolism in late pregnancy (20–40 weeks' gestation).

Hormonal change	Effect	Metabolic change
↑ Human placental lactogen	'Diabetogenic'	Facilitated anabolism during feeding
↑ Prolactin	↓ Glucose tolerance	Accelerated starvation during fasting
↑ Bound and free cortisol	Insulin resistance ↓ Hepatic glycogen stores ↑ Hepatic glucose production	↓ Ensure glucose and amino acids to fetus

From Hollingsworth (1983).

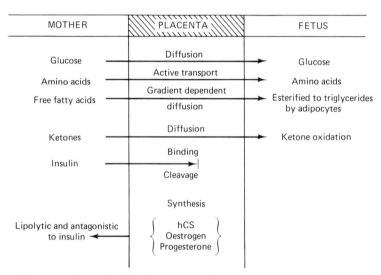

Figure 1. Maternal, placental and fetal integration of fuels for the promotion of fetal growth From Hollingsworth (1983) with permission. hCS = human chorionic somatomannotrophin.

acids are actively transported to the fetus. Free fatty acids cross the placenta in small amounts by gradient-dependent diffusion and are esterified to triglycerides by fetal adipocytes. Insulin, however, is not transported to the fetus, since it binds to microvillus membranes of the placenta in which it is degraded. The role of insulin in placental regulation of metabolic fuels has not been established.

The metabolic alterations in normal pregnancy are therefore diabetogenic and represent a severe stress test of carbohydrate tolerance. Patients with type I diabetes are prone to develop unexplained episodes of hypoglycaemia and ketonuria in the first trimester. During the latter portion of pregnancy, in

Table 5. Maternal complications in diabetic pregnancies.

Hypoglycaemia—first trimester
Ketoacidosis—last trimester
Pre-eclampsia
Pyelonephritis
Polyhydramnios
Hypertension
? worsening of glomerulosclerosis
? onset or worsening of proliferative retinopathy

---

contrast, the likelihood of ketoacidosis is increased. The amount of exogenous insulin increment imposed by pregnancy is comparable, however, to the increase in endogenous insulin in non-diabetic pregnancies (38%). In contrast, type II diabetics are asymptomatic during the first trimester. Although non-insulin dependent diabetics, when not pregnant, do not require exogenous insulin, during gestation their requirements are often higher (100%) than non-pregnant requirements. This group, however, is not prone to ketosis unless stressed by events such as urinary tract infection. It should be noted that although patients are usually older and overweight, type II diabetes may occur in young individuals who are normal weight. Finally, patients with gestational diabetes usually first exhibit hyperglycaemia and glucosuria during the second half of pregnancy. These individuals may be obese or of normal weight. Freinkel and Metzger (1979) have demonstrated that even though diabetes may be mild, patients with gestational diabetes exhibit abnormal alterations in each type of metabolic fuel.

MATERNAL AND FETAL COMPLICATIONS DURING DIABETIC PREGNANCIES

Maternal and fetal complications have been recognized in women with overt diabetes for many years. Maternal complications, listed in Table 5, include hypoglycaemia and ketoacidosis in the first and third trimesters, respectively, and a higher incidence than in non-diabetic pregnancies of pre-eclampsia, pyelonephritis, polyhydramnios and worsening of hypertension. In addition, there has been concern that pregnancy may accelerate diabetic vascular disease, especially retinopathy and glomerulosclerosis. Fetal and neonatal complications, shown in Table 6, include a high incidence of fetal wastage, early delivery, small and large for gestational age infants and congenital malformations. In addition, neonatal complications such as respiratory distress syndrome, hypoglycaemia and jaundice are common.

   A historical overview of maternal and fetal survival was provided by Hare and White (1977) from the Joslin Clinic experience, as shown in Table 7. In the pre-insulin period viable fetal salvage was 40% and maternal survival was 56%. Between 1938 and 1958, in the insulin era, fetal survival rose to 86%, and to 90% by 1974, concurrently with a maternal survival of 100% among all

Table 6. Fetal and neonatal complications in diabetic pregnancies.

Fetal
Increased perinatal death
Early delivery
Macrosomia
Intrauterine growth retardation
Major congenital anomalies

Neonatal
Respiratory distress syndrome
Hypoglycaemia
Hypocalcaemia
Hyperbilirubinaemia

Table 7. Pregnancy and diabetes—Joslin Clinic (viable cases) 1898 to 1975.

Dates	Cases (no.)	Fetal survival (%)	Maternal survival (%)
1898–1917	10	40	66
1924–1938	128	54	
1938–1958	900	86	99
1958–1974	1119	90	
1975	75	94	
Total	2232		

From Hare and White (1977).

diabetes. In a detailed analysis of patients with diabetes complicated by vascular disease, however, they showed that in 1975 the outlook for viable delivery remained reduced within some subgroups of patients (Hare and White, 1977). For example, the incidence of viable survival was 84% in class R, 72% in class F and 81% in class FR, representing women with retinopathy (R), nephropathy (F) or a combination of both vascular abnormalities (FR). Similar results were reported by Pedersen et al (1974). When intrauterine death occurred in these classes, it tended to occur before week 36 of gestation, and the placenta was usually small with vascular insufficiency being potentially causally related.

Regarding maternal and neonatal morbidity in diabetic pregnancies, Kitzmiller and associates (1978) have provided a detailed analysis of 147 patients registered at the pregnancy clinic at the Joslin Diabetes Foundation during 1975 to 1976. As shown in Table 8, the incidence of ketoacidosis, pyelonephritis and pre-eclampsia were low in this meticulously managed group of patients. The incidence of polyhydramnios, however, was high (31%), as in other reports (Pedersen and Pedersen, 1965). There was also a

Table 8. Maternal complications in 147 diabetic women.

Complications	Per cent
Pregnancy headache	2
Ketoacidosis	3
Pyelonephritis	1
General oedema	9
Polyhydramnios	31
Premature labour	6
Pre-eclampsia	5
Transient hypertension	4
Chronic hypertension	5
Thyroid disease	6

From Kitzmiller et al (1978).

Table 9. Frequency of perinatal complications in insulin-dependent diabetic women compared to women with diabetic nephropathy, 1975 to 1978.

	White's classes B,C,D,R		White's class F	
	No.	%	No.	%
n (pregnancies)	232		26	
Polyhydramnios	62	26.7	7	26.9
Delivery < 34 weeks	10	4.3	8	30.8
Fetal death	1	0.4	2	7.7
Intra-uterine growth retardation*	5	2.2	5	20.8
Macrosomia*	94	40.7	3	12.5
Major congenital anomalies	20	8.6	3	11.1
Neonatal				
Respiratory distress syndrome	19	8.2	6	24.0
Hypoglycaemia	113	48.7	11	44.0
Hypocalcaemia	54	23.3	4	16.0
Jaundice, phototherapy	48	20.7	11	44.0
Death	6	2.6	1	4.0
Perinatal survival†		97.0		88.9

* One set of twins excluded from each column.
† Percentage of live-born infants.
From Kitzmiller et al (1981).

high rate of caesarean section, which was performed in 75 women (51%) as a primary or repeat procedure prior to labour. Of 72 women who began spontaneous or induced labour, 46 (64%) were delivered vaginally, 17 (24%) were delivered by caesarean section because of dystocia, and 9 (12.5%) were delivered by section for intrapartum fetal distress.

The frequency and types of fetal complications listed by the same authors are shown in Table 9 for White's classes B, C, D and R. These data show that approximately 40% of neonates were macrosomic. It was proposed that excessive weight gain reflected increased fat deposition caused by fetal hyperinsulinism in response to maternal hyperglycaemia. The causal role of fetal hyperinsulinaemia in the pathogenesis of macrosomia has been confirmed in the Rhesus monkey (Susa, 1979). There was also an 8.6% incidence of major congenital anomalies. Other groups have reported a rate of anomalies that ranges between 8% and 12%, and that are found in all White classes, except class A (Gabbe, 1977). These lesions include anencephaly, meningocoele, transposition of great vessels, ventricular septal defects, caudal regression syndrome and vertebral dysplasia, renal agenesis and anal atresia. It seemed probable to earlier workers that these malformations were caused by the intrauterine environment of the fetus rather than genetic factors, since there is no increase in infants born to diabetic fathers and non-diabetic mothers as compared to normal fathers (Naeve, 1967). Two recent studies have demonstrated that control of maternal blood glucose levels, started before conception and continued through the first weeks of pregnancy, can prevent malformations in diabetic mothers (Fuhrmann et al, 1983; Jovanovic and Jovanovic, 1984). It has also been shown in a preliminary study that intensive glycaemic control results in the normalization of other metabolic fuels, including free fatty acids, branched-chain amino acids, triglycerides, cholesterol and ketones (Reece et al, unpublished data). These data underscore the role of metabolic fuels in normal embryonic development.

Table 9 also indicates an increased incidence of respiratory distress syndrome (RDS) of approximately 8%. This common neonatal complication of diabetic pregnancies was highlighted in an earlier report by Hubbell et al (1965), who reported an overall incidence of 27% in a study of 473 live-born infants of insulin-dependent diabetics at the Boston Hospital for Women from 1959 to 1964. Studies have shown that RDS is the neonatal manifestation of insufficient fetal pulmonary synthesis, storage and release of surface-active phospholipids, and suggest that this abnormality is somehow related to hyperinsulinaemia in the fetus (Epstein et al, 1976).

Other prominent neonatal abnormalities include hyperbilirubinaemia (21%), due presumably to functional prematurity of hepatic enzymes necessary for the conjugation of bilirubin, similar to the incidence of 27% reported by Essex et al (1973). Hypocalcaemia was present at birth in 23% of infants in this series and in 10% of live births in the Pedersen series (Pedersen 1977). The cause of hypocalcaemia has not been established. Finally hypoglycaemia was observed in nearly half the infants (despite a programme of early feeding), due apparently to excessive fetal insulin secretion and termination of placental transfer of glucose after division of the umbilical cord. Although most infants were not symptomatic, symptoms if they did occur included lethargy and could progress to apnoea, tachypnoea, respiratory distress and seizures. Overall, the majority of infants in this series, as in other reports, had significant morbidity. It should be emphasized that studies on long-term physical and psychological development are urgently needed in this group of children.

DIABETIC PREGNANCY COMPLICATED BY NEPHROPATHY

Recent reports have described the outcome of patients with diabetic nephropathy and provide some insight into the question of whether pregnancy accelerates pre-existing vascular disease. Kitzmiller and associates (1981a) reported on the course during and following gestation of 26 women registered in the years 1975 to 1978. Proteinuria was present in all cases; in 75% it was documented prior to conception, while in the remaining patients it was first recognized early in pregnancy. Renal function, assessed by creatinine clearance, was reduced below 70 ml per minute in 8 cases. Management included efforts to normalize blood sugar and to assess fetal well-being during the third trimester. During the course of gestation proteinuria increased in magnitude in most patients, and exceeded 6 g per 24 hours in 58% of cases in the third trimester. Analysis of creatinine clearance levels during gestation and postpartum indicated that renal function remained unchanged. Hypertension worsened in 37% of women with pre-existing hypertension, first occurred during pregnancy in 57% and was most commonly seen in patients with renal insufficiency. Severe hypertension resolved after pregnancy in most subjects. The authors concluded that the long-term decline in renal function postpartum in some patients, during follow-up which ranged from 6 to 35 months, did not differ from the course expected in a population of diabetic patients who had not experienced pregnancy.

Perinatal survival, as shown in Table 9, was 89%. Eighteen infants were examined at a mean age of 20 ± 7.6 months, and all had normal cognitive development, except for one case with major neurologic congenital defects. Compared to classes B, C, D and R, there was a higher incidence of early delivery (31% and 4% respectively) and higher fetal death rate. Macrosomia was less common among infants born to mothers with renal insufficiency because growth retardation was a common complication (21%). In addition, RDS occurred more often than in the general diabetic population, reflecting, in part, early delivery and small-for-gestational age infants.

Reece and associates have demonstrated similar findings on 31 continuing pregnancies with diabetic nephropathy managed at Yale–New Haven Hospital between 1975 and 1984. At initial visit, 8 cases (25.8%) were complicated by nephrotic syndrome (> 3.0 g protein per 24 hours), while 10 cases were associated with mild proteinuria (> 0.5 g per 24 hours). Reduced renal function (serum creatinine (S_c) > 1.2 mg dl^{-1} and/or creatinine (C_{cr}) clearance < 100 ml min^{-1}), associated with proteinuria, was present in 15 (48.3%) pregnancies. Diabetic retinopathy complicated all pregnancies, of which 67.7% had proliferative retinopathy. In 45% of patients, the serum creatinine rose during pregnancy between 15% and 35%, but remained stable or declined in the remaining cases. Most patients had significant increases in proteinuria, and nephrotic syndrome occurred during gestation in 71% of pregnancies. The blood pressure increased in 19 pregnancies by a mean of 15%. As in the Joslin Clinic's experience, worsening changes in renal function, proteinuria and/or hypertension returned shortly after delivery to values similar to that observed in the first trimester. The long-term maternal course was viewed as not differing from the expected course of diabetic nephropathy

Table 10. Perinatal outcome of patients with non-systemic renal disease and patients with diabetes-associated renal disease.

	Pregnant non-diabetics with renal disease (Katz et al, 1981)	Pregnant diabetics with renal disease; White class F or FR (Kitzmiller et al 1981)
No. of patients	121	26
Fetal death	7 (5.7%)	2 (7.7%)
Preterm deliveries	24 (20.0%) (< 36 weeks)	8 (30.8%) (< 34 weeks)
Small for gestational age	27 (24.3%)	5 (20.8%)
Large for gestational age	6 (5.4%)	3 (12.5%)
Adequate for gestational age	78 (70.2%)	18 (69.2%)
Major congenital anomalies	—	3 (11.1%)
Neonatal:		
Respiratory distress syndrome	—	6 (23.0%)
Hypoglycaemia	—	11 (44.0%)
Jaundice, phototherapy	—	11 (44.0%)
Death	6 (4.9%)	1 (4.0%)
Perinatal survival	90%	88.9%

in individuals who had not become pregnant. The fetal survival rate was 94% in this series. Similar findings in patients with diabetic nephropathy have been reported by Jovanovic and Jovanovic (1984) in 8 patients, and by Grenfell et al (1986) in 20 patients.

Table 10 compares the perinatal outcome of patients with non-diabetic renal disease, reported by Katz et al (1980), with the Kitzmiller study (1981a) of pregnant women with diabetic nephropathy. Since these data indicate similar rates of fetal death, preterm deliveries and small-for-gestational-age babies, it seems likely that these fetal complications in the diabetic population may be primarily caused by renal injury and/or associated hypertension. It is of interest that in the series of non-diabetic patients the occurrence of increased proteinuria during the course of pregnancy to nephrotic syndrome levels was observed in the majority of patients. Protein excretion rates returned to levels which approached that of early pregnancy shortly after delivery. Since pregnancy affects protein excretion in patients with pre-existing renal disease, it is not possible to make a diagnosis of pre-eclampsia on the basis of the usual criteria of protein excretion and hypertension. It is proposed that assessment of other systemic manifestations, including liver enzyme abnormalities and coagulation alterations, are useful for establishing the presumed diagnosis of pre-eclampsia.

It should be noted that studies on diabetic nephropathy and non-diabetic primary renal disease in pregnancy have, in general, involved patients with serum creatinine levels below 2 mg dl^{-1}. There is less information on patients with more severe renal insufficiency, although the available data suggest that the course of pregnancy is usually confounded by more severe complications and a higher fetal death rate than in subjects with normal or near-normal renal function (Hayslett, 1985). An account of pregnancy in women with end-stage renal disease, on dialysis treatment and following successful renal transplantation is given in Chapter 15.

In summary, recent experience in patients with diabetic nephropathy, managed with modern perinatal techniques, suggests that pregnancy does not accelerate the course of diabetic glomerulosclerosis. Additional complications during pregnancy may occur in this group, however, as in non-diabetic patients with renal disease, due to the development of nephrotic syndrome with associated peripheral oedema and worsening of hypertension. Since hypertension during pregnancy (in the absence of renal disease) is associated with reduced fetal growth and a higher perinatal death rate (Lin et al, 1982), this factor may play an important role in the higher incidence of perinatal complications in patients with diabetic nephropathy.

GESTATIONAL INFLUENCE ON DIABETIC RETINOPATHY

The influence of pregnancy on diabetic retinopathy has been controversial. Rodman et al (1979) analysed 201 reported cases with background retinopathy. While approximately 10% demonstrated progressive changes during the course of gestation, this incidence was judged not to be higher than expected in a non-pregnant population of diabetic patients. A retrospective evaluation of 64 pregnant diabetics, with and without laser treatment, was performed and showed that in 43 untreated patients with background retinopathy, vascular changes progressed modestly, then regressed in three months postpartum (Kitzmiller et al, 1981b). Among patients with proliferative changes that had been successfully treated prior to pregnancy, or in whom spontaneous regression had occurred prior to pregnancy, retinopathy remained stable. In contrast, the onset of neovascularization in the first trimester rapidly progressed in the second and third trimesters. On the basis of these data it seems that pregnancy may accelerate diabetic retinopathy in some patients. However, with the availability of photocoagulation therapy which can be used throughout pregnancy, *de novo* or worsening proliferative retinopathy can be treated, thus preventing potential adverse effects. Current recommendations include periodic retinal examination at trimester intervals and appropriate laser therapy for proliferative retinal disease. Although there is concern with the possibility of retinal haemorrhage during the Valsalva manoeuvre in the second stage of labour, there is no available data to suggest that maternal retinal complications are significantly altered when patients are delivered by caesarean section. At the Yale–New Haven Hospital caesarean section is not routinely offered to patients with severe diabetic vasculopathy.

MANAGEMENT OF DIABETIC PREGNANCIES

Perinatal mortality (unrelated to congenital anomalies) has gradually improved over the past two to three decades and now approaches levels seen in healthy gravidas. Morbidity, however, remains high, and the incidence of congenital anomalies remains unchanged between 5% and 10% (Kitzmiller et al, 1978; Gabbe, 1977), except in cases where maternal blood glucose control is initiated prior to conception and maintained during the early phase of gestation, as noted above. The cause for improvement is not entirely known, but is accounted for in part by improved methods of fetal monitoring during gestation and modern methods of neonatal care. It seems likely, however, that better control of maternal blood sugar levels has also contributed to the overall improvement. Karlsson and Kjellmer (1972) analysed 180 births by 179 diabetics and reported that reduced perinatal mortality and neonatal morbidity correlated with lower maternal blood glucose levels, measured during hospitalization between 30 and 32 weeks' gestation and delivery. In this analysis, there was a lower incidence of perinatal deaths, jaundice, RDS and malformations among infants born to mothers with mean blood glucose levels less than 100 mg dl^{-1}, than in groups with higher levels. On the basis of these data, most investigators assume that fetal complications are directly or indirectly related to maternal hyperglycaemia, and as a consequence, attempt to normalize blood glucose throughout gestation.

Normal, non-diabetic women in the third trimester of pregnancy have fasting whole blood sugar levels that average 65 mg dl^{-1} (plasma equivalent 75 mg dl^{-1}) and postprandial mean values of 80–90 mg dl^{-1}. Rarely does the whole blood sugar level rise above 100 mg dl^{-1}. To eliminate or reduce the risk factor imposed by maternal hyperglycaemia, efforts were made at the Diabetes in Pregnancy Study Unit at the Yale University School of Medicine to maintain blood sugar levels in diabetics at the same levels as in healthy gravidas (Coustan et al, 1980). In a study of 73 patients in classes B,C,D and F, over the period from 28 weeks' gestation until delivery, mean blood sugar levels below 120 mg dl^{-1} were achieved in 77%, and the mean level for all patients in this series was 108 mg dl^{-1}. This report demonstrates the feasibility of near-normalization of blood sugar in the pregnant diabetic population. Furthermore, in this series (although uncontrolled) the perinatal mortality rate was 4.0%, corrected to 1.4% when deaths from congenital anomalies and birth trauma were excluded. Since the aim of treatment was to reduce the likelihood of fetoplacental dysfunction, it was of interest that in this series deteriorating fetoplacental function was detected in only 2.8%, compared to an incidence of nearly 20% in other recent series where similar control of maternal hyperglycaemia was not achieved.

Our guidelines for managing pregnancy in diabetic women, shown in Table 11 are based on the premise that the majority of fetopathy is caused by maternal metabolic derangement. Therapy aims to maintain fasting plasma glucose levels below 90 mg dl^{-1} and all other plasma glucose levels below 120 mg dl^{-1} throughout gestation, including the first weeks of pregnancy. The value of planned pregnancies is stressed to increase the likelihood of control of maternal blood glucose levels during the early phase of gestation. Fetal monitoring is instituted to establish age, to detect significant congenital anomalies before week 20 of gestation and to determine fetal pulmonary maturity and fetoplacental dysfunction, if any in the last trimester in order to plan delivery. We assume that all pregnancies will go term and delivery will be effected by vaginal route, unless fetal distress, macrosomia or a rapidly

Table 11. Data base for managing diabetic patients during pregnancy.

Mother
Monitor blood glucose levels from finger-stick samples—4 to 5 times daily
Administer insulin via multiple doses or insulin pump
Diet includes 30 to 35 kcal per kg ideal body weight
Laboratory studies on first visit and repeated monthly:
    Serum creatinine, and creatinine clearance if macroproteinuria is present
    Serum urea nitrogen
    Uric acid
    24-hour urine protein excretion, if qualitative test is positive
Maternal serum alpha fetoprotein analysis at 15 weeks as a screen for neural tube defects.
Retinal examination each trimester

Fetal
Level II ultrasound and fetal echocardiogram at 18 to 20 weeks to detect congenital anomalies
Repeat ultrasound examination every 4-6 weeks for fetal growth evaluation
Weekly non-stress test and daily fetal movement counting starting at 33 weeks
Amniocentesis for phosphatidylglycerol before caesarean or induced labour
Delivery at term
Postpartum observation in special neonatal unit

deteriorating maternal condition necessitate early delivery and/or caesarean section. The details of our programme have been reported previously (Coustan, 1980), but are summarized here.

Management of the mother

Blood glucose levels are monitored at home by assays of finger-stick samples, either on indicator strips or on glucose meters. Determination of ketonuria is made by analysis of double-voided urine samples.

Insulin is administered subcutaneously at least twice daily or by insulin pump in doses determined by blood glucose levels. It should be noted that a class A diabetic is regarded as someone with an abnormal glucose tolerance test who does not require insulin to normalize carbohydrate metabolism. If, on a subsequent test, the fasting plasma glucose level is not below 90 mg dl^{-1} and other values are not below 120 mg dl^{-1}, the patient is classified as class B and insulin therapy is instituted.

Diet includes a caloric content of 30 to 35 kcal per kg ideal body weight. The caloric intake is distributed as 24% for breakfast, 30% for lunch, 33% for dinner and 13% before bedtime.

Renal function is assessed at first visit and thereafter at monthly intervals, with creatinine clearance, serum urea nitrogen levels and uric acid levels. A 24-hour urine protein excretion rate is determined if qualitative proteinuria is detected. We have no experience with the measurement of microalbuminuria in these patients. However, since the absence of qualitative proteinuria alone is a positive sign, we doubt if screening for microalbuminuria would be a cost-effective move. A urine culture is performed in each trimester.

An ophthalmologic examination is performed in each trimester to evaluate the retinal status and laser therapy is administered as indicated by examination results.

Blood pressure is recorded on all antepartum visits. Antihypertensive agents are continued if routinely taken prior to conception, or are introduced if hypertension is initially recognized during pregnancy with diastolic levels greater than 100 mmHg. In the latter group the preferred agents include alpha-methyldopa and/or hydrallazine.

In patients with heavy proteinuria in early pregnancy (2.0 g or more per day), a modest sodium-restriction diet (2.0 g sodium) is introduced, whether or not oedema formation is present, to mitigate the rate of anticipated oedema formation as proteinuria increases during the course of pregnancy.

Fetal evaluation

Ultrasound examination is performed between 18 and 20 weeks' gestation to detect major anomalies, giving parents the option for termination. Subsequent ultrasound examination is conducted approximately every four weeks in order to evaluate fetal growth, presence or absence of hydramnios, and fetal weight estimation near term.

An amniocentesis for the presence of phosphatidylglycerol is performed before elective caesarean section or induction of labour to assess pulmonary maturity.

A paediatrician is present at delivery, and all infants are observed for a minimum of six hours in the neonatal special care facility for signs of hypoglycaemia, hypocalcaemia, hyperbilirubinaemia and/or respiratory distress.

Since diabetic pregnancies are associated with a high incidence of maternal and fetal morbidity, and the management of blood sugar during gestation requires a degree of control not ordinarily attempted in the non-pregnant population, we believe that all diabetic patients should be managed in a perinatal clinic with personnel and facilities capable of handling the substantial challenges presented by this group of patients.

SUMMARY

Since the metabolic changes in normal pregnancy are diabetogenic, pregnancy imposes a severe stress on the metabolic milieu of diabetic patients. Moreover many patients with long-standing diabetes have vascular complications including retinopathy, renal insufficiency, nephrotic syndrome and hypertension, that represent separate risk factors for optimal fetal development Recent experience has suggested that maternal hyperglycaemia, and associated fetal hyperinsulinaemia, may represent an important factor in the development of fetal complications.

During the past two to three decades the incidence of perinatal deaths has been reduced in all cases of diabetics to a level that approaches the rate in healthy gravidas when severe congenital anomalies are excluded. Fetal and neonatal morbidity have also been reduced, although rates of congenital anomalies, polyhydramnios and respiratory distress syndrome remain high. In patients with significant vascular complications, especially nephropathy and retinopathy, there is no evidence that pregnancy alters the natural course of these complications. Although the morbidity associated with oedema formation and hypertension is elevated, with meticulous management of patients with diabetic nephropathy, especially in the absence of severe renal insufficiency and/or severe hypertension, pregnancy performance and outcome can be similar to other insulin-dependent diabetics.

REFERENCES

Coustan DR (1980) Recent advances in management of diabetic pregnancy woman. *Clinics in Perinatology* **7**: 299–311.
Coustan DR, Berkowitz RL & Hobbins JC (1980) Tight metabolic control of overt diabetes in pregnancy. *American Journal of Medicine* **68**: 845–852.
Epstein MF, Farrell PM & Chez RA (1976) Fetal lung lecithin metabolism in the glucose-intolerant Rhesus monkey pregnancy. *Pediatrics* **57**: 722–728.
Essex NL, Pyke DA, Watkins PJ et al (1973) Diabetic pregnancy. *British Medical Journal* **4**: 89–93.
Freinkel N & Metzger BE (1979) Pregnancy as a tissue culture experience: the critical complications of maternal metabolism for fetal development. In *Pregnancy Metabolism, Diabetes and the Fetus*, CIBA Foundation Symposium 63 (new series), pp 3–28. Amsterdam: Excerpta Medica.
Fuhrmann K, Reiher H, Semmler K, Fischer F, Fischer M, Glockner E (1983) Prevention of congenital malformations in infants of insulin-dependent diabetic mothers. *Diabetic Care* **6**: 219–233.
Gabbe SO (1977) Congenital malformations in infants of diabetic mothers. *Obstetrics and Gynecology Survey* **129**: 125–132.
Grenfell A, Brundenell JM, Doddridge RMC & Watkins PJ (1986) Pregnancy in diabetic women who have proteinuria. *Quarterly Journal of Medicine* **59**: 379–386.
Hare JW & White P (1977) Pregnancy in diabetes complicated by vascular disease. *Diabetes* **26**: 953–955.
Hayslett JP (1985) Pregnancy does not exacerbate primary glomerular disease. *American Journal of Kidney Diseases* **6**: 273–277.
Hollingsworth DR (1983) Alterations of maternal metabolism in normal and diabetic pregnancies: differences in insulin-dependent, non-insulin-dependent, and gestational diabetes. *American Journal of Obstetrics and Gynecology* **146**: 417–429.
Hubbell JP, Muirhead DM & Drahbaugh JE (1965) The newborn infant of the diabetic mother. *Medical Clinics of North America* **49**: 1035–1052.
Jovanovic R & Jovanovic L (1984) Obstetric management when normoglycemia is maintained in diabetic pregnant women with vascular compromise. *American Journal of Obstetrics and Gynecology* **149**: 617–623.
Karlsson K & Kjellmer I (1972) The outcome of diabetic pregnancies in relation to the mother's blood sugar level. *American Journal of Obstetrics and Gynecology* **112**: 213–220.
Katz AI, Davison JM, Hayslett JP, Singson E & Lindheimer MD (1980) Pregnancy in women with kidney disease. *Kidney International* **18**: 192–206.
Kitzmiller JL, Cloherty JP, Younger MD et al (1978) Diabetic pregnancy and perinatal morbidity. *American Journal of Obstetrics and Gynecology* **131**: 560–580.
Kitzmiller JL, Brown ER, Phillippe M et al (1981a) Diabetic nephropathy and perinatal outcome. *American Journal of Obstetrics and Gynecology* **141**: 741–751.
Kitzmiller JL, Aiello LM, Kaldany A & Younger MD (1981b) Diabetic vascular disease complicating pregnancy. *Clinical Obstetrics and Gynecology* **24**: 107–123.

Lin C, Lindheimer MD, River R & Moa Wad AH (1982) Fetal outcome in hypertensive disorders of pregnancy. *American Journal of Obstetrics and Gynecology* **142:** 255–260.

Naeve C (1967) Congenital malformations in offspring of diabetics. PhD thesis, Harvard University School of Public Health.

National Diabetes Data Group (1979) Classification and diagnosis of diabetes mellitus and other categories of glucose intolerance. *Diabetes* **28:** 1039–1057.

Pedersen J & Pedersen LN (1965) Prognosis of the outcome of pregnancies in diabetics: a new classification. *Acta Endocrinologia* **50:** 70–78.

Pedersen J, Moulstead-Pedersen L & Andersen D (1974) Assessors of fetal perinatal mortality in diabetic pregnancy. *Diabetes* **23:** 302–305.

Pedersen J (1977) *The Pregnancy Diabetic and her Newborn*, 2nd edn. Baltimore; Williams & Wilkins.

Reece EA, Coustan ER, Hayslett JP et al (1987) Diabetic nephropathy: pregnancy performance and feto-maternal outcome. *American Journal of Obstetrics and Gynecology* (in press).

Rodman et al (1979) Diabetic retinopathy and its relationship to pregnancy. In Merketz IR & Adam PAJ (eds) *The Diabetic Pregnancy: A Perinatal Perspective* pp 73–92. New York: Grune & Stratton.

Susa JB, McCormick KL, Widness JA et al (1979) Chronic hyperinsulinemia in the fetal Rhesus monkey. *Diabetes* **28:** 417–429.

White P (1949) Pregnancy complicating diabetes. *American Journal of Medicine* **7:** 609–616.

11

Reflux nephropathy and pregnancy

PAUL JUNGERS
PASCAL HOUILLIER
DOMINIQUE FORGET

The problems associated with pregnancy in patients with reflux nephropathy are of important concern because reflux nephropathy is one of the most frequent renal diseases observed in women of childbearing age. This nephropathy is frequently associated with urinary tract infection, hypertension and/or chronic renal failure (Kincaid-Smith, 1984, 1985), all of which may adversely affect pregnancy outcome. Conversely, the presence of glomerular lesions of the focal segmental hyalinosis and sclerosis type that are consistently present in the most severe forms of reflux nephropathy (with bilateral renal scarring and parenchymal atrophy) justify the fear that maternal renal function may deteriorate in pregnancy (Becker et al, 1985). Currently we have a better understanding of the influences of pregnancy and reflux nephropathy on each other due to recent advances in our knowledge of the pathophysiology underlying renal atrophy and, especially, of the glomerular lesions responsible for the progression to renal failure.

DEFINITION AND PATHOPHYSIOLOGY OF REFLUX NEPHROPATHY

Definition

The term 'reflux nephropathy' refers to renal morphological and functional alterations which relate to present (or past) vesicoureteral reflux. From a semantic point of view, the term 'reflux nephropathy' is virtually synonymous with 'primary chronic non-obstructive atrophic pyelonephritis'. The implicit assumption is that other causes of the pyelonephritic renal atrophy, such as analgesic consumption, urolithiasis, tuberculosis, papillary necrosis or urinary tract obstruction are not present and that the congenital defect of the vesicoureteral junction with or without superimposed urinary tract infection is the cause of the atrophic alterations of the kidneys (Kincaid-Smith, 1984; Rubin et al, 1986). The link between the peculiar radiographic aspect of the kidneys, characterized by enlargement and distortion of the calices ('clubbing') and thinning of the overlying renal cortex ('scarring'), with preferential localization at the upper and lower poles (Moreau et al, 1980) and the existence of a vesicoureteral reflux was first pointed out by Hodson and Edwards (1960) on the basis of radiographic findings in children. The term 'reflux nephropathy' was later proposed by Bailey (1973), who wished to underscore the significance of these associations. Other terms, such as segmental hypoplasia, corticopapillary atrophy or corticomedullary scarring, have been proposed as alternative designations (Rubin et al, 1986).

The pathogenesis of vesicoureteral reflux and renal scarring

Renal parenchymal atrophy is thought to result from the urodynamic consequences of vesicoureteral reflux, and is associated with urinary tract infection (Scott and Stansfeld, 1968; Rolleston et al, 1970; Smellie et al, 1975). Primary vesicoureteral reflux is a congenital defect in which the vesicoureteric junction is incompetent, and during micturition there is regurgitation of urine up to the ureter. Failure of this valve mechanism is due to a shortening of the intravesical portion of the ureter, due to congenital lateral ectopia of the ureteric orifice (Stephens and Lenaghan, 1962) with concomitant alteration in the morphology of the ureteric orifice. The latter tends to have the shape of a stadium, a horseshoe or a golf hole, instead of the normal conic aspect (Lyon et al, 1969).

The degree of reflux, which can be uni- or bilateral, is variable in severity. It can be graded by means of voiding cystourethrography according to the International Reflux Study Committee (Rubin et al, 1986) (Figure 1). Scarring appears in the most severe forms of reflux and, in such cases, may be found in early childhood (Rolleston et al, 1975) or even at birth (Scott, 1987).

As the intravesical portion of the ureter lengthens with growth, vesicoureteral reflux spontaneously tends to disappear with age [in up to 80% of cases (Smellie et al, 1975)], but the abnormal position and configuration of the ureteric orifices often persist (Baker et al, 1966). Thus, endoscopic examination may permit retrospective diagnosis of vesicoureteral reflux in adult patients exhibiting renal scarring on intravenous urography but having no present evidence of vesicoureteral reflux on voiding cystourethrography. The most severe cases of reflux, including those associated with the early appearance of renal scarring, are the least likely to disappear with time, thus accounting for the high frequency of renal scarring observed in adults with persistent severe vesicoureteral reflux (Kincaid-Smith and Becker, 1978).

The formation of renal scars depends on the occurrence of intrarenal reflux, that is urinary backflow into the renal parenchyma through collecting ducts. The importance of intrarenal reflux in the pathogenesis of pyelonephritic scarring has been demonstrated by experimental studies. Hodson and co-workers induced sterile vesicoureteral reflux under high pressure in miniature pigs, and were able to reproduce the type and polar topography of damage observed in patients with clinical reflux. The zones of most intense scarring correlated with the areas shown to have intrarenal reflux on cystography (Hodson et al, 1975a, 1975b). Ransley and Risdon (1978) extended these

I   II   III   IV   V

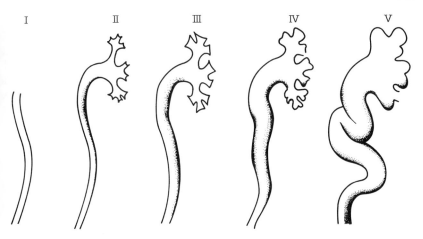

Figure 1. Grades of reflux. International Study Classification: I, ureter only; II, ureter, pelvis and calyces, no dilatation, normal calyceal fornices; III, mild or moderate dilatation and/or tortuosity of ureter and mild or moderate dilatation of renal pelvis but no or slight blunting of fornices; IV, moderate dilatation and/or tortuosity of ureter and moderate dilatation of renal pelvis and calyces. Complete obliteration of sharp angle of fornices but maintenance of papillary impressions in majority of calyces; V, gross dilatation and tortuosity of ureter. Gross dilatation of renal pelvis and calyces. Papillary impressions are no longer visible in majority of calyces. From Rubin et al (1986).

studies and showed that in the multipapillary kidney of young pigs (similar in morphology to that of humans), intrarenal reflux occurred selectively in compound refluxing papillae, which are present predominantly in the upper and lower parts of the kidneys. Thus, the site of scarring appears to be determined by the site of intrarenal reflux (Amar, 1970; Rolleston et al, 1970).

Urine extravasation in the renal interstitium may provoke renal damage either by directly eliciting interstitial fibrosis, or by initiating an autoimmune reaction against the Tamm-Horsfall protein—a normal constituent of the urine formed by the distal tubules (Cotran, 1981). Few question the important contributory role of infection, as new scars occur only in patients with persistent infection and reflux (Edwards et al, 1977; Mihindukulasuriya et al, 1980; Claesson et al, 1981; Huland and Busch, 1984).

There appears to be a direct correlation between the development of renal functional impairment and the degree and extent of renal parenchymal scarring (Malek et al, 1983a; Torres et al, 1983). Thus, surgical repair of the vesicoureteric junction was proposed in the hope of stopping reflux of infected urine and the resultant renal scarring, and to preserve renal growth and function. Some reports suggested that this was the case, at least when antireflux surgery was performed early in life (McRae et al, 1974) and when kidneys had not already been severely damaged (Scott et al, 1986). However, based on most recent studies it appears that when impairment in renal function, hypertension or significant proteinuria is already present, surgical correction of vesicoureteral reflux does not significantly influence the rate of renal atrophy progression, either in children or in adults, even if symptoms related to recurrent urinary tract infection are improved (Torres et al, 1980; Birmingham Reflex Study Group, 1983; Brown et al, 1978; Smellie et al, 1981; Weston et al, 1982; Malek et al, 1983b; Neves et al, 1984). Thus, surgery should be considered only in cases when severe reflux is diagnosed at an early stage, and if it is to be undertaken, it should be performed in infancy or in early childhood (Rolleston et al, 1975). In adults, corrective surgery should only be considered in cases where recurrent pyelonephritic episodes occur despite careful prophylaxis.

Mechanism of progressive renal deterioration: the role of glomerular lesions

Throughout the 1960s, it was generally accepted that tubulo-interstitial lesions were responsible for the relentless progression towards chronic renal failure observed in patients with chronic atrophic pyelonephritis. It has now been clearly established that the progressive deterioration of renal function that occurs in patients with reflux nephropathy is associated with the development of glomerular lesions resembling focal and segmental hyalinosis and sclerosis (or 'glomerulosclerosis') (Cotran, 1982; Steinhardt, 1985). These lesions had been initially described in patients with idiopathic nephrosis (Habib, 1973), but Kincaid-Smith (1975) was the first to draw attention to the association of chronic atrophic pyelonephritis with proteinuria and such glomerular lesions. Other authors subsequently reported focal glomerulo-sclerosis in association with proteinuria, often abundant and in the 'glomeru-lar' range, leading on occasion to the nephrotic syndrome in patients with bilateral reflux nephropathy progressing to end-stage renal failure (Senekjian et al, 1979; Bhathena et al, 1980; Torres et al, 1980), whereas no focal glomerulosclerosis was seen in patients having normal renal function minimal or absent proteinuria and unilateral disease (Cotran, 1982). Patients with unilateral parenchymal scarring usually have a good prognosis but, even in unilateral disease, progression may occur through the development of diffuse glomerular lesions in the contralateral, apparently preserved kidney However, in such cases, proteinuria is usually present (Bailey et al, 1984) Thus, proteinuria is the most significant prognostic feature of progression to renal failure in reflux nephropathy in infants (Bell et al, 1986) and in the adult (Torres et al, 1980; Weston et al, 1982; Torres et al, 1983; Kincaid-Smith 1984; Lorentz and Browning, 1986).

The mechanism by which proteinuria and glomerulosclerosis develop in patients with reflux nephropathy has been partially elucidated, based on the analogy with the morphologically similar lesion observed in animals subjected to severe reduction of nephron mass (Shimamura and Morrison, 1975; Olson et al, 1982). In these animals, micropuncture studies have shown haemodynamic changes in remnant glomeruli, characterized by marked increases in capillary plasma flow and the glomerular transcapillary hydraulic pressure gradient (Deen et al, 1974; Hostetter et al, 1981). It appears that these changes cause progressive mesangial hyalinosis and renal autodestruction (Brenner et al, 1982; Hostetter et al, 1982).

The development of progressive renal failure in reflux nephropathy might thus be explained by a marked and early reduction in the number of functioning nephrons in the scarred areas of the kidneys, the remnant nephrons being subjected to hypertrophy and hyperfiltration. This is probably due to the early age at which scarring occurs in reflux nephropathy, as renal growth and compensatory hypertrophy are more prone to occur in the young (Steinhardt, 1985).

The theory of autodestruction of remnant nephrons through hyperfiltration has received support from the fact that similar lesions focal glomerulosclerosis has also been observed in certain rare conditions which lead to loss of parenchymal renal mass early in life, such as unilateral renal agenesis (Kiprov et al, 1982; Gutierrez-Millet et al, 1986), surgical removal of a kidney for unilateral renal disease (Zucchelli et al, 1983) or bilateral oligomeganephronic hypoplasia (Bhathena et al, 1985), whereas focal segmental glomerulosclerosis is a rather uncommon lesion found in less than 2% of all renal biopsies and, when present, is usually associated with the idiopathic nephrotic syndrome (Velosa et al, 1983).

CLINICAL IMPLICATIONS OF REFLUX NEPHROPATHY IN ADULT WOMEN

Whereas in infants, the sex distribution of vesicoureteral reflux is almost equal (there is a slight excess in boys), after the first year of life 70% of vesicoureteral reflux is observed in girls (Edwards et al, 1977; Scott et al, 1986). The same is true for adults, where the proportion of women with vesicoureteric reflux is 80% or more (Kincaid-Smith and Becker, 1978; Moreau et al, 1980; Arze et al, 1982; Malek et al, 1983a). This preponderance of females among adult patients with reflux nephropathy parallels the fact that, except during the first year of life, lower urinary tract infection is far more common in females and is especially frequent in young, sexually active women.

Almost two-thirds of adult women with reflux nephropathy are under the age of 40 years at the time of presentation. The commonest presenting features are urinary tract infection, hypertension and renal insufficiency, which respectively were observed in 69%, 31% and 12% of cases in a large recent series (Arze et al, 1982). In nearly a third of women with reflux nephropathy clinical symptoms first become apparent during pregnancy, while renal scarring of the type seen with vesicoureteral reflux is the most frequent lesion detected in women screened for pyelonephritis or bacteriuria occurring during gestation (Kincaid-Smith and Bullen, 1965; Williams et al, 1968).

Hypertension is present at presentation in 30–40% of patients (Kincaid-Smith and Becker, 1970; Arze et al, 1982) and positively correlates with the extent of renal scarring (Torres et al, 1983). In more advanced stages of the disease, when marked impairment of renal function is present, hypertension is observed in 80% or more of patients (Torres et al, 1980). The level of

Table 1. Outcome of 254 pregnancies in 104 pregnant patients with reflux nephropathy (Necker Hospital, December 1986).

Outcome of pregnancy	Number
Full-term delivery	178 (all living)
Premature delivery	42 (12 stillbirth or neonatal deaths)
Spontaneous abortion	16
Induced abortion	16
Ectopic pregnancy	2
Total live births	208
Total fetal deaths	46

hypertension is often severe and contributes further to deterioration of renal function.

The most disturbing complication is the frequent development in young women with reflux nephropathy of progressive renal failure, and 10–30% of all adult patients requiring dialysis or transplantation have reflux nephropathy as their primary renal disease (Salvatierra and Tanagho, 1977; Senekjian et al, 1979; Bailey, 1981). Often these patients reach end-stage renal failure under the age of 40 years. Thus, not infrequently impaired renal function and/or hypertension may be present at conception in female patients.

PROBLEMS RELATED TO PREGNANCY IN PATIENTS WITH REFLUX NEPHROPATHY

Considering the high frequency of reflux nephropathy in women of childbearing age, it is surprising that there are so few studies specifically devoted to the problems of this disease occurring in pregnancy. Only two extensive reports bearing on large series of patients have been published to date—one from the Melbourne group (Kincaid-Smith, 1985) and the other from our group at the Necker Hospital (Jungers et al, 1986). Both of these studies have recently been extended. The first series now comprises 345 pregnancies observed in 137 patients (Kincaid-Smith, 1987), and the second 254 pregnancies in 104 women (Jungers et al, 1987). Additionally, some data on the outcome of pregnancy in reflux nephropathy may be found in a report from Newcastle on 79 women who had had 173 pregnancies (Arze et al, 1982).

Influence of reflux nephropathy on the outcome of pregnancy

One consensus derived from the series noted above is that overall, fetal prognosis in reflux nephropathy appears good. In the experience of Arze et al (1982), 81% of the pregnancies were successful, 35% were complicated by hypertension and 33% complicated by urinary tract infection. In their first study of 37 women, Kincaid-Smith (1985) reported a fetal loss rate of 12% in 85 pregnancies; pre-eclampsia and/or urinary tract infection complicated the course of pregnancy in 50% of the cases. In the update of this study, Kincaid-

Smith (1987) reported an overall fetal death rate of 14%, and fetal loss was clearly higher in the group with plasma creatinine levels exceeding 0.11 mmol/l at conception (24% in 118 pregnancies) than in the group with normal renal function (9% in 227 pregnancies). Pre-eclampsia developed in 36% of pregnancies in the group with functional impairment, but in only 13% of pregnancies when renal function was normal (Kincaid-Smith, 1987). Urinary tract infection did not have a major influence on fetal survival, whereas impaired renal function was a key factor in those with an adverse fetal prognosis. This was especially true when the plasma creatinine level at conception or early in gestation was 0.20 mmol/l or more (Becker et al, 1986). Of six pregnancies where plasma creatinine was at these levels, two ended in intrauterine or neonatal death, and four in premature deliveries of infants with very low birthweights (range 1090–1498 g).

In our own series (updated to December, 1986) the fetal death rate corrected for induced abortions was 12.6%, 87.4% of the pregnancies were successful (Table 1), and the mean birthweight was 3080 ± 750 g. The fetal death rate tended to be lower in the 117 pregnancies recorded in the most recent years compared with the 137 gestations reported earlier (11% versus 14%). This reflects primarily a lower mortality rate in prematurely delivered infants and is due to current improvements in obstetric and perinatal care, even though the proportion of premature deliveries had increased in recent years because a higher number of patients with impaired renal function and/or hypertension at conception had been referred to our nephrology unit.

We analysed the respective influences of urinary tract infection (UTI), hypertension and/or impaired renal function on fetal outcome (Houillier et al, 1987, in preparation). UTI complicated 60 pregnancies in 47 patients, two-thirds of whom had histories of previous UTI, including one or more episodes of acute pyelonephritis in half of the cases. In 34 pregnancies, UTI was confined to the lower urinary tract, whereas acute pyelonephritis occurred during 26 pregnancies in 24 patients of whom 62% had experienced previous pyelonephritic episodes. Only one fetal death was observed in this group in the absence of other risk factors such as renal failure or hypertension. Upper UTI was infrequent in women with known impairment of renal function, probably due to the particularly close surveillance of such patients. Recurrence of upper UTI was observed in two patients, despite surgical correction of vesicoureteral reflux prior to pregnancy in eight of the patients. Thus, we agree that even if symptomatic UTI is frequent in pregnant women with vesicoureteric reflux, especially in those with previous bouts of UTI, there is a deleterious effect on fetal outcome in but a very limited number of cases.

By contrast, the influence of renal failure and hypertension appears to be a much greater determinant on fetal prognosis. Significant renal impairment, defined by a plasma creatinine value of 0.135 mmol/l or more, was present at conception or early in gestation in 19 pregnancies (in 14 women), hypertension also being present in 15 instances. Only seven live births occurred in this group (four by preterm caesarean section)—a fetal loss of 63%. Of the 12 pregnancies where hypertension was present at conception or in early gestation, only three ended in live births (in one case hypertension was controlled by treatment; in the other two caesarean section at 35 weeks

Table 2. Fetal outcome in women with reflux nephropathy and impaired renal function at conception or early in pregnancy.

Pcr* range (mmol/l)	Number of pregnancies	Fetal deaths (%)
0.135–0.195	13	7 (53%)
0.20–0.50	6	5 (83%)
	19	12 (63%)

* Plasma creatinine.

resulted in live births, the infants weighing 1800 and 2350 g respectively. Thus, the association of renal failure and hypertension was especially deleterious, with fetal mortality reaching 75%.

The influence of hypertension in the absence of concomitant renal failure was assessed in 24 cases. Of seven pregnancies where hypertension was present at conception or in the first trimester, two ended in fetal death in utero, but five live births occurred in patients whose hypertension was therapeutically controlled (but the birthweight was below 2500 g in three cases). No fetal death was observed in the 14 cases where hypertension occurred late in pregnancy.

A critical problem, with respect to preconception counselling of women with reflux nephropathy, is to decide on the level of renal impairment compatible with a successful fetal outcome. In our series, there were virtually no live births once the plasma creatinine exceeded 0.20 mmol/l at conception (Table 2). In the report of Becker et al (1986), two fetal deaths were observed in six patients whose plasma creatinine early in pregnancy was 0.20–0.35 mmol/l. In four cases live births were effected in mothers who were treated with plasma exchanges and/or heparin in an attempt to slow the progression of renal failure (Becker et al, 1984). However, in these cases there was a rapid decline of maternal renal function to end-stage renal failure after delivery, seemingly implicating pregnancy in this poor outcome (Becker et al, 1986).

Thus the combined experience of two groups suggests that a plasma creatinine level of about 0.20 mmol/l should be considered as the upper limit at which patients with reflux nephropathy should attempt pregnancy. Prognosis is more guarded if they are hypertensive, as is the case in patients with primary glomerular disease (Davison et al, 1985).

The influence of pregnancy on maternal renal function in patients with reflux nephropathy

Whether or not pregnancy may adversely affect the immediate course and remote prognosis of maternal renal disease has long been a matter of controversy in patients with primary renal disease (Becker et al, 1985; Hayslett, 1985; Katz and Lindheimer, 1985). In the case of primary glomerular diseases, a consensus has emerged (Davison et al, 1985), based on the retrospective analysis of several large series of pregnancies reported during the past decade, that pregnancy does not adversely affect the natural course of glomerular disease in women with preserved or mildly decreased renal function and none or minimal hypertension at conception (Katz et al, 1980; Abe et al, 1985; Jungers et al, 1986). However, abnormally rapid deterioration of maternal renal function and/or development of persistent hypertension has been observed in women whose baseline plasma creatinine ranged between 0.15 and 0.25 mmol/l, particularly in those having IgA nephropathy or membranoproliferative glomerulonephritis as underlying disease (Hou et al, 1985; Becker et al, 1985; Imbasciati et al, 1986; Jungers et al, 1986, 1987).

Until recently, data concerning the effects of pregnancy on the course of reflux nephropathy were sparse. Several anecdotal reports had been published which consisted primarily of patients with marked renal impairment at the time of conception who had progressed to end-stage renal failure several months after pregnancy (Orme et al, 1968; Bear, 1976; Johnson et al, 1979). In the Melbourne experience, renal function significantly declined during pregnancy in 8% of women with a plasma creatinine above 0.11 mmol/l, but in only 2% of those with a plasma creatinine below this level (Kincaid-Smith, 1987). However, the adverse effect of pregnancy on the natural course of renal disease was most clearly apparent in the group of patients having a significant renal impairment. There was an abnormally rapid rate of decline of renal function in all six women whose plasma creatinine was in the range of 0.2–0.4 mmol/l in the first trimester of pregnancy, despite adequate control of hypertension. Four of the women developed end-stage renal failure within 2 years of delivery. All of these patients had proteinuria of more than 1 g/day at conception. This accelerated course was in clear contrast with the much slower course observed in 10 other patients in whom neither pregnancy nor uncontrolled hypertension occurred, and in whom it took one or more years to develop from a plasma creatinine level of 0.20 mmol/l to end-stage renal failure (Becker et al, 1986). A similarly slow progression (7 or more years) was also observed in non-pregnant women with reflux nephropathy by Arze et al (1982) in those instances where the data permitted calculation of the time it took to progress from plasma creatinine of 0.20–0.25 mmol/l to end-stage renal failure.

In our initial report we had observed an abnormally rapid deterioration of renal function in only one patient (Jungers et al, 1986). Since then, we have observed 10 further pregnancies in eight patients with moderate impairment of renal function. Among this series of 19 gestations in 14 women whose plasma creatinine ranged from 0.135 to 0.49 mmol/l at conception or in the first trimester of pregnancy, there was an accelerated course, with progression towards end-stage renal failure within 1–4 years postpartum in four patients with a creatinine level ranging between 0.18 and 0.29 mmol/l, and within 6 months in one whose plasma creatinine was 0.49 mmol/l at the start of the pregnancy (Figure 2). All five of these patients also had hypertension and proteinuria. On the other hand, progression of renal failure did not appear to be accelerated in the other nine patients whose plasma creatinine at conception was 0.18 mmol/l or less. Their disease followed the expected natural course of this disease.

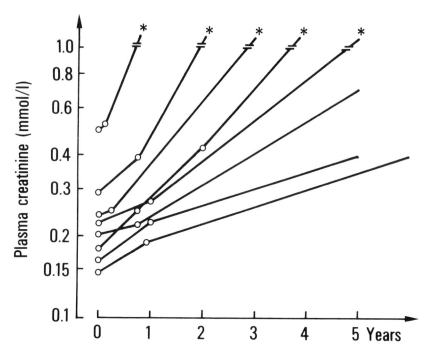

Figure 2. Progression of renal failure from early pregnancy in eight women with reflux nephropathy and a plasma creatinine concentration of 0.18–0.49 mmol/l at conception (*denotes the start of chronic dialysis treatment).

Thus, when combining our data with those of the Melbourne group, it becomes apparent that when pregnancy occurs in a woman with a plasma creatinine level in excess of 0.20 mmol/l (and possibly an even lower value when hypertension is present), there is a clear risk of inducing rapid, irreversible worsening of maternal renal function similar to that observed in patients with primary glomerular diseases.

The mechanisms of such deterioration of renal function related to pregnancy are not fully understood and are possibly multiple. Alteration of the renal parenchyma by infection appears unlikely here because episodes of acute pyelonephritis in pregnancy were rarely observed in women with impaired renal function both in our experience and that of others (Kincaid-Smith, 1987). Severe uncontrolled hypertension, however, is more likely to play a role, causing renal vascular lesions such as hyperplasia of vascular intima. Such lesions were present to a marked degree in renal biopsies taken during pregnancy or within 1 month after delivery in some patients (Becker et al, 1986). The hypercoagulable state which is present in all gravidas, especially in late pregnancy, may provoke acute formation of fibrin thrombi in glomerular capillaries, leading to glomerular crescent formation; on healing, this may convert to a lesion of segmental hyalinosis. Fibrin thrombi were present in glomerular capillaries in renal biopsies performed during pregnancy in some patients with reflux nephropathy (Kincaid-Smith, 1987).

Since sustained physiological hyperfiltration is part of the maternal adaptation to pregnancy, it is tempting to speculate that such hyperfiltration could result in a worsening of pre-existing focal glomerulosclerosis. This hypothesis was supported by the clinical observation that a similar worsening in renal function had been observed in three pregnant patients with primary focal glomerulosclerosis (Taylor et al, 1978), but all of whom were severely hypertensive. In fact, physiological hyperfiltration of pregnancy *per se* has never been proven to induce impairment of renal function or glomerular focal sclerosis in women. Experimentally, an investigation of glomerular function and morphology in pregnant rats demonstrated no persistent abnormality in rats completing five consecutive cycles of pregnancy and lactation (which create a state of persistent hyperfiltration) when compared to age-matched virgin controls (Baylis and Rennke, 1984). If the same holds true for humans, extension of lesions of focal glomerulosclerosis due to pregnancy-induced hyperfiltration is unlikely to occur or play a significant role in the progression of renal disease. In the present state of our knowledge, acute vascular lesions induced by hypertension and intraglomerular fibrin thrombi formation appear to be the most likely mechanisms.

Preconception counselling and management during pregnancy

In view of the preceding data, women with reflux nephropathy who wish to have a family should be allowed to conceive as long as renal function is well preserved and, whenever possible, before the plasma creatinine level has reached 0.18 mmol/l. Patients whose plasma creatinine level is in excess of this value, especially if hypertension is also present (or developed during a previous pregnancy), should be clearly advised of the risks of fetal loss and rapid worsening of their renal function, and, pregnancy should be discour-

---

Table 3. Guidelines for counselling and managing patients with reflux nephropathy who conceive.

Preconception counselling
Consider surgical correction of reflux prior to conception in cases of episodes of upper urinary tract infection despite careful prophylaxis.
Discourage pregnancy when the plasma creatinine level exceeds 0.18 mmol/l, especially when hypertension is also present.

Management of pregnancy
Every patient should be frequently screened for bacteriuria and treated immediately for urinary tract infection.
In women with impaired renal function, the following are required:
 (i) close cooperation between the obstetrician and the physician or the nephrologist;
 (ii) a monthly determination of the plasma creatinine concentration, creatinine clearance, proteinuria and blood pressure;
 (iii) active antihypertensive treatment;
 (iv) reinforced fetal monitoring and preterm delivery when necessary, according to fetal status;
 (v) prolonged surveillance of maternal renal function and blood pressure after delivery.

---

aged (Brown, 1984; Hou, 1985) (Table 3). In women with normal or mildly impaired renal function, special attention should be given to the early detection and immediate treatment of bacteriuria. Surgical correction of reflux before starting pregnancy should be considered in those women exhibiting recurrent urinary tract infection despite prophylactic measures, although this protection is not absolute. When hypertension is present at conception or develops in pregnancy, it should be aggressively controlled by antihypertensive treatment (Davison et al, 1985).

SUMMARY

Reflux nephropathy is one of the most frequent renal diseases encountered in women of childbearing age. Patients with severe bilateral atrophy are the most likely to develop proteinuria, hypertension, focal glomerular sclerosis and progressive chronic renal failure, and those with persistent vesicoureteral reflux are the most likely to suffer recurrent pyelonephritic episodes. Often the disease is clinically latent and first manifests itself in pregnancy, mainly by urinary tract infection but also by proteinuria, hypertension, pre-eclampsia or renal failure.

Pregnancy is most often successful and uneventful whenever renal function is normal or near normal and hypertension is absent at conception. Urinary tract infection accounts for frequent morbidity but rarely results in fetal mortality.

By contrast, when renal function is significantly impaired, that is in patients whose plasma creatinine concentration is in excess of 0.18–0.20 mmol/l at conception, especially when hypertension is also present, there is clearly a high risk of severe fetal growth retardation or intrauterine death. Moreover, there is a striking risk of rapid worsening of renal function and hypertension, with accelerated progression towards end-stage renal failure. Thus, women with reflux nephropathy should attempt to conceive before the plasma creatinine concentration has reached 0.18 mmol/l, and patients with values higher than these should be clearly advised of the high risk for both the pregnancy and the progression of the disease.

REFERENCES

Abe S, Amagasaki Y, Konishi K et al (1985) The influence of antecedent renal disease on pregnancy. *American Journal of Obstetrics and Gynecology* **153:** 508–514.

Amar AD (1970) Calicotubular backflow with vesico-ureteral reflux. *Journal of the American Medical Association* **213:** 293–294.

Arze RS, Ramos JM, Owen JA et al (1982) The natural history of chronic pyelonephritis in the adult. *Quarterly Journal of Medicine* **51:** 396–410.

Bailey R R (1973) The relationship of vesico-ureteric reflux to urinary tract infection and chronic pyelonephritis-reflux nephropathy. *Clinical Nephrology* **1:** 132–141.

Bailey R R (1981) End-stage reflux nephropathy. *Nephron* **27:** 302–307.

Bailey R R, Swainson CP, Lynn K L & Burry AF (1984) Glomerular lesions in the 'normal' kidney in patients with unilateral reflux nephropathy. *Contributions to Nephrology* **39:** 126–131.

Baker R, Maxted W, Maylath J & Shuman I (1966) Relation of age, sex and infection to reflux. Data indicating high spontaneous cure in the pediatric population. *Journal of Urology* **95:** 27–32.

Baylis C & Rennke HR (1984) Repetitive pregnancy: a physiologic model of hyperfiltration? *Clinical Research* **32:** 441A.

Bear RA (1976) Pregnancy in patients with renal disease. A study of 44 cases. *Obstetrics and Gynecology* **48:** 13–16.

Becker GJ, Ihle BU, Fairley KF, D'Apice AJF & Kincaid-Smith P (1984) Plasma exchange in pregnancy complicated by renal failure due to reflux nephropathy. *Clinical and Experimental Hypertension* (B) **3:** 329 (abstract).

Becker GJ, Fairley KF & Whitworth JA (1985) Pregnancy exacerbates glomerular disease. *American Journal of Kidney Diseases* **6:** 266–272.

Becker GJ, Ihle BU, Fairley KF, Bastos M & Kincaid-Smith P (1986) Effect of pregnancy on moderate renal failure in reflux nephropathy. *British Medical Journal* **292:** 796–798.

Bell FG, Wilkin TJ & Atwell JD (1986) Microproteinuria in children with vesicoureteric reflux. *British Journal of Urology* **58:** 605–609.

Bhathena DB, Weiss JH, Holland NH et al (1980) Focal and segmental glomerular sclerosis in reflux nephropathy. *The American Journal of Medicine* **68:** 886–892.

Bhathena DB, Julian BA, McMorrow RG & Baehler RW (1985) Focal sclerosis of hypertrophied glomeruli in solitary functioning kidneys of humans. *American Journal of Kidney Diseases* **5:** 226–232.

Birmingham Reflux Study Group (1983) Prospective trial of operative versus non operative treatment of severe vesicoureteric reflux: two years observation in 96 children. *British Medical Journal* **287:** 171–174.

Brenner BM, Meyer TW & Hostetter TH (1982) Dietary protein intake and the progressive nature of kidney disease: the role of hemodynamically mediated glomerular injury in the pathogenesis of progressive glomerular sclerosis in aging, renal ablation, and intrinsic renal disease. *New England Journal of Medicine* **307:** 652–659.

Brown RS (1984) Case records of the Massachusetts General Hospital. *New England Journal of Medicine* **310:** 1176–1181.

Brown CB, Cameron JS, Turner DR et al (1978) Focal segmental glomerulosclerosis with rapid decline in renal function ('malignant FSGS'). *Clinical Nephrology* **10:** 57–61.

Claesson I, Jacobsson B, Jodal U & Winberg J (1981) Compensatory kidney growth in children with urinary tract infection and unilateral renal scarring: an epidemiologic study. *Kidney International* **20:** 759–764.

Cotran RS (1981) Pathogenetic mechanisms in the progression of reflux nephropathy: the roles of glomerulosclerosis and extravasation of Tamm–Horsfall protein. In *Proceedings of the 8th International Congress of Nephrology, Athens*, pp 374–381. Basel (Switzerland): Karger.

Cotran RS (1982) Glomerulosclerosis in reflux nephropathy. *Kidney International* **21:** 528–534.

Davison JM, Katz AI & Lindheimer MD (1985) Pregnancy in women with renal disease and renal transplantation. *Proceedings of the European Dialysis and Transplant Association* **22:** 439–459.

Deen WM, Maddox DA, Robertson CR & Brenner BM (1974) Dynamics of glomerular ultrafiltration in the rat. VII. Response to reduced renal mass. *American Journal of Physiology* **227:** 556–562.

Edwards D, Normand ICS, Prescod N & Smellie JM (1977) Disappearance of vesicoureteric reflux during long-term prophylaxis of urinary tract infection in children. *British Medical Journal* **ii:** 285–288.

Gutierrez-Millet V, Nieto J, Praga M et al (1986) Focal glomerulosclerosis and proteinuria in patients with solitary kidneys. *Archives of Internal Medicine* **146:** 705–709.

Habib R (1973) Focal glomerular sclerosis. *Kidney International* **4:** 355–361.

Hayslett JP (1985) Pregnancy does not exacerbate primary glomerular disease. *American Journal of Kidney Diseases* **6:** 273–277.

Hodson CJ & Edwards D (1960) Chronic pyelonephritis and vesico-ureteric reflux. *Clinical Radiology* **11:** 219–231.

Hodson CJ, Maling TMJ, McManamon PJ & Lewis MG (1975a) The pathogenesis of reflux nephropathy (chronic atrophic pyelonephritis). *British Journal of Radiology* **48:** (supplement 13) 1–26.

Hodson J, Maling TMJ, McManamon PJ & Lewis MG (1975b) Reflux nephropathy. *Kidney International* **8:** S50–S58.

Hostetter TH, Olson HG, Rennke HG, Venkatachalam MA & Brenner BM (1981) Hyperfiltration in remnant nephrons: a potentially adverse response to renal ablation. *American Journal of Physiology* **241:** F85–F93.

Hostetter TH, Rennke HG & Brenner BM (1982) Compensatory renal hemodynamic injury: a final common pathway of residual nephron destruction. *American Journal of Kidney Diseases* **1:** 310–314.

Hou S (1985) Pregnancy in women with chronic renal disease. *New England Journal of Medicine* **312:** 836–839.

Hou S, Grossman SD & Madias NE (1985) Pregnancy in women with renal disease and moderate renal insufficiency. *American Journal of Medicine* **78:** (1987) 185–194.

Houillier P, Forget D, Henry-Amar M, Grünfeld JP & Jungers P (1987) Reflux nephropathy and pregnancy (in preparation).

Huland H & Busch R (1984) Pyelonephritic scarring in 213 patients with upper and lower urinary tract infections: long-term follow up. *Journal of Urology* **132:** 936–939.

Imbasciati E, Pardi G, Capetta P et al (1986) Pregnancy in women with chronic renal failure. *American Journal of Nephrology* **6:** 193–198.

Johnson TR, Lorenz RP, Menon KMJ & Nolan GH (1979) Successful outcome of a pregnancy requiring dialysis. *Journal of Reproductive Medicine* **22:** 217–218.

Jungers P, Forget D, Henry-Amar M et al (1986) Chronic kidney disease and pregnancy. *Advances in Nephrology* **15:** 103–141.

Jungers P, Forget D, Houillier P, Henry-Amar M & Grünfeld JP (1987) Pregnancy in IgA nephropathy, reflux nephropathy and focal glomerular sclerosis. *American Journal of Kidney Diseases* **9:** 334–338.

Katz AI & Lindheimer MD (1985) Does pregnancy aggravate primary glomerular disease? *American Journal of Kidney Diseases* **6:** 261–265.

Katz AI, Davison JM, Hayslett JP, Singson E & Lindheimer MD (1980) Pregnancy in women with kidney disease. *Kidney International* **18:** 192–206.

Kincaid-Smith P (1975) Glomerular and vascular lesions in chronic atrophic pyelonephritis and reflux nephropathy. *Advances in Nephrology* **5:** 3–17.

Kincaid-Smith P (1984) Vesicoureteral reflux and reflux nephropathy. In Suki WN and Massry SG (eds) *Therapy of Renal Diseases and Related Disorders*, pp 235–254. Boston/The Hague: Martinus Nijhoff Publishers.

Kincaid-Smith P (1985) Pregnancy-related renal disease. In Seldin DW and Giebisch G (eds) *The Kidney: Physiology and Pathophysiology*, pp 2043–2058. New York: Raven Press.

Kincaid-Smith P (1987) Renal disease in pregnancy. Three controversial areas: mesangial IgA nephropathy, focal glomerular sclerosis and reflux nephropathy. *American Journal of Kidney Diseases* **9:** 328–333.

Kincaid-Smith P & Becker GJ (1970) Reflux nephropathy in the adult. In Hodson J and Kincaid-Smith P (eds) *Reflux Nephropathy*, pp 21–27. New York: Masson Publishing.

Kincaid-Smith P & Becker G (1978) Reflux nephropathy and chronic atrophic pyelonephritis: a review. *Journal of Infectious Diseases* **138:** 774–780.

Kincaid-Smith P & Bullen M (1965) Bacteriuria in pregnancy. *Lancet* **i:** 395–399.

Kiprov DD, Colvin RB & McCluskey RT (1982) Focal and segmental glomerulosclerosis and proteinuria associated with unilateral renal agenesis. *Laboratory Investigation* **46:** 275–281.

Lorentz WB & Browning MC (1986) Vesicoureteral reflux, proteinuria and renal failure. *Journal of Urology* **135:** 559–562.

Lyon RP, Marshall S & Tanagho EA (1969) The ureteral orifice: its configuration and competency. *Journal of Urology* **102:** 504–509.

Malek RS, Svensson JP & Torres VE (1983a) Vesicoureteral reflux in the adult. I. Factors in pathogenesis. *Journal of Urology* **130:** 37–40.

Malek RS, Svensson J, Neves RJ & Torres VE (1983b) Vesicoureteral reflux in the adult. III. Surgical correction: risks and benefits. *Journal of Urology* **130:** 882–886.

McRae CU, Shannon FT & Utley WLF (1974) Effect on renal growth of reimplantation of refluxing ureters. *Lancet* **i:** 1310–1312.

Mihindukulasuriya JCL, Maskell R & Polak A (1980) A study of fifty-eight patients with renal scarring associated with urinary tract infection. *Quarterly Journal of Medicine* **49:** 165–178.

Moreau JF, Grenier R, Grünfeld JP & Brabant J (1980) Renal clubbing and scarring in adults: a retrospective study of 110 cases. *Urologic Radiology* **1:** 129–135.

Neves RJ, Torres VE, Malek RS & Svensson J (1984) Vesicoureteral reflux in the adult. IV. Medical versus surgical management. *Journal of Urology* **132:** 882–885.

Olson JL, Hostetter TH, Rennke HG, Brenner BM & Venkatachalam MA (1982) Altered glomerular permselectivity and progressive sclerosis following extreme ablation of renal mass. *Kidney International* **22:** 112–126.

Orme BM, Ueland K, Simpson DP & Scribner BH (1968) The effect of hemodialysis on fetal survival and renal function in pregnancy. *Transactions of the American Society for Artificial Internal Organs* **14:** 402–404.

Ransley PG & Risdon RA (1978) Reflux and renal scarring. *British Journal of Radiology* **51:** (supplement 14) 1–35.

Rolleston GL, Shannon FT & Utley WLF (1970) Relationship of infantile vesicoureteric reflux to renal damage. *British Medical Journal* **i:** 460–463.

Rolleston GL, Shannon FT & Utley WLF (1975) Follow-up of vesico-ureteric reflux in the newborn. *Kidney International* **8** (supplement 4): S59–S64.

Rubin RH, Tolkoff-Rubin N & Cotran RS (1986) Urinary tract infection, pyelonephritis, and reflux nephropathy. In Brenner BM & Rector FC (eds) *The Kidney*, 3rd edn, pp 1085–1141. Philadelphia: WB Saunders.

Salvatierra OJr & Tanagho EA (1977) Reflux as a cause of end stage kidney disease: report of 32 cases. *Journal of Urology* **117:** 441–443.

Scott JES (1987) Fetal ureteric reflux. *British Journal of Urology* **59:** 291–296.

Scott JES & Stansfeld JM (1968) Ureteric reflux and kidney scarring in children. *Archives of Disease in Childhood* **43:** 468–470.

Scott DJ, Blackford HN, Joyce MRL et al (1986) Renal function following surgical correction of vesico-ureteric reflux in childhood. *British Journal of Urology* **58:** 119–124.

Senekjian HO, Stinebaugh BJ, Mattioli CA & Suki WN (1979) Irreversible renal failure following vesicoureteral reflux. *Journal of the American Medical Association* **241:** 160–162.

Shimamura T & Morrison AB (1975) A progressive glomerulosclerosis occurring in partial five-sixths nephrectomized rats. *American Journal of Pathology* **79:** 95–101.

Smellie J, Edwards D, Hunter N, Normand ICS & Prescod N (1975) Vesico-ureteric reflux and renal scarring. *Kidney International* **8** (supplement 4): S65–S72.

Smellie JM, Edwards D, Normand ICS & Prescod N (1981) Effect of vesicoureteric reflux on renal growth in children with urinary tract infection. *Archives of Disease in Childhood* **56:** 593–596.

Steinhardt GF (1985) Reflux nephropathy. *Journal of Urology* **134:** 855–859.

Stephens FD & Lenaghan D (1962) The anatomical basis and dynamics of vesicoureteral reflux. *Journal of Urology* **87:** 669–674.

Taylor J, Novak R, Christiansen R & Sorensen ET (1978) Focal sclerosing glomerulopathy with adverse effects during pregnancy. *Archives of Internal Medicine* **138:** 1695–1696.

Torres VE, Velosa JA, Holley KE et al (1980) The progression of vesicoureteral reflux nephropathy. *Annals of Internal Medicine* **92:** 776–784.

Torres VE, Malek RS & Svensson JP (1983) Vesicoureteral reflux in the adult. II. Nephropathy, hypertension and stones. *Journal of Urology* **130:** 41–44.

Velosa JA, Holley KE, Torres VE & Offord KP (1983) Significance of proteinuria on the outcome of renal function in patients with focal segmental glomerulosclerosis. *Mayo Clinic Proceedings* **58:** 568–577.

Weston PMT, Stone AR, Bary PR, Leopold D & Stephenson TP (1982) The results of reflux prevention in adults with reflux nephropathy. *British Journal of Urology* **54:** 677–681.

Williams GL, Davies DKL, Evans KT & Williams JE (1968) Vesicoureteric reflux in patients with bacteriuria in pregnancy. *Lancet* **ii:** 1202–1205.

Zucchelli P, Cagnoli L, Casanova S, Donini S & Pasquali S (1983) Focal glomerulosclerosis in patients with unilateral nephrectomy. *Kidney International* **24:** 649–655.

12

Renal pathology in pre-eclampsia

LILLIAN W. GABER
BENJAMIN H. SPARGO
MARSHALL D. LINDHEIMER

Hypertension developing for the first time during pregnancy may be due to a variety of causes. In most instances it represents a disease specific to gestation (e.g. pre-eclampsia) or essential hypertension (which may only become manifest several decades later). In other cases, the rise in blood pressure is due to exacerbation of an underlying renal disease, alone or with superimposed pre-eclampsia. Very rarely it is due to secondary causes such as renal artery stenosis, primary aldosteronism, or phaeochromocytoma. With the exception of these last examples, treatment is usually similar. Still, knowledge of the exact cause is extremely useful, given the varying impact of different disease states on the outcome of future pregnancies, as well as the remote cardiovascular and renal prognosis of the patient. This chapter focuses on the renal lesion of pre-eclampsia, stressing several unresolved controversies concerning its morphology.

BACKGROUND

The literature concerning high blood pressure during pregnancy is controversial and confusing. One reason for this is the difficulty of distinguishing by clinical criteria alone the various aetiologic causes described above. These difficulties are best illustrated in two reports where the aetiology of the hypertension complicating pregnancy was established by renal biopsy. In one study, in which the physicians recorded their impressions prior to the biopsy, an exact diagnosis was made on clinical grounds in only 58% of the patients (Pollak and Nettles, 1960). Our own institution's experience comprising 176 patients biopsied between 1958 and 1976, summarized in Table 1, is similar (Fisher et al, 1981). These women were biopsied because their gestations were complicated by hypertension, and in most instances the clinician thought the patient had pre-eclampsia (or 'toxaemia'), since proteinuria and oedema were usually present. Such a diagnosis was incorrect in a quarter of the nulliparas and in over 50% of the multiparas. In addition, a surprisingly large number had unsuspected parenchymal renal disease. Even more recently, Ihle et al

Table 1. Renal pathology in 176 hypertensive patients.

Diagnosis	Number of patients	Primigravidas	Multiparas
Pre-eclampsia	96	79	17
with nephrosclerosis	13	6	7
with renal disease	3	1	2
with both	2	1	1
Nephrosclerosis	19	3	16
with renal disease	4	2	2
Renal disease	31	12	19
Normal histology	8	0	8

* Biopsy material (obtained between 1958 and 1976) was considered adequate if it contained eight glomeruli for light microscopic analysis and three for electron microscopic analysis. From Fisher et al (1981) with permission.
† Only glomerular endotheliosis on biopsy.

(1987) suggested that the majority of pregnant patients classified as pre-eclamptic whose hypertension manifests prior to gestational week 37 have another glomerular disease. The caveat behind such information is that all women developing hypertension for the first time during pregnancy require close postpartum scrutiny. Some may eventually require evaluation for underlying renal disease, including performance of a renal biopsy.

THE RENAL LESION OF PRE-ECLAMPSIA

The nature of the renal lesion in pre-eclampsia was a subject of considerable controversy during the first sixty years of this century. Lohlein (1918) was the first to recognize that the kidney, especially the glomerulus, was involved in the pre-eclamptic process. His observations were restricted to autopsy material, and he was impressed with the presence of glomerular hypercellularity and enlargement, as well as basement membrane thickening. Lohlein considered these changes to be inflammatory and regarded the lesion as a form of glomerulonephritis. This claim was disputed by Fahr (1920), who also studied autopsy material only, and who described mainly 'degenerative' changes, focusing on decreases in the number of endothelial cells. He termed the lesion 'eclamptic glomerulonephrosis'. Bell (1932), one decade later, taking advantage of newer histochemical techniques, described what appeared to be glomerular basement membrane thickening, and cited this change as the primary pathologic feature of pre-eclampsia. The latter view predominated until as late as 1962, when Allen labelled the glomerular lesion as 'acute membranous nephropathy' (Allen, 1962). His conclusion, however, was not accepted unanimously, for others like Sheehan (1950) and McManus (1959) had always disputed the presence of basement membrane thickening. Sheehan attributed the light-microscopic interpretation of 'thickening' to the deposition of subendothelial fibrils, while McManus described oedema of the glomerular tuft producing reticulation of the intercapillary space with occasional extension into the capillary wall. Sheehan was also the first pathologist to consider endothelial cell swelling as the primary glomerular lesion of pre-eclampsia.

Dieckmann et al (1957), among the first to utilize material obtained by renal biopsy, noted many of the same changes originally described in autopsy material including glomerular enlargement, cellular swelling, basement membrane thickening, and decreasing vascularity. They also attempted clinical–pathological correlations, comparing morphological changes with disease severity and outcome. However, it was the introduction of electron microscopy techniques, which permit better visualization and localization of glomerular components, that led to our present state of the art. Farquahar (1959) and Spargo et al (1959) described the ultrastructural pathology characteristic of pre-eclampsia, emphasizing endothelial vacuolization and hypertrophy of the cytoplasmic organelles. Spargo and colleagues referred to these lesions by the now widely accepted term 'glomerular capillary endothe- liosis', stating that the changes described were specific and pathognomonic of pre-eclamptic nephropathy and were not present in any other renal disease. The advent of immunohistology has also added to our concept of the pre- eclamptic lesion. However, several controversies (discussed below) still remain to be resolved. These include observations by some that the glomerular lesions may also be proliferative; the nature of the changes within or in the area of the basement membrane; alterations involving the juxtaglomerular apparatus; and whether or not tubular and/or vascular lesions are part of 'pure pre-eclampsia'. The most recent debate, however, relates to the coexistence of focal glomerular sclerosis in renal biopsies obtained from pre- eclamptics; do such lesions predate or result from the disease? These and other aspects of the renal lesions in pre-eclampsia are discussed below.

Morphological changes

There is only one major autopsy series of women dying from pre-eclampsia or eclampsia (the convulsive phase of the disorder) (Sheehan and Lynch, 1973). Gross inspection proved unrevealing and provided only non-specific informa- tion. It is of interest that the senior author (Sheehan) performed most of the autopsies 15 minutes to 2 hours postpartum, and these histologic examin- ations represent an extremely valuable source of material for those who wish to understand the pathology of pre-eclampsia.

Light-microscopic examination of the kidney

Pre-eclampsia affects primarily the glomerulus, and contrary to the older literature it is a combination of glomerular alterations and not a single feature that permits differentiation of pre-eclamptic nephropathy from other renal lesions causing hypertension in pregnancy. The glomerular lesions are diffuse in nature (relating perhaps to the severe and generalized vasomotor distur- bances that may occur in this disease), a characteristic that differentiates pre-

974   L. W. GABER, B. H. SPARGO AND M. D. LINDHEIMER

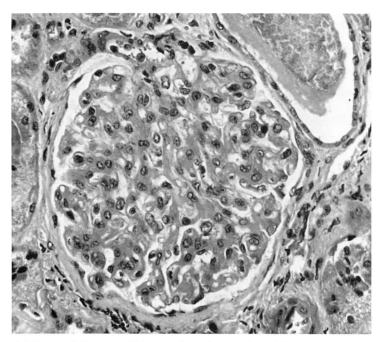

Figure 1. Micrograph from a renal biopsy performed on a patient with pre-eclampsia, displaying the characteristic light-microscopic features of the glomerular lesion. The glomerulus is moderately enlarged, and the capillary lumina are bloodless and obstructed by hypertrophied intracapillary cells (H & E, × 520).

eclamptic nephropathy from the zonal patterns of other disorders, such as subcapsular ischaemic changes in hypertensive nephrosclerosis, or early juxtaglomerular localization in focal segmental glomerulosclerosis.

The most striking light-microscopic feature of the kidney in pre-eclampsia is the presence of diffusely enlarged and bloodless glomeruli (Figure 1). The increase in glomerular size, alone, does not differentiate this lesion from other hypertensive disorders; Sheehan and Lynch (1973), for example, noted a 10% increase in glomerular diameter when gestation was complicated by high blood pressure, irrespective of the underlying pathology. In pre-eclampsia, however, the most reactive glomeruli could be twice normal size.

The enlargement of the glomeruli in pre-eclampsia is characterized by the maintenance of normal amounts of stroma and cells. This feature distinguishes pre-eclamptic nephropathy from other conditions where glomerular enlargement due to increments in cells or matrix is observed, such as glomerulonephritis and diabetic glomerulopathy. It should be noted that some have claimed proliferation to be a feature of the pre-eclamptic lesion; however, evaluation of glomerular cellularity by various counting techniques reveals the absence of, or at best minimal, hypercellularity (Sheehan and Lynch, 1973).

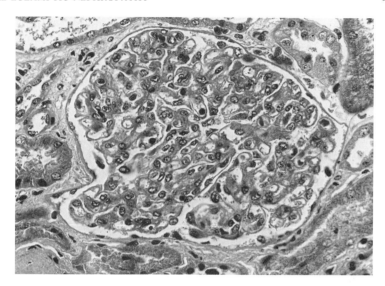

Figure 2. An example of an enlarged, bloodless glomerulus, typical of pre-eclamptic nephropathy. A few glomerular capillaries herniate for a short distance into the proximal tubule ('pouting') (H & E, × 550).

Closer inspection of the glomerulus in pre-eclampsia reveals the following. The enlarged glomerular tuft contains voluminous intracapillary and mesangial cells which alter the gross appearance of the capillary loops, another feature that aids in differentiating pre-eclampsia from other disorders. Some of the peripheral capillary loops acquire a 'cigar-shaped' configuration, having become longitudinally expanded by the swollen intracapillary cells. Still others, presumably at an early stage of the lesion, are distended with intracapillary fibrils and swollen cells, and have dilated tips (ballooning).

The expanded cellular elements may result in herniation of several capillary loops into the proximal tubule, a phenomenon labelled as 'pouting' (Figure 2). This is one of the most dramatic changes in the renal morphology of pre-eclamptics. Ischaemic changes, ballooning and foam cells appear to be more common in these herniated tufts than in the remainder of the glomerulus. It is important to note that 'pouting' itself is not pathognomonic for pre-eclampsia, and can be seen in other conditions where glomeruli are enlarged, especially in acute glomerulonephritis. In these latter diseases, however, the frequency of pouting is minimal, while in pre-eclampsia it occurs in 50% of the glomeruli, and in some instances the capillary loops herniate as much as 200 μm into the proximal tubule (although the mean is usually 30–50 μm) (Sheehan and Lynch, 1973).

'Stem laddering' and 'beading' are two other, albeit infrequent, alterations in loop pattern. They were originally described by Sheehan and Lynch in postpartum patients and probably represent a healing phase of pre-eclamptic nephropathy. The lesions are characterized by loops which are dilated and traversed by bands of fibrils intersecting the swollen endocapillary cells, giving a ladder-like appearance, or there may be sequential narrowing and dilatation of the loops like a string of beads (Sheehan and Lynch, 1973; Sheehan, 1980).

The hypertrophied endothelial cells and, to a lesser extent, mesangial cells contain more cytoplasmic particulate as well as a heterogeneous array of lipid-filled and fluid-filled vacuoles. This pattern of cytoplasmic changes is readily appreciated in osmium-fixed, toluidine blue-stained, 1 μ sections viewed by light microscopy (Taylor and Spargo, 1986). The cytoplasm of some of these cells becomes foamy, or can be largely displaced by the vacuoles, in which case grape-like clusters are observed. The 'foam cells' are similar to those present in 'lipoid nephrosis', and may relate to the occurrence in many pre-eclamptics of nephrotic-range proteinuria. Cholesterol clefts, situated within the stroma or in an intracellular location, may also be present, but are usually observed in biopsies performed later in the puerperium, suggesting that they are formed during the reparative phase of the lesion (Spargo et al, 1976).

The glomeruli in pre-eclamptic nephropathy are virtually obstructed, and appear devoid of red blood cells. In fact, 'bloodless glomeruli' are another major feature of pre-eclampsia, and are due to intracapillary cell hypertrophy as well as to peripheral interposition of mesangium, both of which encroach upon the capillary cell lumen. Despite this apparent obstruction of the glomerular capillaries, congested and even preinfarcted glomeruli may be seen, albeit rarely, in severely affected kidneys (Spargo et al, 1976).

These bloodless-looking glomeruli are of interest in view of the fact that renal haemodynamics are so well preserved in pre-eclampsia (Lindheimer and Katz, 1986). Glomerular filtration and renal plasma flow do decrease, but the decrements of 25–35% below values measured in normal gestation are still at or above non-pregnant levels. However, on rare occasions, pre-eclampsia has evolved into acute tubular and even cortical necrosis, developments more consistent with the lesions described above.

Although intravascular coagulation is implicated in the development of pre-eclampsia, intraglomerular thrombosis is infrequent in renal biopsies obtained from women with pure pre-eclampsia. When present, it is usually associated with a clinically severe case, especially where pre-eclampsia is superimposed on (or complicated by) other obstetrical and renal diseases, such as endotoxin shock, abruptio placentae or nephrosclerosis (Sheehan and Lynch, 1973).

As mentioned above, the mesangium is affected by pre-eclampsia, its cellular element demonstrating histologic alterations similar to those of endothelial cells. On occasion, the expanded mesangial matrix and enlarged mesangial cells extend out into the peripheral capillary loops, and become insinuated between the endothelial cells and basement membrane. This process of mesangial interposition leads to pseudothickening and splitting of the basement membrane, and is one reason why pre-eclampsia was previously mislabelled as a form of membranous nephropathy. Mesangial interposition was not a common feature in our earlier biopsy series (Fisher et al, 1981), but has been observed more often in biopsies performed after 1980, reflecting, perhaps, the fact that our experience is now skewed towards material from patients with very severe disease. This process of mesangial interposition, however, is described with even greater frequency by other investigators, and

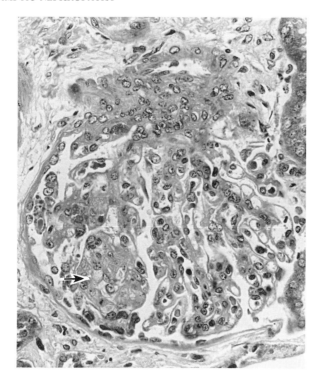

Figure 3. Renal biopsy from a pre-eclamptic woman. The endothelial and mesangial cells are not increased in number but are swollen, thus obstructing the capillary lumina. These features, though generalized within the glomerular tuft, are most pronounced segmentally and near foam cells (arrow). Note the large hyaline droplets in the epithelial cells (H & E, × 550).

is considered to contribute to the encroachment on the lumen of peripheral capillaries and to result in a 'double contoured' appearance of the basement membrane (Tribe et al, 1979; Kincaid-Smith, 1973; Sheehan and Lynch, 1973).

The role of epithelial cells is not clear, as most investigators (including ourselves) observe only non-specific changes that are probably related to proteinuria, including the presence of cytoplasmic, PAS-positive protein transport droplets (Figure 3). Epithelial cell proliferation as well as crescents have been observed in some unusually severe cases. These epithelial crescents, however, are more frequent in multigravidas and elderly primigravidas (Sheehan and Lynch, 1973; Sheehan, 1980), leading to speculation that they might be related to an underlying renal disease rather than pure pre-eclampsia (which typically affects young nullipara).

Kincaid-Smith et al (1986) have claimed that granulated visceral epithelial cells are specific for pre-eclamptic nephropathy and that the degree of granulation relates to disease severity and proteinuria. These authors have also equated these granulated epithelial cells with 'peripolar cells', suggesting they have a secretory role. We disagree.

Peripolar cells, described in the glomeruli of sheep are located in the hilum and contain abundant cytoplasmic granules. These cells, which may be related to the juxtaglomerular apparatus, apparently discharge their granules into the urinary space when the animal is subjected to sodium depletion (Hill et al, 1983). In contrast, the epithelial cell granules in pre-eclamptic nephropathy are spheroidal and lysosomal in nature, lacking any of the features of either normal secretory granules or those seen in certain forms of pathology (e.g. intraepithelial laminated inclusions in Fabry's disease) (Spargo et al, 1980).

The epithelial granules of pre-eclamptic nephropathy not only lack secretory features but resemble those observed in biopsies from patients with nephrotic syndrome irrespective of cause. Thus we believe the granules to be non-specific, and present in any disease where increased permeability of the filtration barrier to protein is present (protein overload), especially when accompanied by vasospasm and ischaemia. This may impair the ability of the visceral epithelium to transport protein, leading to the accumulation of large protein reabsorption droplets.

Extraglomerular lesions are not a feature of pre-eclamptic nephropathy and when present are non-specific. Tubulointerstitial changes appear related to the degree of proteinuria, as large protein transport droplets are formed in the proximal convoluted tubules in approximately 50% of cases. Fatty changes are rare, and when present are localized to a few tubules in a given biopsy. Tubular dilatation and flattening of the epithelial lining can occur in the most severe cases of pre-eclampsia.

The effects of pre-eclampsia on the renal vasculature are disputed. This is because investigators attempting to describe the pathology of these vessels are hindered by limitations of sampling, in which tissue from medium and large intrarenal arteries is present only occasionally. The nature and the significance of hyaline arteriolosclerosis (HA), observed on occasion in biopsies from young gravidas, has been disputed. This lesion is characterized by insudative trapping of a homogeneous, PAS-positive material in the wall of arterioles (Figure 4a). It is our experience that this intramural leakage of proteinaceous material indicates injury of the vessel wall and is seen in other conditions such as hypertensive nephrosclerosis, diabetic nephropathy and focal glomerulo-sclerosis (Spargo et al, 1980; Lee and Spargo, 1985). Unfortunately, it is still not clear if HA is caused by the acute hypertension associated with pre-eclampsia, or whether it is an indication of pre-existing hypertensive nephrosclerosis. Differentiation between these conditions is significant for the remote prognosis of pre-eclamptic patients. Contrary to the controversial significance of insudative trapping within the arterioles, the presence of intimal fibrosis and widening, reduplication of the elastic lamina, sclerosis of the media and lumen narrowing are undisputed features of hypertensive nephrosclerosis (Figure 4b). Endothelial cell changes similar to those seen in the glomeruli, with swelling and vacuolization of the cortical arterioles, have been described (Pollak and Nettles, 1960), but we have not seen such lesions In fact we consistently note that endothelial cell reactions stop abruptly at the junction of the afferent arterioles.

(a)

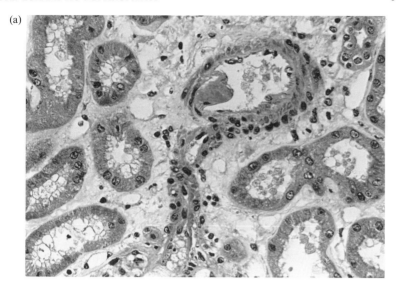

(b)

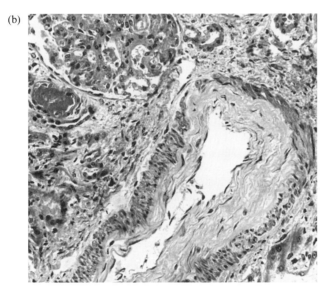

Figure 4. (a) An example of hyaline arteriolosclerosis, characterized by insudative trapping within the vessel wall (H & E, × 450). (b) Renal biopsy from a patient with pre-eclampsia superimposed on hypertensive nephrosclerosis. The interlobular artery is sclerotic. The intima is greatly expanded with increased amounts of stroma (H & E, × 550).

Medial hypertrophy of both renal and extrarenal vessels, which is a reversible lesion, is also reported in pre-eclamptic patients and could be an adaptation to the elevated blood pressure. Of importance is a report by

Aalkjaer et al (1985) correlating circulating angiotensin II (AII) levels, in vitro vascular reactivity and vascular morphology. These authors noted smooth-muscle hypertrophy in the omental vessels which were hyper-responsive to AII, concluding that the structural alteration was a consequence of the acute blood-pressure rise associated with pre-eclampsia.

An interesting group of patients with surprising findings on their renal biopsies has been described by Pollak and Nettles (1960), Smythe et al (1964), Peyser et al (1978) and Fisher et al (1981). The women tend to be quite young, usually black, and have a family history of hypertension. These patients, normotensive earlier in pregnancy, present late in gestation with high blood pressure, which often normalizes in the puerperium. Surprisingly, despite this clinical presentation, their renal biopsies may contain evidence of hyaline arteriosclerosis only, and although their blood pressure may normalize postpartum, those followed-up eventually develop essential hypertension (Peyser et al, 1978; Fisher et al, 1981). Thus it appears that nephrosclerosis can precede the development of frank hypertension in some instances. Also, these cases illustrate why authors must be careful when ascribing nephrosclerotic changes to the transient elevations of blood pressure during pre-eclampsia, especially when more advanced nephrosclerotic lesions are present (e.g. intimal and medial sclerosis, or reduplication of the internal elastica).

Whether or not pre-eclampsia affects the juxtaglomerular apparatus is controversial. Of interest is a report in which a decreased number of renin-containing cells (demonstrated by immunofluorescent techniques) were observed in postpartum renal biopsies from women with gestational hyper-tension (Nochy et al, 1984). The significance of this observation is limited, as a relatively small number of patients was biopsied and (for obvious reasons) there was no comparable material from subjects with normotensive ges-tations. Furthermore, these observations contrast with the older literature; Altchek et al (1968) observed that the number and size of the juxtaglomerular cells were increased, while the macula densa was small and atrophic. All the above findings, however, may be non-specific as the size and number of juxtaglomerular cells may be altered by several other glomerular and vascular diseases as well as by salt intake. The latter was not documented in any of the cited reports.

Electron microscopy

The characteristic features of pre-eclampsia are best demonstrated by electron microscopy, and the diagnosis can be uncertain if ultrastructural examination of the biopsy material is omitted. Farquahar (1959), Spargo et al (1959), Pirani et al (1963) and Faith and Trump (1966) were amongst the first to focus on the electron-microscopic interpretation of pre-eclamptic nephropathy. The major ultrastructural alterations of pre-eclamptic glomeruli are localized in the endothelial cells, and to a lesser extent in the mesangial cells (Figure 5). The cytoplasmic organelles are hypertrophied, particularly the lysosomes which undergo marked enlargement and vacuolization due to the accumu-lation of free neutral lipids (which, if associated with fluid, display sharp interfaces) (Figure 6). Myelin-like figures may be present, which if membrane-

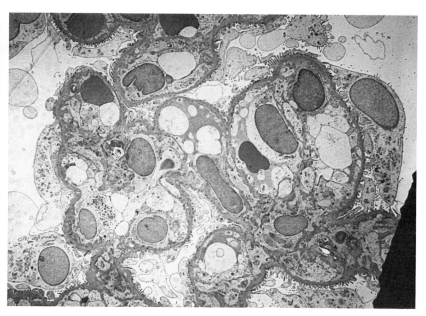

Figure 5. Electron micrograph of a renal biopsy demonstrating swelling and vacuolization of the intracapillary cells ('glomerular capillary endotheliosis'), causing obstruction of the capillary lumina. Clusters of intracytoplasmic lipid droplets are noted (upper right). Note that epithelial foot processes are preserved (× 6300).

bound are caused by phagocytosed phospholipids, but if free in the cytoplasm are due to prolonged fixation of the free neutral lipids. Occasionally cholesterol clefts are noted in the mesangium and the intracapillary cells, especially if the biopsy is performed after a considerable postpartum interval.

Cytoplasmic vacuolization has also been attributed to extensive folding of the cytoplasmic membrane producing multiple cytofolds and pseudovesicles (Faith and Trump, 1966). The endothelial fenestrae are inconspicuous due to the hypertrophied intracapillary cells, a process that may alter the filtration barrier. Intracytoplasmic fibrils may be present, but only occasionally (Spargo et al, 1959). These endothelial and mesangial cell changes are apparently reactive in nature rather than proliferative or degenerative, and thus were termed 'glomerular capillary endotheliosis' by Spargo et al (1959). 'Intracapillary cell swelling' in another term, best used to describe advanced lesions, especially when the cytoplasmic reactive changes are so marked that the origin of the obstructing cells can no longer be determined (Figure 7).

Spargo indicated that 'glomerular capillary endotheliosis' was unique and pathognomonic for pre-eclampsia, a view that has been challenged. Robson (1976), for example, stated that similar lesions occur in biopsies obtained from non-gravid subjects with a variety of glomerular diseases, as well as in essential hypertension; while Lopez-Llera and Rubio (1965) and Thompson et al (1972) have claimed that renal lesions similar to those of pre-eclampsia

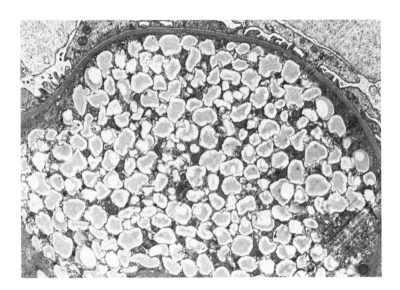

Figure 6. Electron micrograph depicting enlarged obstructing endothelial cells, containing numerous droplets of neutral fat which displace the cytoplasmic organelles (× 11 000).

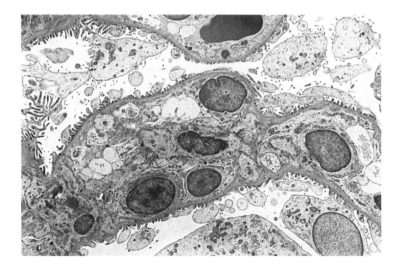

Figure 7. Electron micrograph from a patient with pre-eclampsia, demonstrating a 'cigar-shaped' capillary loop which is longitudinally expanded, and whose capillary lumen is bloodless and obstructed by hypertrophied intracapillary cells (× 7000).

were present in a number of normotensive patients presenting with abruptio placentae. In these latter cases, however, pre-eclampsia may have been masked by the massive bleeding characteristic of abruption. Also, in all these reports the extent and severity of these glomerular changes are certainly less than in pre-eclampsia. Finally, glomerular capillary endotheliosis has been observed in renal biopsies from hypertensive women with abdominal pregnancy (M.D. Lindheimer and B.H. Spargo unpublished data) and hydatidiform mole (Sanchez-Torres et al, 1965; Curry et al, 1975). However, these represent special forms of pre-eclampsia.

Another important ultrastructural feature is the presence of subendothelial and sometimes mesangial electron-dense deposits that are fibrillary or granular. The nature of this material is disputed; some authors claim it represents immune complexes, while we and others believe it represents fibrin or fibrinogen-related products. Our view is supported by immunologic studies demonstrating variable amounts of fibrin in pre-eclamptic glomeruli (Vassalli et al, 1963; Morris et al, 1964) and by the occasional demonstration of fibrin tactoids with their characteristic periodicity in the mesangium, and subendothelial and urinary spaces (Fisher et al, 1981). Additionally, several structural proteins of the basement membrane have been shown to be produced in excess and to accumulate along the basement membrane (Foidart et al, 1983).

Faith and Trump (1966), Kincaid-Smith (1973) and Seymour et al (1976) describe circumferential interposition of mesangial cell cytoplasm and mesangial matrix along the inner aspect of the glomerular basement membrane. This process, as mentioned previously, contributes to the 'double contour' appearance of the basement membrane which in itself is of normal thickness and texture. Extracellular and intracellular fibrils may be present, forming a coarse, intracellular network or thin lamina that runs parallel to the basement membrane (Spargo et al, 1959). This may be another reason why some describe a 'double contour' appearance. These fibrils are probably produced by the mesangial cells and are seen wedged between them and the endothelial cells. Although proteinuria is a consistent finding in pre-eclampsia and is often nephrotic in range, epithelial foot process effacement is infrequent, and when present it is focal and limited. Cytoplasmic changes similar to but less extensive than those seen in endothelial cells can be shown in epithelial cells as well.

Immunohistology

The goal of immunohistochemical studies is to identify the mesangial and subendothelial deposits and, by characterizing the components of these deposits, to elucidate the underlying pathogenetic mechanism. Unfortunately this has not been achieved in pre-eclampsia. Although a similar pattern of immunoglobulin and fibrin deposition is present in the material of most investigators, the frequency of these findings is inconsistent and the interpretation of their meaning controversial. Most of the disagreements revolve around the intensity and significance of IgM and IgG staining, as well as that of fibrin.

Table 2. Immunofluorescence in biopsies demonstrating glomerular endotheliosis

	Frequency of glomerular deposition	
	All cases	Greater than 1 +
Fibrin	20 of 45	8 of 45 (18%)
AHG*	5 of 10	1 of 10 (10%)
IgC	10 of 43	3 of 43 (7%)
IgM	23 of 45	16 of 45 (36%)
IgA	6 of 43	2 of 43 (5%)
IgE	9 of 36	2 of 36 (6%)
C3	8 of 40	1 of 40 (3%)
C4	15 of 36	10 of 36 (28%)

* Antihaemophilic globulin.
From Fisher KA, Luger A, Spargo BH, and Lindheimer MD (1981) Hypertension in pregnancy: clinical-pathological correlations and late prognosis. *Medicine* **60:** 267–276. Reproduced with permission of Williams and Wilkins.

Petrucco et al (1974) observed IgM in the peripheral capillaries and mesangium in the glomeruli of biopsies from pre-eclamptic patients. IgG was present in most instances, while complement was detected in the afferent arterioles of severe cases. Seymour et al (1976) reported diffuse peripheral granular IgM frequently associated with the complement components C3 and C1q. Both groups of investigators interpreted their findings as evidence of activation of the classic complement pathway in a manner similar to immune complex trapping in glomerulonephritis. Seymour also noted decreased levels of C3 in sera obtained from hypertensive gravidas, further evidence in support of his theory. However, non-specific fixation of plasma proteins, or localized non-specific activation of complement during the course of intravascular coagulation, are alternative explanations for the complement deposition. In addition, decrements in C3 levels are not customarily observed in pre-eclampsia. The view that pre-eclampsia might be an immunologically triggered disease has recently been revived, however, by Foidart and his colleagues (1986), who have observed circulating antibodies to laminin in the blood of pre-eclamptic subjects.

Table 2 summarizes our observations (Fisher et al, 1981) concerning the incidence and role of immunoglobulins in pre-eclampsia. IgG was present in only 10 of 43 biopsies, and in only 3 was the intensity of staining greater than 1 +. IgM was present more often (23 of 45 biopsies) but stained 2 + or higher in only 36% of the cases. Ultrastructurally, electron-dense deposits were quite infrequent, which is not what would be anticipated if the observed fluorescence represented immune deposits. In our opinion immunoglobulins were more likely to be present in the kidneys of the most severely pre-eclamptic women, especially those with heavy proteinuria, an observation consistent with an insudative origin for these findings.

Vassalli et al (1963) were among the first to observe fibrin or fibrin-like material in the renal biopsies of pre-eclamptic women, findings present in all their material. This led them to suggest that fibrin may initiate the swelling of the glomerular cells. In support of this, Fisher et al (1969) demonstrated ferritin in biopsies from pre-eclamptic women, suggesting a haematogenous derivation of the subendothelial, electron-dense deposits via a process of intravascular coagulation. Petrucco et al (1974) and Seymour et al (1976) also observed glomerular fibrin in all the biopsies from pre-eclamptic women. Our data do not confirm these findings and thus do not support an aetiological role for fibrin in the genesis of the pre-eclamptic lesion. For instance, fibrin-like material was demonstrated by immunofluorescence in only 20 of 45 biopsies, and stained greater than 1 + in only 8 of them (Table 2). Antihaemophilic globulin staining was sought for in 10 biopsies and was present in 5 of them, only 1 staining over 1 +. Moreover, both fibrin and anti-haemophilic globulin were present in material from women without pre-eclampsia, but whose biopsies had changes consistent with nephrosclerosis. Our immunologic findings are also consistent with the low frequency of fibrin-like tactoids and electron-dense deposits in the biopsies of all 96 patients with glomerular endotheliosis only (Fisher et al, 1981). Reasons why our findings disagree with others—but not with all: see Fisher et al (1981)—are not clear; one possibility is that we may have biopsied women with a broader spectrum of disease, while other investigators have focused on a population with more severe disorders, including heavy proteinuria and overt coagulation defects.

Matrix proteins and structural components of the glomerular basement membrane such as laminin, fibronectin, type IV collagen and proteoglycan may also be detected by immunohistological techniques (Foidart et al, 1983). Under normal conditions, type IV collagen, located mainly in the mesangium and lamina densa of the basement membranes, forms the scaffolding of the glomerular matrix; while laminin, a glycoprotein present in both the mesangial and subendothelial regions, facilitates adhesion of the epithelial and endothelial cells to the type IV collagen. Fibronectin, located almost exclusively in the mesangial matrix, may have a regulatory role in the production of collagen by epithelial or mesangial cells.

In pre-eclampsia there is an increase in the density of staining for all the proteins described above. Also, fibronectin staining is present in the basement membrane, as well as in the mesangium. Foidart et al (1983) also noted that fibronectin and fibrinogen had similar distribution patterns. This finding of excess production of glomerular matrix proteins may explain observations such as the narrowing of capillary lumina, inconsistent basement membrane thickening and altered basement membrane permeability. The structural proteins, especially fibronectin, may also relate to certain subendothelial and mesangial deposits described by various investigators. These interesting findings by Foidart et al (1983) require confirmation.

Focal segmental glomerulosclerosis and pre-eclampsia

Recently, several investigators have described focal segmental glomerulo-sclerosis (FSGS) in association with pre-eclampsia, suggesting that FSGS was a consequence of the latter disease (Heaton, 1985; Kida et al, 1985; Nochy et al, 1986a, 1986b). If this were true it would alter the benign prognostic implication of pure pre-eclampsia (see below) and might suggest that clinicians have not been sufficiently aggressive in controlling the rise in blood pressure, or have utilized antihypertensive agents that failed to decrease glomerular pressure, which might conceivably be high during this disease. The importance of these issues led us to re-evaluate our most recent biopsy experience (Gaber and Spargo, 1987).

In a study designed to investigate associations between FSGS and pre-eclampsia, we reviewed 20 consecutive postpartum biopsies performed for hypertension complicating pregnancy. This group differed from our series of 176 cases spanning 1958 to 1976 and published by us in 1981 (Fisher et al, 1981). In essence, criteria had changed; starting during the late 1970s renal biopsies were only performed on 'atypical' and 'severe' cases, while the original 1958–76 group represented a more heterogeneous population. In reviewing our material we specifically searched for focal segmental glomerulosclerosis in pre-eclampsia, attempting to derive its clinical significance. We therefore step-sectioned the biopsies and reviewed an average of 20 glomeruli per patient in a specific attempt to document FSGS. Our data are summarized in Table 3. In this group of women with severe disease, 7 of 20 biopsies (35%) disclosed some evidence of focal segmental glomerulosclerosis involving a few lobules of glomeruli (Figure 8). These glomeruli demonstrated segmental collapse of the peripheral capillary loops, sclerosis and folding of the basement membrane, decreased number of endothelial and mesangial cells and expansion of the mesangial matrix. Epithelial cell proliferation was present in 4 out of the 7 biopsies. An intriguing finding was the presence of arteriolosclerosis in 5 of the 7 cases (71%), and tubular loss and interstitial condensation in the other 2. Tubular atrophy and interstitial fibrosis were also evident in this material, indirect evidence of a chronic injury antedating the 'pre-eclamptic' complication. Another atypical feature was the presence of epithelial crescents in 4 of these 7 biopsies. This persistent occurrence of vascular lesions when FSGS was seen, classified this group as suffering from hypertensive nephrosclerosis, and suggests that focal segmental glomerulosclerosis is not a feature of pure pre-eclampsia, but an indicator of underlying nephrosclerosis.

Our data suggest, therefore, that FSGS when present antedated pregnancy or was due to haemodynamic factors earlier in gestation (e.g. hyperfiltration and hypertension of another aetiology, the latter associated with increased glomerular pressure). Our own studies (Fisher et al, 1981) concerning the remote prognosis of pre-eclampsia support this view. As discussed later in this chapter, on re-examination the incidence of remote hypertension in women whose renal biopsies contained lesions of glomerular intracapillary swelling only, was no different than that expected in the population at large. In contrast, most of those with nephrosclerosis, with or without superimposed pre-eclampsia, had developed sustained hypertension. It should be borne in mind, however, that all these conclusions are based on selective data, and considerably more research is required to resolve the postulated relationship between FSGS and pre-eclampsia.

Table 3. Clinical pathological correlations in 20 women with pre-eclamptic gestations.

Patient	Age	Race	Parity	Onset of hypertension (gestational week)	Indication for renal biopsy	Biopsy performed (postpartum day)	Total number of glomeruli	PIN	FSG	Global sclerosis	Cellular crescents	Tubulo-interstitial changes	Vascular lesions
1	28	B	M	32	Severe pre-eclampsia (HELLP syndrome)—persistent postpartum hypertension	15	3	+	—	—	—	—	—
2	27	W	M	25	Early onset of severe pre-eclampsia with HELLP syndrome	11	17	++	—	6%	—	+	++
3	26	B	M	32	Hypertension with marked nephrotic proteinuria	10	26	++	8%	8%	—	+	++
4	32	B	M	28	Early onset of severe pre-eclampsia	7	29	++	—	—	—	+	—
5	19	B	N	34	Persistent postpartum hypertension	11	33	++	7%	—	9%	+	++
6	19	W	M	34	Eclampsia and persistent postpartum hypertension	7	20	++	4%	—	4%	+	+
7	20	B	N	29	Early onset of pre-eclampsia	6	37	++	—	—	—	—	—
8	30	W	N	33	Persistent postpartum hypertension	21	4	++	—	—	—	—	—
9*	18	B	N	19	Early onset of pre-eclampsia and eclampsia	5	66	+++	2%	3%	—	+	NA
10*	19	B	M	24	Early onset of severe pre-eclampsia	8	113	++	—	—	—	+	+
11	22	B	M	22	Early onset of severe pre-eclampsia	10	17	+	—	—	—	—	—
12	21	B	N	33	Persistent postpartum hypertension	6	19	—	—	—	—	—	—
13	18	B	N	32	Severe pre-eclampsia	5	5	++	10%	—	20%	+	NA
14	25	B	N	28	Early onset of nephrotic syndrome and hypertension	7	50	+++	—	—	—	—	—
15	18	B	N	37	Postpartum hypertension and seizures in a diabetic patient	9	30	+	—	—	—	—	—
16	15	B	M	28	Early onset pre-eclampsia	6	13	++	—	8%	—	—	+
17	18	B	M	32	Severe hypertension and nephrotic proteinuria	5	20	++	—	—	—	+	+
18	23	B	M	27	Early onset of severe pre-eclampsia	6	20	+++	10%	—	—	—	+
19	36	W	N	34	Persistent postpartum hypertension and nephrotic range proteinuria	4	36	++	10%	—	10%	+	+
20	17	B	N	39	Persistent postpartum hypertension	7	20	+	—	—	—	—	+

Abbreviations: B = black; W = caucasian; N = nullipara; M = multipara; HELLP syndrome = acronym for haemolysis, elevated liver enzymes and low platelet counts; PIN = pregnancy-induced nephropathy (i.e. pre-eclampsia changes only: glomerular capillary swelling +, ++, +++ = mild, moderate and severe respectively); NA = inadequate material for diagnosis. *Patients 9 and 10 are the same woman biopsied after successive hypertensive gestations. From Gaber and Spargo (1987) with permission.

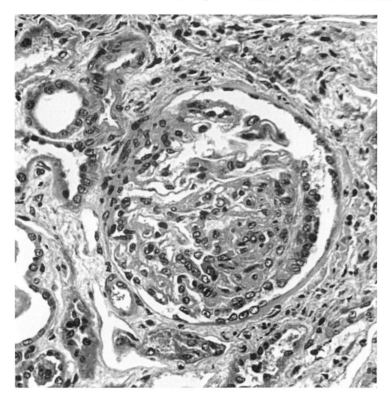

Figure 8. Photomicrograph of a glomerulus displaying segmental collapse of the peripheral capillaries and sclerosis. Note also proliferation of visceral and capsular epithelium (H & E, × 550).

Pre-eclampsia and the thrombotic microangiopathies

There are variants of pre-eclampsia (for example, the 'HELLP' syndrome; an acronym for haemolysis, elevated liver enzymes and low platelet count) which may be difficult to differentiate from several other aggressive thrombotic microangiopathies, such as thrombotic thrombocytopaenic purpura (TTP) and the haemolytic uraemic syndrome (HUS). Some link these diseases together aetiologically, even suggesting similar renal pathology. We do not agree with the latter contention.

In TTP (which may be a unique systemic disease, or associated with other entities such as systemic lupus erythematosus) microthrombi are found in biopsy material from many organs, as well as the kidney (Ambrose et al, 1985). Arteriolar lumina are obstructed by fibrin–platelet thrombi, often associated with segmental aneurysmal dilatation of the vessel wall and substantial fibrin deposition. In contrast, pre-eclampsia is characterized by predominantly, if not exclusively, glomerular lesions. Also, intraglomerular thrombi are infrequent, usually observed when biopsies are performed in patients with severe disease (Spargo et al, 1980).

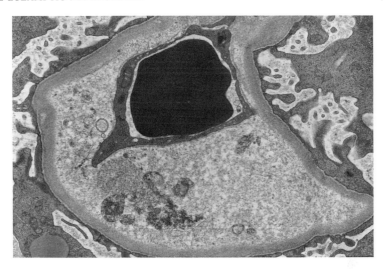

Figure 9. Electron micrograph of a renal biopsy from a woman with haemolytic uraemic syndrome. The endothelial cell is 'blistered off' and the subendothelial space is expanded by the accumulation of debris (× 20 000).

The histopathology of HUS is also quite different from pre-eclamptic nephropathy. In the former disease the primary lesion is insudation of fibrin and red cells, with or without thrombosis. Renal lesions in HUS are classified as arteriolar, glomerular or a combination of both. Distinction between these subtypes is of prognostic importance. Women with arterial thrombotic microangiopathy do poorly, while glomerular subtypes are associated with a virtually 100% recovery rate (Loirat et al, 1984). The intrarenal arteries are obstructed due to intimal proliferation, as well as to intramural haemorrhage, or to intimal and subintimal fibrin deposition. Mucoid degeneration and necrosis of the vessel wall is seen occasionally, and is usually associated with severe disease.

Aneurysmal dilatation of the afferent arterioles, similar to that described in TTP, is a feature of the renal lesion in HUS. This is occasionally accompanied by endothelial cell proliferation, a process which may result in the formation of 'glomeruloid bodies'. Other lesions include decreased glomerular vascularity, intraglomerular thrombi, segmental collapse and, on occasion, epithelial crescents.

The most impressive glomerular feature of HUS, which is best demonstrated ultrastructurally, is the pronounced widening of the subendothelial space, a phenomenon that causes blistering of the endothelium (Figure 9). Fibrin tactoids, proteinaceous debris, granular deposits and red blood cells all accumulate in the spaces underneath the elevated endothelium. On occasion, endothelial swelling may be observed; but the vacuolization, as well as lipid accumulation and cytofolds, are never as florid as in pre-eclamptic nephropathy. Although the subendothelial space may be widened in pre-eclampsia, the extent of this widening is not as severe as that seen in HUS, which we have previously characterized as 'blister formation'. Finally, and of importance to the differential diagnosis, pathology in pre-eclampsia is limited to the glomeruli; lesions stop abruptly at the junction between the glomerulus and the preglomerular arterioles.

Evaluation and reversibility of the renal lesion

The natural history of pre-eclamptic nephropathy, as well as questions of its reversibility and/or residual lesions, are incompletely understood, as shown by the controversy concerning FSGS and pre-eclampsia discussed above. This is because only limited information is provided by serial biopsies, and most other information was obtained by evaluating the renal lesion in relation to the onset of proteinuria. Furthermore, as late as 1987, there were no known animal models with kidney pathology resembling pre-eclampsia in humans.

Sheehan and Lynch (1973) attempted to correlate the lesion with the onset of abnormal proteinuria, noting that 'glomerular lesions', including intracapillary cell swelling, intraglomerular fibril formation and ballooning of the capillary loops, seemed to occur one to one-and-a-half days after the appearance of increased urinary protein excretion. Proximal tubular cells containing hyaline droplets were also seen at this time. Herniation of the glomerular tuft (pouting) and foam cells were more apt to be present in specimens obtained three to five days after the proteinuria was detected, while glomerular ectasia, congestion and infarction, as well as crescents, were late and unusual phenomena, usually occurring when the disease had been present one week or more. These estimates, however, are both crude and suspect. First, the initial glomerular pathology most likely predated the development of proteinuria and there may have been a variable period of 'microalbuminuria'; that is, excretion of abnormal quantities of albumin when qualitative and quantitative proteinuria were still at values considered normal. In general, however, it appears that the glomerular lesions accentuate if the disease is permitted to continue.

Reversibility of pre-eclamptic nephropathy

Healing begins within 48 hours after delivery and complete resolution of the glomerular lesions is said by some to occur by four to five weeks postpartum (Fadel et al, 1969; Sheehan and Lynch, 1973; Oe et al, 1986). Others have claimed that in some cases periods as long as six months are necessary (Dennis et al, 1968; Furukawa et al, 1983). Studies of remote cardiovascular prognosis of women who had eclampsia, or who had biopsy evidence of pure pre-eclampsia (discussed below), support the view that pre-eclamptic lesions are completely reversible (Bryans, 1966; Chesley, 1980). Others have questioned the benign nature of pre-eclamptic nephropathy, reporting lesions such as lobular hyalinization, capsular adhesions (Sheehan and Lynch, 1973) and persistent basement-membrane thickening (Pollak et al, 1956). Aber (1978) and Burden et al (1979) have described radiologic evidence of structural and functional changes in the interlobar, lobar and arcuate arteries in the kidneys of patients with gestational hypertension examined three months following delivery. This group of patients had had severe pre-eclampsia, often of the early onset variety. Interestingly, however, renal biopsies had failed to show morphologic lesions in the cortical vessels. Aber (1978) speculated that his observations represented complications of severe pre-eclampsia. However, the possibility that these alterations had in fact antedated the pregnancy could not be excluded. That this might have been so is suggested by the fact that 50% of his patients later developed hypertension, which is an incidence approaching that noted by us in patients with pre-existing nephrosclerosis who had superimposed pre-eclampsia.

REMOTE PROGNOSIS

This section explores the remote prognosis of pre-eclampsia–eclampsia—and again we meet controversy. One view is that pre-eclamptics have an increased incidence of cardiorenal disorders later in life, related perhaps to the duration of the disease in pregnancy. Certainly, those who have proposed recently that pre-eclampsia is a cause of FSGS would favour such a view. Others disagree, claiming that the remote cardiovascular prognosis of women who had pre-eclampsia is benign, and that those who manifested hypertensive cardiovascular disorders later in life were destined to develop essential hypertension anyway. The validity of the second view seems to have been established by Bryans and Torpin (1949; Bryans, 1966) and Chesley et al (1976; Chesley, 1978), the latter group having performed one of the most thorough epidemiologic surveys ever published. Dr Chesley and his associates periodically examined 267 of 270 women surviving eclampsia during the years 1931 to 1951; the last examination of those still alive was reported in 1976. Thus the clinical course of some of these women was followed for as long as 40 years after their eclamptic episode (Chesley et al, 1976). It should be noted here that in the absence of renal biopsy, a survey of eclamptics (women who convulsed) is very likely to yield a population likely to have had pure or superimposed pre-eclampsia, thus obviating the problems of diagnosis based on clinical criteria alone.

Chesley observed that the remote mortality in white patients who convulsed as nulliparas was not greater than that of age-matched, unselected women, whereas white multiparas who convulsed had a remote mortality two to five times that expected. The prevalence of later hypertension was increased in those who had been eclamptic as multigravidas, and this increment seemed to account for their higher death rate. In contrast the prevalence of high blood pressure, or the distribution of systolic and diastolic levels in women eclamptic as nulliparas, was also similar to those reported in several large epidemiologic surveys. In addition, women eclamptic as nulliparas, but who manifested high blood pressure in one or more subsequent gestations, had a higher prevalence of remote hypertension than the nulliparous eclamptics who remained normotensive in all later pregnancies. The authors therefore concluded that eclampsia is neither a predictive sign nor is it a cause of essential hypertension, and suggested that women eclamptic as multiparas were more apt to have *both* pre-eclampsia–eclampsia and latent essential hypertension—the latter responsible for their prognosis later in life. Similar conclusions were reached by Bryans and Torpin (1949; Bryans, 1966), who studied a large group of black women with eclampsia.

Others (references cited in Chesley, 1978; Fisher et al, 1981) who have observed an increased incidence of remote hypertension in 'toxaemic' women have criticized the conclusions of Chesley and Bryans and their respective colleagues, stating that such studies use reference populations and fail to survey 'control groups' of normotensive gravidas. Chesley, however, has responded that because pregnancy often induces transient increments in the blood pressure of initially normotensive women destined to have essential hypertension later in life, the choice of only normotensive gravidas as controls creates a population with an abnormally low remote incidence of high blood pressure. If such were the case, then eclamptics (who are presumably a less selected population) would always demonstrate more hypertension when re-examined years later in life.

Our own studies support Chesley's thesis (Fisher et al, 1981). We re-examined 53 biopsy-proved pre-eclamptic black gravidas an average of 68 months after their index pregnancies, and found their incidence of high blood pressure (9%) to be similar to an age-matched and race-matched group of women selected from the survey of the National Institutes of Health. Each pre-eclamptic patient was also compared with a woman matched for age, race and parity, whose normotensive gestation occurred within six months of the index pre-eclamptic's pregnancy. The latter group had an incidence of remote hypertension that was abnormally lower than the biopsied pre-eclamptics or the population at large. Thus, restricting comparisons to women normotensive during pregnancy only would have led to the erroneous conclusion that pre-eclamptics have a higher incidence of remote hypertension. In fact, normotension throughout one or more pregnancies suggests that a woman is apt to remain normotensive for life.

SUMMARY

Pre-eclampsia affects the kidney both functionally and morphologically. Renal haemodynamics decrease and urinary protein excretion increases, in part due to lesions affecting the glomerulus, where a combination of changes produces a characteristic appearance and permits differentiation of pre-eclamptic nephropathy from other glomerular alterations associated with hypertension in pregnancy. In pre-eclampsia the glomerulus is diffusely enlarged and bloodless, due not to proliferation, but to hypertrophy of the intracapillary cells. These alterations, best described ultrastructurally, include hypertrophy of the cytoplasmic organelles in endothelial and occasionally mesangial cells, particularly the lysosomes, which undergo marked enlargement and vacuolization (due to accumulation of free neutral lipids). These reactive changes have been termed 'glomerular capillary endotheliosis'. Other lesions, observed occasionally, include subendothelial and mesangial elec-tron-dense deposits, as well as interposition of mesangial cell cytoplasm or mesangial matrix along an otherwise normal basement membrane.

Some investigators have described immunohistologic findings (presence of IgM, IgG and fibrin) which they believe specific for pre-eclampsia, and others have claimed the disease may cause focal segmental glomerulosclerosis (FSGS). We believe the immunohistologic findings are non-specific and insudative, and that FSGS when present predates the pre-eclamptic complica-tion. Finally, the renal lesions appear fully reversible and the disease has no remote cardiorenal effects on its patients.

Acknowledgements

We thank Mrs Penny Papadatos and Mrs LeDung Ray for their excellent secretarial help. Some of the work described here was supported by grants from the National Institutes of Health (HD5575, RR55, as well as a Career Investigator Award to B.H.S.) and the American Heart Association.

REFERENCES

Aalkjaer C, Danielsen H & Johannesen P (1985) Abnormal vascular function in pre-eclampsia: a study of isolated resistance vessels. *Clinical Science* **69:** 477–482.

Aber GM (1978) Intrarenal vascular lesions associated with pre-eclampsia. *Nephron* **21:** 297–309.

Allen AC (1962) *The Kidney: Medical & Surgical Diseases.* New York: Grune & Stratton.

Altchek A, Albright NL & Sommers SC (1968) The renal pathology of toxaemia of pregnancy. *Obstetrics and Gynecology* **31:** 595–607.

Ambrose A, Welham RT & Cefalo RC (1985) Thrombotic thrombocytopenic purpura in early pregnancy. *Obstetrics and Gynecology* **66:** 267–272.

Bell ET (1932) Renal lesions in the toxemias of pregnancy. *American Journal of Pathology* **8:** 1–41.

Bryans Jr CI (1966) The remote prognosis of toxemia of pregnancy. *Clinics in Obstetrics and Gynecology* **9:** 973–990.

Bryans Jr CI & Torpin R (1949) A follow-up study of two hundred forty-three cases of eclampsia for an average of twelve years. *American Journal of Obstetrics and Gynecology* **58:** 1054–1065.

Burden RP, Boyd WN & Aber GM (1979) Structural and functional changes in the renal circulation after complicated pregnancy. *Nephron* **24:** 183–192.

Chesley LC (1978) *Hypertensive Disorders in Pregnancy.* New York: Appleton-Century-Crofts.

Chesley LC (1980) Hypertension in pregnancy: definitions, familial factors and remote prognosis. *Kidney International* **18:** 234–240.

Chesley LC, Annitto JE & Cosgrove RA (1976) Long-term follow-up study of eclamptic women, sixth periodic report. *American Journal of Obstetrics and Gynecology* **124:** 446–459.

Curry SL, Hammond CB, Tyrey L, Creasman WT & Parker RT (1975) Hydatidiform mole: diagnosis, management and long-term follow-up of 347 patients. *Obstetrics and Gynecology* **45:** 1–8.

Dennis EJ, McIver FA & Smythe CM (1968) Renal biopsy in pregnancy. *Clinics in Obstetrics and Gynecology* **11:** 473–486.

Dieckmann WM, Potter EL & McCartney CP (1957) Renal biopsies from patients with toxemia of pregnancy. *American Journal of Obstetrics and Gynecology* **73:** 1–16.

Fadel HE, Sabour MS, Mahram M, Seif El-Din D & El-Mahalawi MN (1969) Reversibility of the renal lesion and functional impairment in pre-eclampsia diagnosis by renal biopsy. *Obstetrics and Gynecology* **33:** 528–534.

Fahr T (1920) Uber Neirenveranderunger bei Eklampsie. *Zentralblatt Für Gynakologie* **44:** 991–993.

Faith GC, & Trump BE (1966) The glomerular capillary wall in human kidney disease, acute glomerulonephritis, systemic lupus erythematosus, pre-eclampsia-eclampsia. *Laboratory Investigation* **15:** 1682–1719.

Farquahar M (1959) Review of normal and pathologic glomerular ultrastructures. *Proceedings of the Tenth Annual Conference on the Nephrotic Syndrome*. New York: National Kidney Disease Foundation.

Fisher ER, Pardo V, Paul R & Hayashi TT (1969). Ultrastructural studies in hypertension. IV Toxemia of pregnancy. *American Journal of Surgical Pathology* **55:** 109–131.

Fisher KA, Luger A, Spargo BH & Lindheimer MD (1981) Hypertension in pregnancy: Clinical-pathological correlations and late prognosis. *Medicine* **60:** 267–276.

Foidart JM, Nochy D, Nusgens B et al (1983) Accumulation of several basement membrane proteins in glomeruli of patients with pre-eclampsia and other hypertensive syndromes of pregnancy: Possible roles of renal prostaglandin and fibronectin. *Laboratory Investigation* **49:** 250–259.

Foidart JM, Hunt J, Lapiere CM et al (1986) Antibodies to laminin in preeclampsia. *Kidney International* **29:** 1050–1057.

Furukawa T, Shigematsu H, Aizawa T, Oguchi H & Furuta S (1983) Residual glomerular lesions in postpartal women with toxemia of pregnancy. *Acta Pathologica Japonica* **33:** 1159–1169.

Gaber LW & Spargo BH (1987) Pregnancy induced nephropathy: the significance of focal segmental glomerulosclerosis. *American Journal of Kidney Disease* **9:** 317–323.

Heaton JM (1985) Persistent renal damage following pre-eclampsia. A renal biopsy study of 13 patients. *Journal of Pathology* **147:** 121–126.

Hill PA, Coghlan JP, Scoggins BA & Ryan GB (1983) Ultrastructural changes in the sheep renal juxtaglomerular apparatus in response to sodium depletion or loading. *Pathology* **15:** 463–473.

Ihle BU, Long P & Oats J (1987) Early onset pre-eclampsia: recognition of underlying renal disease. *British Medical Journal* **294:** 79–81.

Kida H, Takeda S, Yokoyama H, Tomosugi N, Abe T & Hattori N (1985) Focal segmental glomerulosclerosis in pre-eclampsia. *Clinical Nephrology* **24:** 221–227.

Kincaid-Smith PS (1973) The similarity of lesions and underlying mechanisms in pre-eclampsia-toxemia and post partum renal failure. In Kincaid-Smith P, Mathew TH & Becker EL (eds) *Glomerulonephritis: Morphology, Natural History and Treatment*, pp 1013–1025. New York: John Wiley.

Kincaid-Smith PS, North RA, Becker GJ & Fairley FK (1986) Proteinuria during pregnancy. In Andreucci VE (ed.) *The Kidney in Pregnancy*, pp 133–164. Boston: Martinus Nijhoff.

Lee HS & Spargo BH (1985) Significance of renal hyaline arteriosclerosis in focal segmental glomerulosclerosis. *Nephron* **41:** 86–93.

Lindheimer MD & Katz AI (1986) The kidney in pregnancy. In Brenner BM & Rector FC (eds) *The Kidney*, 3rd edn, pp 1253–1295. Philadelphia: WB Saunders.

Lohlein M (1918) Zur Pathogense der Neirenkrankheiten; nephritis und nephrose mit besonderer Berücksichtigung der Nephropathia gravidarum. *Deutsche Medizinische Wochenschrift* **44:** 1187–1189.

Loirat C, Sonsino E & Varga Moreno A (1984) Hemolytic uremic syndrome: an analysis of the natural history and prognostic features. *Acta Pediatrica Scandinavica* **73:** 505–514.

Lopez-Llera M & Rubio G (1965) Severe abruptio placentae, toxemia of pregnancy and renal biopsy. A clinicopathologic study. *American Journal of Obstetrics and Gynecology* **93:** 1144–1150.

McManus JFA (1950) *Medical Diseases of the Kidney*, pp 103–109. Philadelphia: Lea & Febiger.

Morris RH, Vassalli P, Beller F & McCluskey R (1964) Immunofluorescent studies of renal biopsies in the diagnosis of toxemia of pregnancy. *Obstetrics and Gynecology* **24:** 32–46.

Nochy D, Bariety J, Camilieri JP, Barres D, Carvol P & Menard J (1984) Diminished number of renin-containing cells in kidney biopsy samples from hypertensive women immediately postpartum: an immunomorphologic study. *Kidney International* **26:** 85–87.

Nochy D, Gaudry C, Hinglais Rouchen M & Bariety J (1986a) Can focal segmental glomerulosclerosis appear in preeclampsia? *Advances in Nephrology* **15:** 71–85.

Nochy D, Hinglais N, Jacquot C et al (1986b) *De novo* focal glomerular sclerosis in preeclampsia. *Clinical Nephrology* **25:** 116–121.

Oe PL, Ooms ECM, Uttendorjsky OT et al (1980) Postpartum resolution of glomerular changes in edema-proteinuria-hypertension gestosis. *Renal Physiology* **3:** 375–379.

Petrucco OM, Thompson NM, Laurence JR & Weldon MV (1974) Immunofluorescent studies in renal biopsy in preeclampsia. *British Medical Journal* **1:** 473–476.

Peyser MR, Toaff R, Leiserowitz DM, Avirm A & Griffen B (1978) Late follow-up in women with nephrosclerosis diagnosed at pregnancy. *American Journal of Obstetrics and Gynecology* **132:** 480–485.

Pirani CL, Pollak VE, Lannigan R & Folli G (1963) The renal glomerular lesions of pre-eclampsia: electron microscopic studies. *American Journal of Obstetrics and Gynecology* **87:** 1047–1070

Pollak VE & Nettles JB (1960) The kidney in toxemia of pregnancy; a clinical and pathological study based on renal biopsies. *Medicine* **39:** 469–526.

Pollak VE, Pirani CL & Kark RM (1956) Reversible glomerular lesions in toxemia of pregnancy. *Lancet* **ii:** 59–62.

Robson JS (1976) Proteinuria and the renal lesion in preeclampsia and abruptio placentae. In Lindheimer MD, Katz AI & Zuspan FS (eds) *Hypertension in Pregnancy*, pp 61–73. New York: John Wiley.

Sanchez-Torres F, Santamaria A, Rocha H & Gomez JA (1965) Renal changes in hydatidiform mole with toxemia. *American Journal of Obstetrics and Gynecology* **92:** 498–505.

Seymour AE, Petrucco OM, Clarkson AR et al (1976) Morphological evidences of coagulopathy in renal complications of pregnancy. In Lindheimer MD, Katz AI & Zuspan FS (eds) *Hypertension in Pregnancy*, pp 139–153. New York: John Wiley.

Sheehan HL (1950) Pathologic lesions in the hypertensive toxaemias of pregnancy. In Hammond J, Browne FJ & Wolenstenholm GEW (eds) *Toxaemias of Pregnancy, Human and Veterinary*, Philadelphia: Blackiston.

Sheehan HL (1980) Renal morphology in pre-eclampsia. *Kidney International* **18:** 241–252.

Sheehan HL & Lynch JB (1973) *Pathology of Toxaemia of Pregnancy*. Baltimore: Williams & Wilkins.

Smythe CM, Bradham WS, Dennis EJ, McIver FA & Howe HG (1964) *Journal of Laboratory and Clinical Investigation* **63:** 562–573.

Spargo BH, McCartney C & Winemiller R (1959) Glomerular capillary endotheliosis in toxemia of pregnancy. *Archives of Pathology* **13:** 593–599.

Spargo BH, Lichtig C, Luger AM, Katz AI & Lindheimer MD (1976) The renal lesion in pre-eclampsia. In Lindheimer MD, Katz AI & Zuspan FD (eds) *Hypertension in Pregnancy*, pp 129–137. New York: John Wiley.

Spargo BH, Seymour AE & Ordonez NG (1980) *Renal Pathology with Diagnostic and Therapeutic Implications*. New York: John Wiley.

Taylor J & Spargo BH (1986) Pathology of the kidney in pre-eclampsia. In Andreucci VE (ed.) *The Kidney in Pregnancy*, pp 47–63. Boston: Martinus Nijhoff.

Thompson D, Peterson WG, Smart GE, MacDonald M & Robson JS (1972) The renal lesions of toxaemia and abruptio placentae studied by light and electron microscopy. *Journal of Obstetrics and Gynaecology of the British Commonwealth* **79:** 311–320.

Tribe CR, Smart GE, Daurics DR & Mackenzie JC (1979) A renal biopsy study in toxaemia of pregnancy. *Journal of Clinical Pathology* **32:** 681–692.

Vassalli P, Morris RH & McCluskey RT (1963) The pathogenic role of fibrin deposition in the glomerular lesions of toxemia of pregnancy. *Journal of Experimental Medicine* **118:** 467–479.

13

Reproductive endocrinology in uraemia

VICTORIA S. LIM

Reproductive function is impaired in patients with severe renal insufficiency. In women, this is characterized by anovulation and decreased fertility; in men, by reduced testosterone production and impaired spermatogenesis. This chapter looks at the mechanisms behind these defects, and the therapeutic alterations that may ameliorate some of the problems, focusing on our own research in this area.

OVARIAN DYSFUNCTION

Ovarian dysfunction among premenopausal women undergoing haemodialysis treatment is quite prevalent. In a recent survey at our unit, we found that only about 25% of our haemodialysis patients have regular menses, approximately 50% are totally amenorrhoeic, and the rest have irregular menses ranging from occasional spotting to frequent dysfunctional uterine bleeding.

The pathogenesis of ovarian dysfunction in patients with renal insufficiency has been elucidated, and is believed to be due to a functional defect involving hypothalamic regulation of gonadotropin secretion (Lim et al, 1980; Handelsman, 1985). Table 1 summarizes basal hormonal values in women undergoing haemodialysis treatment compared to those of normal controls. Plasma levels of oestradiol and progesterone are not different in dialysis patients and normal women during the follicular phase of the menstrual cycle. However, oestradiol in dialysis patients generally does not reach the level seen during normal midcycle peaks. Similarly, progesterone levels in these women are much lower than those seen during the luteal phase of normally menstruating women. While plasma follicle-stimulating hormone (FSH) is normal, plasma luteinizing hormone (LH), in contrast, is significantly elevated in the renal patients, giving rise to lower FSH/LH ratios, a finding commonly seen in the prepubertal state. Even though the mean plasma LH is higher in uraemic patients than in normal women during the follicular phase, it is far below the level observed in normal women during the midcycle LH surge. Plasma prolactin is four times higher in uraemic women than in normal women, and no correlation between plasma concentrations of prolactin and FSH or LH is discernible.

Table 1. Ovarian hormonal profile in normal and uraemic women*.

Group	Oestradiol pg ml^{-1}	Progesterone ng ml^{-1}	FSH mIU/ml^{-1}	LH mIU/ml^{-1}	Prolactin ng ml^{-1}
Chronic renal failure					
Premenopausal	63.9 ± 8.2	0.6 ± 0.2	13.4 ± 1.5	18.6 ± 1.5	41.4 ± 5.8
	(17)	(17)	(17)	(17)	(17)
P	NS	NS	NS	<0.001	<0.001
Postmenopausal	<40	0.4 ± 0.1	196.0 ± 41.0	205.0 ± 20.0	
	(7)	(7)	(7)	(7)	
P	<0.001†	<0.01	<0.001	<0.001	
Normal					
Follicular	80.1 ± 5.4	0.7 ± 0.1	15.0 ± 1.0	10.9 ± 1.0	11.7 ± 1.1
	(15)	(12)	(12)	(12)	(12)
Midcycle	239.3 ± 21.4	2.4 ± 0.6	24.2 ± 3.3	55.7 ± 16.1	
	(9)	(5)	(5)	(5)	
Luteal	141.8 ± 15.1	10.1 ± 1.4	12.0 ± 1.7	10.9 ± 1.4	
	(12)	(11)	(11)	(11)	

* Plasma concentrations of oestradiol, progesterone, follicle-stimulating hormone (FSH), luteinizing hormone (LH) and prolactin are represented as means $\pm$ SEM. Numbers in parentheses indicate the number of subjects. P values were obtained by comparing the levels in premenopausal and postmenopausal uraemic women, respectively, to those obtained from normal subjects during the follicular phase of the ovarian cycle. NS = not significant.
† P value obtained by Fisher's exact test as all patients in this group had values of less than 40 pg ml^{-1}.
From Lim et al (1980).

Further important features, not included in Table 1, are:

1. Patients who are totally amenorrhoeic tend to have lower plasma oestradiol.
2. Plasma prolactin levels are generally normal in patients who have regular menses, and markedly elevated in those with amenorrhoea, especially those with galactorrhoea.

Serial daily measurements of ovarian and pituitary hormones revealed that most women with renal insufficiency have an anovulatory pattern characterized by oscillation of both LH and FSH without discernible peaks. This lack of ovulation is further confirmed by a persistently low plasma progesterone (Figure 1(b) and (c)). Of the seven premenopausal women that we studied, only one had regular menses and she had a normal ovulatory pattern of hormone secretion (Figure 1a).

Clomiphene administration in azotaemic patients, as in normally menstruating women, resulted in a noticeable rise in plasma LH and, to a lesser extent, FSH (Figure 2). Clomiphene is an anti-oestrogen compound that competes with oestrogen for receptors at the hypothalamus, resulting in an increased secretion of luteinizing hormone-releasing hormone (LH–RH) and, secondarily, a rise in plasma LH and FSH. Thus the pituitary is capable of responding to LH–RH adequately, and the negative feedback loop between ovarian steroids and gonadotropin secretion appears to be intact.

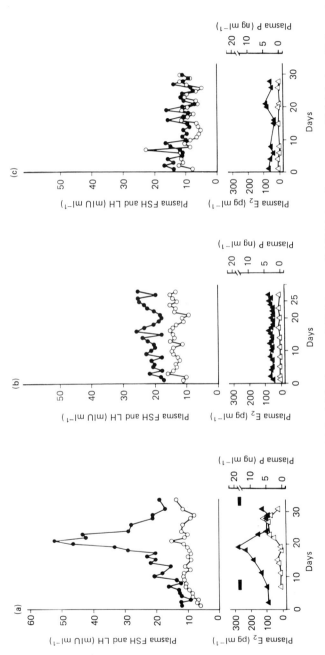

Figure 1. Plasma follicle-stimulating hormone (FSH) (○), luteinizing hormone (LH) (●), oestradiol (E₂) (▲), and progesterone (P) (△) during a 30-day period in three women with chronic renal failure. (a) Normal ovulatory pattern; (b) acyclic anovulation; (c) acyclic anovulation. From Lim et al (1980).

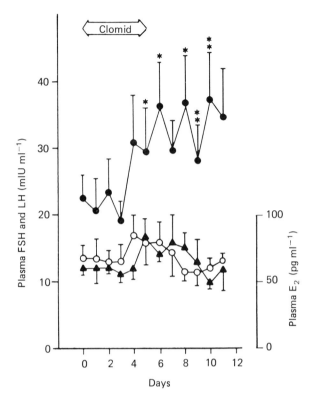

Figure 2. Hormonal responses to clomiphene citrate in seven women with chronic renal failure. Plasma luteinizing hormone (LH) (●) and, to a lesser extent, follicle-stimulating hormone (FSH) (○) as well as oestradiol (E₂) (▲) rose above baseline. *$P < 0.05$; **$P < 0.01$, as compared to the basal value by paired t test. From Lim et al (1980).

Administration of exogenous LH-RH to renal patients also produces a significant rise in LH and FSH, confirming our hypothesis that the pituitary responds normally to its trophic hormone (Schalch et al, 1975). Oestrogen replacement in postmenopausal women undergoing haemodialysis treatment effectively suppresses both LH and FSH to normal levels, proving again that the negative feedback relationship between ovarian steroids and gonadotropins remains intact.

In view of these findings, we believe the absence of cyclicity in renal patients to be hypothalamic in origin. We consider low oestrogen secretion (oestradiol is lower than that seen during midcycle in normally menstruating women) to be a potential pathogenetic factor because of its known positive feedback effect on the hypothalamo-pituitary axis. Oestrogen supplementation with doses calculated to achieve oestrogen peak in the midcycle (oestradiol 2.5 μg kg⁻¹ every 12 hours orally for four consecutive days), however, failed to induce a rise in serum LH (Figure 3). In normal premenopausal women during the follicular phase, similar doses of oestradiol result in a remarkable surge of

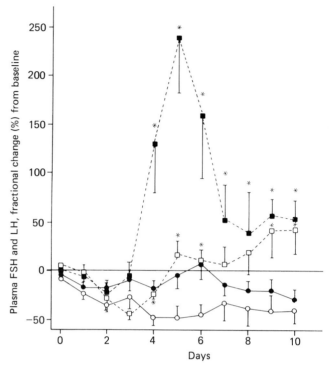

Figure 3. Plasma gonadotropin responses to ethinyl oestradiol in four normal women and eight uraemic patients. Both plasma follicle-stimulating hormone (FSH) (□ = normal; O = uraemic) and luteinizing hormone (LH) (■ = normal; ● = uraemic) are presented as percentage changes from baseline. Uraemic patients showed a markedly blunted response to ethinyl oestradiol. * Indicates *P* values ranged from <0.05 to <0.001. From Lim et al (1980).

LH to levels greater than 200% above baseline. During the reproductive years, gonadotropin secretion in women is believed to consist of tonic and cyclic components. The former regulates basal gonadotropin secretion and is governed by an oestradiol negative feedback, the latter is dependent on the priming action of oestrogen on the hypothalamus. Heightened oestrogen secretion during the midcycle is responsible for the increased secretion of the gonadotropin-releasing hormone, resulting in a subsequent LH surge. In patients with renal failure, the negative feedback relation between oestrogen and the tonic component of LH release appears normal; the cyclic component of gonadotropin secretion, however, is impaired. This, we think, is responsible for the prevalence of anovulation and the failure of LH to rise in response to oestradiol stimulation.

The hormonal derangements described here are not specific for renal insufficiency, and are seen in association with a number of acute and chronic conditions, classically in patients with anorexia nervosa and in women undergoing intensive athletic training. These changes are functional in the sense that successful renal transplantation restores ovarian function.

HYPERPROLACTINAEMIA

Hyperprolactinaemia is prevalent in patients with renal insufficiency, especially those women who are totally amenorrhoeic. In our earlier survey, serum prolactin was elevated in about 50% of the dialysis population. This elevation is, in part, due to impaired prolactin degradation, as demonstrated by the decrease in metabolic clearance rate and the prolongation of the plasma disappearance rate of ^{131}I-prolactin. More importantly, there is a component of hypersecretion as well (Sievertson et al, 1980). The calculated secretion rate was at least three times higher in renal patients. Furthermore, there was no correlation between the metabolic clearance rate and the plasma concentration of prolactin, suggesting that increased production is the more important determinant of hyperprolactinaemia during renal insufficiency. As prolactin is normally under tonic inhibition by dopaminergic mechanisms, persistent elevation in renal patients suggests disturbed dopamine metabolism either in the hypothalamus or elsewhere in the central nervous system. The observation that, in renal patients, neither L-dopa oral administration nor dopamine infusion was able to suppress plasma prolactin levels adequately, indicates that pituitary lactotrophs may be resistant to dopaminergic suppression (Lim et al, 1979). This resistance could represent either qualitative or quantitative changes of the lactotrope receptors or a derangement in postreceptor metabolism. The presence of this pituitary hyporesponsiveness made it difficult, if not impossible, to substantiate a central defect with the test methods currently available.

As prolactin is known to inhibit gonadotropin secretion, the possibility that hyperprolactinaemia may account for the commonly observed gonadal dysfunction in dialysis patients appears to be an attractive hypothesis. While we were able to suppress prolactin to normal level with long-term bromocriptine treatment in four women on haemodialysis, only one showed resumption of cyclicity and ovulation (Figure 4) (Lim and Frohman, 1983). Thus, the pathogenesis of ovarian dysfunction in uraemia is complex and multifactorial. The biologic significance of hyperprolactinaemia in renal patients remains unclear.

TESTICULAR DYSFUNCTION

In many male dialysis patients, testosterone production is reduced and spermatogenesis is defective; the true incidence of these disturbances however, is not known. Clinically, impotence and decreased libido are common. The pathogenesis of impotence in uraemia is multifactorial Although neuropathy and vascular insufficiency of the pelvic organs may cause impotence, they should not lead to decrements in libido and fertility Many of the medications taken by the dialysis patients may decrease sexual potency, and nutritional inadequacy, particularly zinc deficiency, has been implicated as the aetiology of uraemic hypogonadism. The latter assumption suffers from the fact that plasma zinc is only minimally reduced and there is no evidence of tissue zinc depletion. Moreover, with few exceptions, zinc

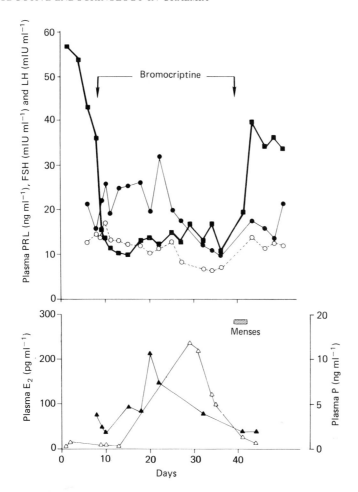

Figure 4. Effect of bromocriptine treatment (2.5 mg orally twice a day) on hyperprolactinaemia and amenorrhoea in a haemodialysis patient. Plasma prolactin levels were decreased to normal range. She subsequently had ovulatory menses. Plasma prolactin (PRL) (■); follicle-stimulating hormone (FSH) (○); luteinizing hormone (LH) (●); progesterone (P) (△); oestradiol (E_2) (▲). From Lim and Frohman (1983).

supplementation has failed to produce favourable responses. Thus, psychologic stress and endocrinologic disturbances are the most likely cause of sexual dysfunction in patients with renal insufficiency.

The best study correlating sexual dysfunction and mental depression to renal failure was reported by Procci et al (1981). In their study, sexual function was assessed by history and by measurement of nocturnal penile tumescence (NPT), and mental depression was quantitated by psychiatric interviews. They studied two groups of patients with renal insufficiency, one before and the other after initiation of maintenance dialysis treatment, and compared the results with those obtained from age-matched, normal control subjects, as well as age-matched patients with normal renal function but with a variety of other chronic illnesses. They noted a positive correlation between frequency of sexual intercourse and the magnitude of NPT. Both groups of renal patients had greater reduction of libido and potency as reflected by the lower frequency of sexual intercourse and greater decrement of NPT. The renal patients also had an increased incidence of major depression. Patients with mental depression, however, did not necessarily have more erectile dysfunction, thus dissociating mental depression from impaired sexual activity, at least in this group of renal patients. Furthermore, other investigators have reported that treatment of haemodialysis patients with tricyclic antidepressants failed to improve sexual function. In summary, current evidence suggests that sexual dysfunction in patients with renal insufficiency is, in part, organic in nature.

Decreased fertility in renal patients is reflected by defective spermatogenesis; seminal fluid analysis usually shows depressed sperm counts and a low fraction of motile sperms. Testicular morphology varies from mild maturation arrest to germinal cell aplasia. The most commonly observed characteristics are preservation of early spermatogenesis and depletion of the more mature forms, notably the spermatids. These features are typical of hormonal deficiency because the earlier stages of spermatogenesis are not hormone dependent. In contrast, damage induced by cytotoxic agents is usually characterized by disappearance of the earlier stages of spermatogenesis.

In the circulation, testosterone-binding globulin levels are normal, yet both total and free testosterone are reduced, as is plasma dihydrotestosterone. Despite this, LH is only modestly elevated and FSH is usually normal; the latter is elevated only in patients who have azoospermia. Stimulation with clomiphene citrate or with human chorionic gonadotropin (HCG) increases plasma testosterone (Handelsman, 1985; Lim and Fang, 1975). Holdsworth et al (1977), who studied 35 patients with creatinine clearance of less than 4 ml min^{-1}, found low plasma testosterone and reduced spermatogenesis accompanied by elevated plasma LH and FSH. They noted a blunted response to HCG in the renal patients. While four days of HCG treatment in normal controls resulted in a fourfold rise of plasma testosterone, in the renal patients the increase was only double. Thus, testicular steroidogenesis appears to be less efficient in the presence of uraemia; a greater than normal amount of LH is needed to achieve a physiologic level of testosterone. These data were taken as evidence supporting a primary testicular dysfunction.

A single defect in the testis, however, cannot explain the following observations. First, there is a significant positive correlation between serum LH and testosterone (Lim et al, 1978). Those renal patients with higher LH also have greater amount of circulating testosterone. This is in contrast to non-uraemic subjects in whom serum LH and testosterone are reciprocally correlated (Figure 5). Second, in a longitudinal study of dialysis patients, we noted a predictable rise of FSH following successful renal transplantation. The magnitude of the increment was quite marked, and the elevation was sustained for many months; when sperm counts approached normal values,

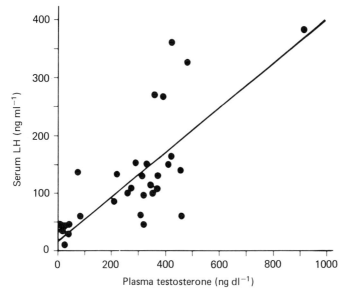

Figure 5. Relationship between plasma LH and testosterone. The line of least square linear regression, derived from 31 blood samples of 19 men with chronic renal failure, shows a positive correlation between these two hormones ($y = 0.39x + 16.9$, $r = 0.759$, $P < 0.0001$). From Lim et al (1978).

FSH then declined (Figure 6) (Lim and Fang, 1975). These observations led us to hypothesize that testicular dysfunction in dialysis patients is, at least in part, due to a central defect in the regulation of gonadotropin secretion. As in the case of female patients, the pituitary appears normal; thus, the putative defect must be located at the hypothalamus, involving regulation of LH-RH secretion.

TREATMENT OF URAEMIC HYPOGONADISM

In women with renal insufficiency, ovarian dysfunction does not appear to cause serious problems other than infertility, and perhaps decreased libido. However, the persistent oestrogen secretion and the lack of ovulation result in hormonal imbalance with metromenorrhagia and, less frequently, cystic ovaries. Dysfunctional uterine bleeding usually responds to progestational agents such as medroxy progesterone acetate 10 mg orally daily for the last 10 days of each month. Rupture of ovarian cysts (including bloody dialysate in patients on chronic ambulatory peritoneal dialysis) (Harnet et al, 1987) has been reported in a few patients on dialysis.

Contraception should be discussed with every female dialysis patient of child-bearing age. This is especially true now that dialysis has improved considerably and patients are, in general, healthier than a decade ago. As a result of this improvement, fertility may be increased. Random measurements

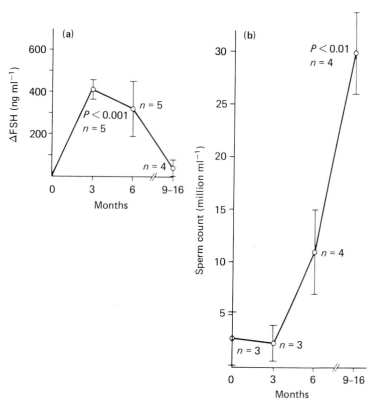

Figure 6. Changes in FSH (a) and sperm counts (b) after renal transplantation. Means and standard errors (shown in bars) are obtained from the number of patients (*n*) included in each study period. The zero time values were arbitrarily taken from the last determinations preceding transplantation. *P* values comparing pre- and post-transplantation data were calculated by paired *t*-test for FSH and by Student's *t* test for sperm counts. From Lim and Fang (1975).

of plasma oestrogen, progesterone or gonadotropins are not helpful in characterizing the ovulatory pattern. If a patient is totally amenorrhoeic (no menses for six months or more), contraceptive precaution is unnecessary.

Patients receiving androgenic hormone for anaemia are generally amenorrhoeic and anovulatory. If menses are present, whether regular or irregular, contraception is advisable. This policy may be viewed as overly cautious, as the likelihood of pregnancy is small. One should, however, be cognizant of the fact that pregnancy in a dialysis patient is an extremely complicated situation, requiring vigilant control of blood pressure and aggressive dialysis management. Despite vigorous effort, fetal growth is often retarded. The method of contraception is a matter of choice for each individual. There is no contraindication to the use of oral contraceptive agents as long as blood pressure is well controlled. In fact, oestrogen supplementation may improve libido and retard the development of osteoporosis. Moreover, because of its suppressive effect on gonadotropin secretion, an oral contraceptive may also prevent cystic changes in the ovary.

In male patients, impotence requires medical attention. If nocturnal penile tumescence is normal, the subjects need reassurance and psychotherapy. If nocturnal penile tumescence is decreased, potential causative factors should be searched for and treated accordingly. Depot testosterone injections can be given to normalize serum testosterone. Generally, a replacement dose of 200 mg of depot testosterone given intramuscularly once every two weeks is adequate. Bromocriptine may be given to patients who have elevated serum prolactin and impotence. The use of bromocriptine is limited by its hypotensive effect. It is advisable to start with a low dose and gradually increase to 2.5 mg orally b.i.d. Treatment should be discontinued after three months and the situation reassessed. Zinc deficiency, if documented, could easily be replaced by oral zinc sulphate.

Short-term treatment with clomiphene citrate and human chorionic gonadotropin has been reported to improve potency and libido, albeit anecdotally (Lim and Fang, 1976). If central defect is the predominant factor, reproductive function could be normalized by administration of rapidly metabolized gonadotropin agonist, or LH-RH itself, administered in a pulsatile manner. In non-renal patients whose infertility is central in origin, ovulation induction has been demonstrated following LH-RH infusion every 60–120 minutes. In males, spermatogenesis has been successfully induced by LH-RH administration subcutaneously every two hours. This type of treatment, though theoretically possible, has never been tried in patients with renal insufficiency, partly because it is not always desirable to restore fertility in this group of subjects. As the technique of dialysis improves, and patients are healthier, such a need may conceivably arise in the future.

REFERENCES

Handelsman DJ (1985) Hypothalmic-pituitary gonadal dysfunction in renal failure, dialysis and renal transplantation. *Endocrine Reviews* 6: 151–182.

Harnett JD, Gill D, Corbett L, Parfrey PS, Gault H (1987) Recurrent haemoperitoneum in women receiving continuous ambulatory peritoneal dialysis. *Annals of Internal Medicine* 107: 341–343.

Holdsworth S, Atkins RC & DeKrester DM (1977) The pituitary-testicular axis in men with chronic renal failure. *New England Journal of Medicine* 296: 1245–1249.

Lim VS & Fang VS (1975) Gonadal dysfunction in uremic men: a study of the hypothalamo-pituitary-testicular axis before and after renal transplantation. *American Journal of Medicine* 58: 655–662.

Lim VS & Fang VS (1976) Restoration of plasma testosterone levels in uremic men with clomiphene citrate. *Journal of Clinical Endocrinology and Metabolism* 43: 1370–1377.

Lim VS & Frohman LA (1983) Pathogenesis of hyperprolactinemia in chronic renal failure. In Tolis G, Stefones C, Mountokalakes T & Labrie F (eds) *Prolactin and Prolactinomas*, pp 265–276. New York: Raven Press.

Lim VS, Auletta F & Kathpalia S (1978) Gonadal dysfunction in chronic renal failure. *Dialysis & Renal Transplantation* 7(9): 896–902.

Lim VS, Kathpalia SC & Frohman LA (1979) Hyperprolactinemia and impaired pituitary response to suppression and stimulation in chronic renal failure: reversal after transplantation. *Journal of Clinical Endocrinology and Metabolism* 48: 101–107.

Lim VS, Henriques C, Sievertson G & Frohman LA (1980) Ovarian function in chronic renal failure: evidence suggesting hypothalamic anovulation. *Annals of Internal Medicine* **93:** 21–27.

Procci WR, Goldstein DA, Adelstein J et al (1981) Sexual dysfunction in the male patient with uremia: a reappraisal. *Kidney International* **19:** 317–323.

Schalch DS, Gonzales-Barcena D, Kastin AJ, Landa L, Lee LA & Schally A (1975) Plasma gonadotropins after administration of LH-releasing hormone in patients with renal and hepatic failure. *Journal of Clinical Endocrinology and Metabolism* **41:** 921–925.

Sievertson GD, Lim VS, Nakawatase C et al (1980) Metabolic clearance and secretion rates of human prolactin in normal subjects and in patients with chronic renal failure. *Journal of Clinical Endocrinology and Metabolism* **50:** 846–852.

14

Peritoneal dialysis and haemodialysis in pregnancy

SUSAN HOU

Pregnancy is unusual in women with moderate renal insufficiency and very rare in women with end-stage renal disease treated with peritoneal dialysis or haemodialysis. However, as the length of survival increases and the quality of life improves for patients with chronic renal failure, decreased fertility and increased fetal loss continue to bar women with renal failure from child bearing and parenthood at a time when adoption by a woman with a serious medical illness is all but impossible. The first two sections of this chapter will review the literature describing the experience with dialysis in pregnant women. The third section will address specific management issues.

As of the summer of 1987, there are at least 28 individual case reports of successful pregnancies in women dialysed during pregnancy for renal failure (Herwig et al, 1965; Orme et al, 1968; Mitra et al, 1970; Confortini et al, 1971; Unzelman et al, 1973; Ackrill et al, 1975; Marwood et al, 1977; Nemoto et al, 1977; Leader et al, 1978; Ringenbach et al, 1978; Sanchez-Casajus et al, 1978; Sheriff et al, 1978; Thompson et al, 1978; Johnson et al, 1979; Naik et al, 1979; Kobayashi et al, 1981; Lee et al, 1981; Savdie et al, 1982; Kioko et al, 1983; Redrow et al, 1987). Case reports are heavily skewed towards reporting successful outcomes, and there are only five cases (Pepperell et al, 1970; Cattran and Benzie, 1983; Redrow et al, 1987) which report the details of unsuccessful pregnancies. Furthermore, estimates of the likelihood of pregnancy succeeding in a woman with renal failure is based on two surveys (Registration Committee of EDTA, 1980; Roxe and Parker, 1985).

As of 1978, 115 pregnancies were reported in the 13 000 women of child-bearing age followed by the European Dialysis and Transplant Association. Forty-five women had therapeutic abortions, and of the remaining 70 women, 16 carried the pregnancy to viability (23%). As of 1982, the registry was updated and 35 successful pregnancies were reported, 15 of whom became pregnant prior to starting dialysis, while data was no longer collected on failed gestations (Challah et al, 1986). Roxe and Parker (1985) have collected data on women in the United States undergoing haemodialysis who became pregnant after starting dialysis. They reported 43 pregnancies in 35 of these women, 26 of whom had not been electively terminated. These pregnancies led to six live births (19.2%) (one set of twins). We can presume that both surveys which attempted to look at the denominators (the total number of pregnancies) were still weighed towards recording successful gestation. Also, because of the tendency of women with end-stage renal disease to have menstrual irregularities, pregnancies that end in early spontaneous abortions may go unnoticed by the health care team. Thus, at most, one-fourth of the pregnancies resulted in surviving infants.

Although the estimated success rate for pregnancies among dialysis patients was 19–23%, there appeared to be two groups. Of the 33 cases described in the literature, 17 conceived prior to starting dialysis. The mean length of time on dialysis for the 16 who conceived while on dialysis was 29 months (range 1–108 months), and residual renal function was noted in six cases. Four of the five pregnancy failures described in the literature occurred in the group that had started dialysis prior to conception. The likelihood of success for a long-term dialysis patient without residual renal function is probably much less than 23%.

MATERNAL RISKS

There have been no maternal deaths reported in women who were dialysed during pregnancy. However, hypertension and bleeding, which are common complications of pregnancy in dialysis patients, constitute a risk which could result in a maternal death if extreme vigilance is not employed.

Decline in renal function

As noted above, nearly half of the women who have been dialysed during pregnancy conceived prior to the initiation of dialysis. In this group, worsening of renal function may have resulted from the pregnancy. In 1985, we reported on a group of 23 women with moderate renal insufficiency (serum creatinine > 1.4 mg/dl) who became pregnant (Hou et al, 1985). A third of these women experienced a decline in renal function that was faster than would have been expected from the natural history of the underlying renal disease. These deteriorations in renal function did not reverse, and generally progressed after delivery. Surian et al (1984), using the slope of the reciprocal of the serum creatinine to define more precisely the natural history of the disease and its acceleration during pregnancy, confirmed our findings. More recently, Becker et al (1986) reported rapid deterioration of renal function in six women with reflux nephropathy and moderate renal insufficiency who became pregnant. They were compared to 10 control women who had reflux nephropathy and who did not become pregnant. Decline in renal function was significantly slower in the control group.

Hypertension

Of the 32 pregnant dialysis patients in the literature, 20 were noted to be hypertensive as defined by a diastolic blood pressure of 90 mmHg or above, or by the use of antihypertensive medications. In nine of these women, the

Table 1. Highest blood pressure measurements in 32 pregnant dialysis patients.

Highest blood pressure measurement (mmHg)	Number	Percentage
< 140/90	6	19
≥ 140/90 but < 170/140	10	31
≥ 170/110 but ≤ 170/130	5	16
≥ 170/130	4	13
Taking antihypertensive medications, BP not mentioned	1	3
BP not mentioned	6	19

diastolic blood pressure rose to 110 mmHg or above, and four had diastolic pressures of 130 mmHg or greater. Blood pressure was noted to be normal in six women, and no mention is made of blood pressure in six other cases (Table 1). A wide range of medication was used to control high blood pressure, including methyldopa, hydralazine, clonidine, propranolol, metoprolol, reserpine, prazosin, labetalol and nifedipine.

Anaemia and bleeding problems

Haemorrhage and abruptio placentae appear to be more common in patients than in the general population. The anaemia associated with renal failure increases the danger of bleeding episodes that may occur as a result of obstetric problems. In women with renal insufficiency the hematocrit decreases during pregnancy, even without evident blood loss, as it appears that plasma volume increases but red cell mass does not. Over a third of case reports mention that patients required transfusion due either to progressive anaemia or to bleeding episodes. It was initially hoped that chronic ambulatory peritoneal dialysis (CAPD), which is performed without the use of heparin, would decrease such problems as bleeding and abruptio placentae, but this has not been borne out. Abruptio placentae has already been noted once in the six reported patients who have been treated exclusively with CAPD during pregnancy.

Other maternal problems

Problems with clotting of vascular access have been noted in a number of pregnancies (Redrow et al, 1987). In some patients they represent the continuation of problems which were present prior to conception. In others it is possible that the hypercoagulable state that accompanies gestation may have played a role. Since dialysis is frequently begun earlier in the course of chronic renal disease than it would be were the patient not pregnant, and the frequency of dialysis is often increased in women already treated with maintenance dialysis, the effect of uraemia on platelet function is minimal in these women. In essence, normalization of the bleeding time may actually make access thrombosis more likely.

Table 2. Gestational age at birth.

Weeks of gestation	Number	Percentage
⩾ 36	10	33
33–35	8	26
28–32	9	30
< 28	2	6.7

The effect of pregnancy and fetal calcium requirements on materna osteodystrophy has not been systematically studied. In one case repor maternal bone disease worsened during pregnancy and fetal skeletal calcifica tion was less complete than expected for gestational age (Pepperell et al, 1970) In another, note is made of congenital rickets in the infant (Savdie et al, 1982)

Pregnancy is a recognized cause of sensitization to transplant antigens anc may make it more difficult to find a donor kidney with a negative cross-matcł (Sanfilippo et al, 1982). Once pregnancy occurs, it is not clear whethei termination of the gestation will prevent sensitization.

Pregnancy in a dialysis patient may also increase the risk of severe emotional stress. Often the pregnancy has occurred after years of infertility and the patient is usually requested to undertake a time-consuming regimer which consists of increased dialysis and blood pressure monitoring with but a small chance of successful completion of the pregnancy. Second-trimestei spontaneous abortions are common, and neonatal deaths continue to occui and none of the modifications in dialytic regimens have reliably preventec these late pregnancy losses. This too is a cause of psychological stress.

RISKS TO THE FETUS

Fetal or neonatal death

Pregnancy loss can occur at any time during pregnancy. First-trimester losse: are probably underestimated as the diagnosis is frequently made late Placental insufficiency occurs late in gestation. Abnormalities found in the placenta include abruptio, infarction and microscopic areas of fibrosis Second-trimester spontaneous abortions are common, and neonatal death: secondary to prematurity occur.

Prematurity

Prematurity was common as 20 of the 29 infants born alive were of less than 36 weeks gestation. The distribution of gestational age is summarized in Table 2 The most common reason for early delivery was premature labour, whick accounted for nine (45%) of the premature deliveries (see Table 3). Premature labour also occurred during an additional nine pregnancies but did no provide sufficient reason for delivery. Transient contractions were common

Table 3. Cause for premature delivery.

Cause	Number	Percentage
Premature labour	9	45
Fetal distress	3	15
Ruptured membranes	1	5
Hypertension	2	10
Haemorrhage	4	29
Intrauterine growth retardation	1	5

with dialysis and after placement of peritoneal dialysis catheters. In three patients, there were causes for premature labour which were not necessarily the result of renal disease, i.e. polyhydramnios in two cases and an incompetent cervix in another. Other reasons for premature delivery included abruptio placentae or bleeding problems in four cases, fetal distress in three, ruptured membranes in one, hypertension in two and intrauterine growth retardation in one. In some of these premature deliveries several factors seem to have been causative.

In many instances, premature labour began during dialysis, but it was unclear whether dialysis itself caused premature labour. Premature labour occurs in women with renal insufficiency who are not on dialysis (Hou et al, 1985) and has been noted in peritoneal dialysis as well as in haemodialysis patients. However, haemodialysis is accompanied by a decrease in progesterone levels of about 10%, and this decrement may precipitate labour (Johnson et al, 1979).

Growth retardation

The weights of infants born at various gestational ages (29 live births and one stillbirth) are recorded in Figure 1. Eight of the infants were below the tenth percentile at birth, with an additional six at the tenth percentile. Ten were between the tenth and fiftieth percentile, and only five were above the fiftieth percentile. Many of the infants were exposed to severe hypertension. None of the babies who were above the fiftieth percentile were born to mothers who experienced severe hypertension. Of the eight infants who were below the tenth percentile, five were exposed to severe hypertension. One of the remaining four mothers had mild hypertension, one was not hypertensive, and in the other two maternal blood pressure is not mentioned.

Other fetal complications

Most of the difficulties experienced by the infants resulted from prematurity. In all infants in whom blood urea nitrogen and serum creatinine were measured, cord blood levels approached maternal levels at birth. This led to an osmotic diuresis in the neonatal period.

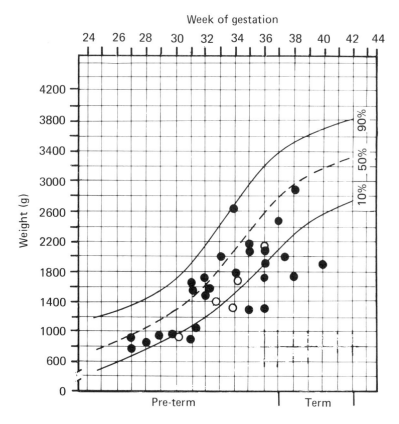

Figure 1. Comparison of fetal weight versus gestation age in 30 infants born to women who were dialysed during pregnancy. The 10, 50, and 90% confidence bands represent the expected normal weight for the gestational age. ●, Haemodialysis; ○, CAPD.

Additionally, one infant was born with a poorly calcified skeleton and a second was born with congenital rickets; both problems were felt to be the result of the derangement of maternal calcium and phosphorus metabolism (Pepperell et al, 1970; Savdie et al, 1982).

Detailed follow-up of intellectual function in these infants who have been exposed to an azotaemic intrauterine environment has not been carried out. It will be difficult to separate the effects of azotaemia from the effects of prematurity and other diseases such as lupus erythematosus and diabetes. Apgar scores were recorded in 17 babies. Six had 1-minute Apgar scores of 5 or less while scores at 5 minutes were 6 or more. Congenital anomalies did not appear to be increased.

MANAGEMENT

Diagnosis of pregnancy

Pregnancy in women on chronic dialysis is often diagnosed late. The majority of dialysis patients have amenorrhoea or irregular periods, and gastrointestinal symptoms are common. A high index of suspicion is required to make the diagnosis in the first trimester and to avoid X-rays for the evaluation of gastrointestinal symptoms. In 14 of the 16 women reported to have conceived on dialysis, duration of gestation at diagnosis was noted. The mean gestational age at diagnosis was 16.5 weeks. Six were diagnosed in the second trimester and one in the third trimester. Urine pregnancy tests are either unreliable or unobtainable in patients receiving dialysis, and diagnosis must be made through measurement of the serum β-subunit of human chorionic gonadotrophin (HCG) or by ultrasound. Since HCG is made in small quantities by other cells and excreted in part by the kidney, HCG levels may be high in dialysis patients who are not pregnant, and borderline values will have to be repeated. Schwartz et al (1985) measured β-HCG levels in 52 samples from 19 women and 4 men on dialysis. The mean values were within the normal range, but 32% of the measurements were above this range. Seven of the women had at least one elevated reading, and in two women values were ten-fold higher than the upper limit of normal. Since HCG is partly excreted by the kidney, quantitative HCG measurements will often be high for gestational age and may be in the range associated with molar pregnancy. Gestational age is best assessed by ultrasound, which will also exclude a mole in pregnancies with very high HCG levels.

Deterioration in renal function

Almost one-half of the patients dialysed during pregnancy did not require dialysis prior to pregnancy. When a woman with renal insufficiency experiences a decline in renal function during pregnancy, she needs to be assessed for reversible causes of renal failure. Nephrotoxic drugs should be avoided, including non-steroidal anti-inflammatory agents and aminoglycosides. Several cases of reversible obstruction during pregnancy have been described (Homans et al, 1981). Polyhydramnios, single kidney or transplanted kidney make the risk of obstruction higher. When obstruction is caused by the pregnancy it may be relieved by turning the patient to the side opposite the single kidney or, in the case of polyhydramnios, by periodic removal of amniotic fluid. If obstruction occurs secondary to other causes, percutaneous nephrostomy tubes or stents can be placed in pregnant women by a urologist experienced in performing such procedures. Pre-eclampsia is probably the most common cause of reversible renal failure in pregnant women. Diagnosis can be problematic as most of the clinical parameters followed are distorted by the underlying renal disease. It is rarely necessary to do a biopsy to distinguish between pre-eclampsia and other causes of worsening renal function. The decision whether to terminate the pregnancy can usually be decided on the basis of whether the blood pressure can be controlled.

Standard practice in the past was to recommend termination of the pregnancy when renal function deteriorated, with the hope that the deterioration could be reversed. Our experience has been that once a decline in renal function occurs, it may progress after termination of the pregnancy, or at best stabilize. The decision as to whether to terminate the pregnancy to protect renal function is best made before the decline in renal function. Once renal function has begun to deteriorate, the patient cannot be assured that termination will help renal function and that delivery of a pre-viable fetus is justified. Often, the underlying disease is one that is destined to progress, and pregnancy merely hastens the time at which dialysis is needed. If renal function worsens at a time later than 32 weeks when fetal survival without long-term problems is likely, it is reasonable to deliver the baby prematurely for combined maternal and fetal indications.

Prophylactics on intensified dialysis

It has become common practice to begin dialysis in pregnant women before it would otherwise be necessary for the health of the mother. In patients who conceive while on dialysis, an increase in the frequency of dialysis is usually prescribed. Unless pregnancy in dialysis patients becomes more common than it is now, this practice will not be subjected to prospective randomized studies. Although few cases have been reported detailing the management of dialysis patients with unsuccessful pregnancies in at least some of those patients, dialysis frequency has been increased and control of azotaemia has been good (Redrow et al (1987). By the same token, there are case reports of successful pregnancies in patients with advanced azotaemia who have not been dialysed (Naranjo et al, 1978). However, there are several arguments in favour of initiating dialysis early and intensifying dialysis. We know that fetal outcome is poor on regimes that merely keep the mother free of uraemic symptoms, and residual renal function is common in women with successful pregnancies. It is reasonable to hypothesize that the baby's chance of survival would be improved if the intrauterine environment could be made less azotaemic, even though it is unclear how renal failure leads to the placental pathology that is often seen. The initiation of dialysis may make blood pressure control easier, as hypertension in women with renal failure frequently has a component that is caused by hypervolaemia. Daily dialysis enables the patient to follow a more liberal diet. The amount of fluid that needs to be removed at each treatment is smaller so that the risk of hypotension during dialysis will be lower.

There is little evidence that haemodialysis is harmful to the baby. Fetal monitoring during haemodialysis has been described in two patients. Sanchez-Casajus (1978) described fetal monitoring during haemodialysis treatment. During one dialysis treatment, the baby developed fetal distress when maternal hypotension occurred. A second patient, described by Redrow et al (1987) was dialysed three to four times weekly from 26 to 38 weeks gestation. Fetal monitoring performed during dialysis demonstrated a single episode of fetal distress that was not associated with maternal hypotension. We have generally started dialysis when the serum urea nitrogen (SUN) is between 80 mg/dl and 100 mg/dl and we have not been able to discontinue dialysis following delivery. Once dialysis is initiated, we have tried arbitrarily to keep the SUN below 50 mg/dl. This goal was attainable in women who started dialysis after conception and who had some residual renal function, but was more difficult in women without residual renal function. Often, in these women, daily dialysis is needed to keep the SUN lower than 50 mg/dl. Most nephrologists have found that SUN increases in the third trimester, and increased dialysis is needed to maintain the same SUN and creatinine level (Confortini et al, 1971). By term, fetal urea production averages 540 mg/day and must be removed by maternal dialysis.

Modifications of haemodialysis prescription

For women treated with haemodialysis during pregnancy, the dialysis prescription should be modified to approximate as nearly as possible normal physiology. Serum urea nitrogen should be maintained below 50 mg/dl if possible, even if daily dialysis is required. Daily dialysis with standard dialysate composition may result in hypokalaemia, particularly if nausea accompanies the pregnancy. We monitor predialysis chemistries weekly and raise dialysate potassium to 3–3.5 mEq/l if necessary. Daily dialysis will result in uptake of more alkali than necessary to offset daily acid production. Dialysate alkali concentration should be lowered as needed to maintain the serum bicarbonate in the 18–22 mEq/l range to offset the respiratory alkalosis that occurs in pregnant women. There is no information concerning acetate metabolism in pregnant women, and the use of bicarbonate containing dialysate should be used if practical. The effects of pregnancy on maternal calcium and phosphorus metabolism in dialysis patients are not known. There is some production of 1,25-dihydroxy cholecalciferol ($1,25(OH)_2D_3$) by the fetus and placenta, but it is not clear by how much intestinal calcium absorption is increased (Weisman et al, 1978). We usually start with a 1 g oral calcium supplementation and a 0.25 μg of $1,25(OH)_2D_3$ at the beginning of pregnancy. We use a dialysate containing 3.5 mEq/l of calcium. We measure serum calcium and phosphorus weekly. If serum calcium is low, we confirm the hypocalcaemia with a measurement of ionized calcium, and increase oral calcium if it is truly low. If hypercalcaemia occurs, we stop $1,25(OH)_2D_3$ and calcium supplements and dialyse with a low calcium bath (usually 1–2 mEq/l) until serum calcium is below 11 mg/dl. We then restart calcium supplements at a lower dose and hold $1,25(OH)_2D_3$ unless serum calcium drops. We use a dialysate sodium concentration of 134 mEq/l to bring about the mild hyposmolarity seen in pregnancy. Avoidance of hypotension during dialysis is of paramount importance. Daily dialysis minimizes the amount of fluid that needs to be removed during each treatment and lowers the risk of hypotension. Blood pressure can be supported by the usual administration of saline, and in non-diabetics by the administration of hypertonic glucose. In instances where fluid overload occurs in spite of daily dialysis, hypotension can be avoided by the liberal use of isolated ultrafiltration. The amount of heparin used should be minimized and given by constant infusion. Although heparin does not cross the placenta, its use has been associated with fetal loss and even maternal death in other settings (Hall et al, 1980). We have not found it practical to dialyse patients entirely without heparin.

Mode of dialysis: CAPD in pregnancy

Since 1976, chronic ambulatory peritoneal dialysis (CAPD) has emerged as a major form of treatment for patients with end-stage renal disease, including many young, active patients. This type of dialysis combines the established technique of instilling dialysate through a permanent indwelling peritoneal catheter into the peritoneum with prolonged dwell times. With this technique, between $1\frac{1}{2}$ and 3 litres of dialysate are instilled through the catheter four or more times daily and left for 4–8 hours, after which the fluid is removed and replaced by fresh dialysate. Urea and other waste products are removed by diffusion into the dialysate. Volume removal is achieved by including glucose in different concentrations as the osmotically active substance that pulls fluid into the peritoneal cavity to be discarded with the spent dialysate. There are six reports in the literature of patients treated exclusively with CAPD during pregnancy. Cattran and Benzie (1983) describe a woman who conceived while treated with CAPD; the gestation ended with an intrauterine fetal death at 30 weeks. A successful pregnancy in a woman who started CAPD at 10 weeks gestation has been reported by Kioko et al (1983). Redrow et al (1987) described a remarkable cluster of four patients who had been treated with CAPD during pregnancy. Two of the patients started CAPD after conception and two conceived while being treated with CAPD. Three out of the four pregnancies were successsful. An additional three women who conceived on CAPD were pregnant at the time of writing. The maintenance of a constant intrauterine environment and the avoidance of hypotension associated with rapid fluid shifts are potential advantages offered by CAPD. Blood pressure appears to be easier to control in CAPD patients. The placement of a peritoneal dialysis catheter, even late in gestation, can usually be accomplished without difficulty although mechanical difficulties with the catheter have been described (Redrow et al, 1987). Towards term, instillation of the standard $1\frac{1}{2}$–2 litres may become uncomfortable for the patient and it may become necessary to do more frequent exchanges with a smaller volume. Caesarean section was required in all three of the successful pregnancies reported by Redrow et al (1987) and in the one pregnancy reported by Kioko (Kioko et al, 1983). The peritoneal catheter was left in place, and there was no difficulty in resuming CAPD 24–72 hours after delivery. Our current recommendation for patients undergoing a caesarean section on CAPD is to drain the peritoneum prior to surgery, remove the tubing and cap off the catheter. During the first 24 hours, the catheter is irrigated with 500 ml of 4.25% dianeal containing 2000 units of heparin. CAPD can be resumed after 24 hours, starting with 1000 ml exchanges and gradually increasing to 2000 ml exchanges by the third postpartum day. If there is leakage from the incision, CAPD should be discontinued and the patient treated with haemodialysis as needed for 1–2 weeks. The catheter should be flushed daily with 50 ml of heparinized dianeal to keep the catheter patent. The problems of hypertension, prematurity and fetal distress have not been eliminated by the use of CAPD. As noted, there was one stillbirth at 30 weeks. Three of the four successful pregnancies were terminated prior to 36 weeks because of fetal distress or intrauterine growth retardation. However, although experience with CAPD is very limited, the outcome of patients on haemodialysis during pregnancy is sufficiently poor that more extensive use of CAPD is warranted to determine whether it is possible to improve upon the disappointing track record of haemodialysis.

Blood pressure control

There is considerable debate over what degree of hypertension should be treated during pregnancy either for the sake of the fetus or for the sake of the mother. In treating the woman whose renal failure is severe enough to require dialysis, it behoves us to forgo the argument and treat hypertension early and aggressively, recognizing that this group of women has a substantial risk of developing life-threatening blood pressure elevation. We recommend teaching the patient to take her own blood pressure at home, as abrupt increases may occur. We recommend treating any blood pressure over 140/90 mmHg with antihypertensive drugs if the blood pressure cannot be lowered by fluid removal during dialysis. Methyldopa in doses of up to four grams daily has been used in pregnant women for over 25 years, and long-term ill-effects have not been described. Ounsted and her colleagues (1980) have done careful follow-up of children whose mothers were treated with methyldopa during pregnancy and have compared them with normotensive and untreated hypertensive controls. In most areas of development the children of mothers treated with methyldopa were not significantly different from controls. In areas where differences were significant, the children of mothers treated with methyldopa performed slightly less well than children of normotensive controls and better than children of untreated hypertensive controls. However, methyldopa frequently causes central nervous system side-effects such as fatigue and depression. Moreover, since methyldopa causes hepatitis in a small percentage of patients, its use can make the assessment of transaminase elevations in the third trimester more difficult. None the less, methyldopa still represents the standard against which other antihypertensive drugs should be measured. Beta adrenergic antagonists have enjoyed increasing use in the treatment of hypertension. Initial use of them in pregnant women led to case reports of apnoea, bradycardia and hypoglycaemia in infants exposed to β-adrenergic blocking agents in utero (Gladstone et al, 1975). Intrauterine growth retardation has been noted (Pruyn et al, 1979) and there has been concern based on animal work that these drugs interfere with the ability of the fetus to withstand anoxic stress (Cottle et al, 1983). Since many diseases treated with β-adrenergic blocking agents are associated with fetal distress and intrauterine growth retardation, it is difficult to assess if these are truly adverse actions of these agents, except in prospective randomized trials. Gallery et al (1979) carried out a randomized comparison of the β-adrenergic blocking drug, oxyprenolol, with methyldopa and observed no differences in fetal loss. They did note, however, that infants born to mothers treated with oxyprenolol were significantly heavier than infants born to mothers taking methyldopa. Rubin et al (1983), in a placebo-controlled trial, found atenolol was effective in controlling blood pressure and in avoiding premature pregnancy termination for hypertension. Atenolol induced brady-cardia in the infants which was not clinically significant. Limited studies have been carried out with both clonidine (Horvath et al, 1985) and labetolol and in them no fetal problems were uncovered (Jouppila et al, 1986). Hydralazine, used both orally and intravenously, has been found to be safe in pregnancy. Oral hydralazine can be added to a sympatholytic agent if blood pressure control is inadequate.

Two new categories of drugs have become popular in the treatment of hypertension in the general population: calcium channel blockers and angiotensin-converting enzyme inhibitors. Nifedipine has been used both acutely and chronically for pregnancy-associated hypertension without serious ill-effects (Walters and Redman, 1984). It often remains effective when the response to combined methyldopa and hydralazine is inadequate. We feel that captopril is contraindicated in pregnancy. Animal data in rabbits demonstrate that captopril decreases placental prostaglandin production and placental blood flow (Ferris and Weir, 1983). When rabbits were treated with captopril 2.5 mg/kg/day, only 20% of fetuses survived, and when the dose was increased to 5.0 mg/kg/day, only 7.5% of fetuses survived. The frequency of fetal demise was so striking that we recommend avoiding the use of captopril until further data are available.

In summary, our approach when medication is needed is to begin treatment with methyldopa 1 g daily in two divided doses. If a large dose is not tolerated the daily dose can be divided into four doses. β-Adrenergic blocking drugs, labetolol (a combined alpha and beta antagonist) and clonidine, are acceptable alternatives. Methyldopa can be increased to a total dose of three grams. If blood pressure remains elevated, hydralazine can be added in daily doses of 200 mg and even up to 400 milligrams, but there is a 10% incidence of drug-induced lupus erythematosus with these higher doses. If blood pressure control is still unsatisfactory, nifedipine in doses starting from 10 mg three times daily and increasing to 30 mg three times daily can be used in place of hydralazine.

When the patient develops hypertensive crisis, seizures or diastolic blood pressure over 110 mmHg when taking maximal oral medications and dialysed to ideal weight, the pregnancy should be terminated. Maternal safety must take precedence over concern about prematurity and possible fetal side-effects. The patient can be treated with intravenous hydralazine while preparing for delivery. If there is an inadequate response to hydralazine, 10–30 milligrams of nifedipine can be used. If blood pressure is not controlled by hydralazine and nifedipine, diazoxide can be used in successive doses of 30 milligrams of intravenous push. In the setting of emergency where other drugs have failed, nitroprusside can be used, despite reports of accumulation of cyanide in the fetus (Naulty et al, 1981; Stempel et al, 1982). Termination of the pregnancy will almost invariably make the blood pressure control easier.

Benzodiazepine and phenobarbital are preferable to magnesium for the prevention of seizures, as magnesium can only be removed by dialysis if levels rise too high.

Treatment of premature labour

Premature labour is the most frequent single cause of prematurity in infants of dialysis patients. Since it does appear that placental abruption occurs more frequently in dialysis patients, premature labour should prompt an assessment for underlying causes of uterine irritability. The use of β-adrenergic agonists is relatively contraindicated in women with renal disease, but terbutaline in repeated doses of 0.25 milligrams can be given subcutaneously if the patient is not hypertensive. Redrow et al (1987) have treated CAPD patients with magnesium for control of premature labour. They gave a loading dose of 4 grams, given intravenously, and then added magnesium to the dialysate to give a concentration of 5 mEq/l. If serum magnesium exceeded 5 mEq/l, it was lost in the dialysate, preventing dangerous levels. Despite the safety and ease of treatment found by Redrow et al (1987) we recommend extreme caution with the use of magnesium in dialysis patients as toxicity occurs occasionally when healthy pregnant women are treated with magnesium. We have a limited but favourable experience with the use of nifedipine in the treatment of premature labour. We start with doses of 10 mg three times daily. Nifedipine has been well tolerated even in women whose pre-treatment systolic blood pressure is below 100 mmHg. Nifedipine and magnesium should not be used together.

Diet

Home haemodialysis and CAPD patients should be seen weekly and others at each dialysis treatment. We prescribe a high protein diet (1–1.2 grams of protein per kilogram). High protein diet is particularly important in CAPD patients, who may suffer protein losses in the dialysate. In them, protein allowance may be increased to 1.5 g/kg. Daily dialysis or an increased number of exchanges in CAPD patients usually makes fluid and potassium restriction unnecessary. The patient is examined weekly for evidence of volume overload and electrolytes, and the serum urea nitrogen, creatinine level and haematocrit are checked. We generally allow the weight to increase by 0.5–1 kg/month during the first 6 months and by 0.25–0.5 kg/week during the last trimester. Blood pressure recording and an examination follow, and the target weight is adjusted as dictated by the examination. Water-soluble vitamins which can be lost in dialysate are supplemented. Iron stores are assessed by serum ferritin levels, and iron supplements are given to those who are not iron overloaded.

Correction of anaemia

Anaemia usually worsens during pregnancy as the plasma volume increases and the red cell mass stays constant. We have transfused pregnant women to keep the haematocrit in the range of 25%. Although it has been suggested that anaemia does not affect the fetus adversely unless the haemoglobin is below 6 grams (Leven et al, 1982), the risk of bleeding complications and the likelihood of caesarean delivery are of sufficient concern that it is prudent to maintain the haemoglobin level above 7.5 grams%. It is hoped that when recombinant DNA erythropoietin becomes universally available, transfusions will rarely be necessary for dialysis patients.

Infectious complications

Infants born to hepatitis antigen-positive dialysis patients should be treated with hepatitis B immunoglobulin and Hepatovax (hepatitis B vaccine) immediately after birth. Hepatovax should be repeated at one and six months of age to avoid developing the hepatitis B carrier state with its risks of cirrhosis and hepatocellular carcinoma (Beasley et al, 1983). There is currently no way to prevent transplacental infection with $HTLV_3$ in carriers.

Pregnant dialysis patients are as much at risk for peritonitis and graft infections as are non-pregnant dialysis patients. These infections can be life-threatening for the mother and they should be treated with whatever combination of antibiotics and surgical procedures is necessary to protect the mother's life. Penicillin derivatives and cephalosporins are generally considered safe for the fetus. Aminoglycosides cross the placenta and theoretically put the fetus at risk for ototoxicity or renal toxicity. Ototoxicity has been reported with kanamycin. There is little information about vancomycin use in pregnancy, but we have used it without ill-effects. Tetracyclines and chloramphenicol should not be used.

Fetal monitoring

Antenatal testing with twice weekly non-stress testing or oxytocin challenge tests should be started early as there is a chance of fetal survival. We recommend twice weekly testing because stillbirths have been reported within a week of a reassuring non-stress test. In women treated with β-adrenergic blocking agents for hypertension, fetal bradycardia may occur without fetal distress. When an oxytocin challenge test is used to assess fetal well-being there is some risk that it will precipitate premature labour in this high-risk group, but it may be necessary when non-stress tests are difficult to interpret. Periodic ultrasound should be carried out to assess fetal growth.

Timing of delivery

There is not yet enough experience to know whether antenatal monitoring will consistently identify fetal distress in pregnant dialysis patients. Serious maternal and fetal complications are sufficiently common that elective delivery at 34–36 weeks may be the safest course for mother and child. At present, in the absence of specific indications, delivery earlier than 34 weeks with risk of greater problems associated with prematurity is not justified.

In summary, pregnancy in women with renal insufficiency and end-stage renal disease, while uncommon, is definitely possible, and such women should not assume that they are infertile. For the woman who is dialysed during pregnancy, the risks to the mother can be minimized by aggressive blood pressure control and prompt treatment of bleeding episodes. Intensive dialysis should be undertaken to maintain chemistries that are as near normal as possible. Our current state of knowledge suggests a success rate that is no better than 20–25%. The success of a small series of CAPD patients who have become pregnant suggests that in the future the dismal statistics cited above will improve.

While transplantation offers the best chance of child-bearing for women with end-stage renal disease, such a course is not always possible. Thus, we no longer discourage women on dialysis from becoming pregnant if they understand that the likelihood of success is low and that risks are present, and if they are willing to follow the time-consuming regimen we feel is necessary for their safety. We hope that, in time, increased experience with pregnant dialysis patients will lead to more successful outcomes and that the possibility of parenthood will be added to the improved quality of life in these women.

Addendum

Subsequent to the preparation of this chapter, we have had the opportunity to follow four additional pregnancies. Three of these pregnancies in CAPD patients resulted in two live births. The other pregnancy in a haemodialysis patient ended in spontaneous abortion at 15 weeks. Data from these pregnancies did not otherwise substantially change the data described in this report.

REFERENCES

Ackrill P, Goodwin FJ, Marsh FP, Stratton D & Wagman H (1975) Successful pregnancy in a patient on regular dialysis. *British Medical Journal* ii: 172–174.

Beasly RP, Lee GCY, Roan CH et al (1983) Prevention of perinatally transmitted hepatitis B virus infections with hepatitis B immune globulin and hepatitis B vaccine. *Lancet* ii: 1099–1102.

Becker GJ, Ihle B, Fairley K, Bastos M & Kincaid-Smith P (1986) Effect of pregnancy on moderate renal failure in reflux nephropathy. *British Medical Journal* 292: 796–798.

Cattran DC & Benzie RJ (1983) Pregnancy in a continuous ambulatory peritoneal dialysis patient. *Peritoneal Dialysis Bulletin* 3: 13–14.

Challah S, Wing A & Broyer M (1986) Successful pregnancy in women on regular dialysis treatment and women with a functioning transplant. In Andreucci VF (ed.) *The Kidney in Pregnancy*, pp 185–194. The Hague: Martinus Nijhoff.

Cottle MKW, Van Petten GR & Muyden P (1983) Maternal and fetal cardiovascular indices during fetal hypoxia due to cord compression in chronically cannulated sheep responses to timolol. *American Journal of Obstetrics and Gynecology* 146: 678–685.

Confortini P, Galanti G, Ancona G et al (1971) Full term pregnancy and successful delivery in a patient on chronic hemodialysis. *Proceedings of the European Dialysis and Transplant Association* 8: 74–80.

Ferris TF & Weir EK (1983) Effect of captopril on uterine blood flow and prostaglandin E synthesis in the pregnant rabbit. *Journal of Clinical Investigation* 71: 809–815.

Gallery EDM, Saunders DM, Hunyor SN & Gyory AZ (1979) Randomized comparison of methyldopa and oxyprenolol for treatment of hypertension in pregnancy. *British Medical Journal* i: 1591–1594.

Gladstone GR, Hordot A & Gersony WM (1975) Propranolol administration during pregnancy: effects on the fetus. *Pediatrics* 86: 962–964.

Hall JG, Pauli RM & Wilson KM (1980) Maternal and fetal sequellae of anticoagulation. *American Journal of Medicine* 68; 122–140.

Herwig KR, Merrill JP, Jackson RL & Oken DE (1965) Chronic renal disease and pregnancy. *American Journal of Obstetrics and Gynecology* 92: 1117–1121.

Homans DC, Blake GD, Harrington JT & Cetrullo CL (1981) Acute renal failure caused by ureteral obstruction by a gravid uterus. *Journal of the American Medical Association* 246: 1230–1231.

Horvath JS, Phippard A, Korda A et al (1985) Clonidine hydrochloride—a safe and effective antihypertensive agent in pregnancy. *Obstetrics and Gynecology* 66: 634–638.

Hou S, Grossman S & Madias N (1985) Pregnancy in women with renal disease and moderate renal insufficiency. *American Journal of Medicine* 78: 185–194.

Johnson TR, Lorenz RP & Menon KMJ (1979) Successful outcome of a pregnancy requiring dialysis. *Journal of Reproductive Medicine* 22: 217–218.

Jouppila P, Kirkinen P, Koivula A & Ylikorkalao (1986) Labetolol does not alter the placental and fetal blood flow or maternal prostanoids in pre eclampsia. *British Journal of Obstetrics and Gynaecology* 93: 543–547.

Kioko M, Shaw KM, Clarke AD & Warren DJ (1983) Successful pregnancy in a diabetic patient treated with continuous ambulatory peritoneal dialysis. *Diabetes Care* 6: 298–300.

Kobayashi H, Matsumoto Y, Otsubo O, Otsubo K & Naito T (1981) Successful pregnancy in a patient undergoing chronic hemodialysis. *Obstetrics and Gynecology* 57: 382–386.

Leader L, Strasburg ER, Baillie P & Keeton RD (1978) Hemodialysis in pregnancy. *South African Medical Journal* 53: 871–872.

Lee SH, Wang TC, Lee TY, Chen FY & Chien TY (1981) Successful pregnancy in a patient on hemodialysis. *Journal of Formosan Medical Association* 80: 136–140.

Burrow GN & Ferris TF (ed.) (1982). *Medical Complications During Pregnancy*, pp 62. Philadelphia: WB Saunders.

Marwood RP, Ogg CS, Coltart TM & Klopper AI (1977) Plasma oestrogens in pregnancy associated with chronic haemodialysis. *British Journal of Obstetrics and Gynaecology* 84: 613–617.

Mitra S, Vertes V, Roza O & Berman LB (1970) Periodic hemodialysis in pregnancy. *American Journal of Medical Science* 259: 333–339.

Naik RB, Clark AD & Warren DJ (1979) Acute proliferative glomerulonephritis with crescents and renal failure in pregnancy successfully managed by intermittent haemodialysis. *British Journal of Obstetrics and Gynaecology* 86: 819–822.

Naranjo P, Prats D & Rodrigo A (1978) Insuficiencia renal avanzada y embarazo. *Revista Clinica Espanola* 149: 509–512.

Naulty J, Cefalo RC & Lewis PE (1981) Fetal toxicity of nitroprusside in the pregnant ewe. *American Journal of Obstetrics and Gynecology* 139: 708–711.

Nemoto R, Sugiyama Y, Kuwahara M, Kato T & Tsachida (1977) Successful delivery of a patient on hemodialysis for acute renal failure. A case report and review of the literature. *Journal of Urology* 118: 673–674.

Orme BM, Ueland K, Simpson DP & Scribner BH (1968) The effect of hemodialysis on fetal survival and renal function in pregnancy. *Transactions of the American Society for Artificial Internal Organs* 14: 402–404.

Ounsted MK, Moar VA, Good FJ & Redman CWG (1980) Hypertension during pregnancy with and without specific treatment: the development of the children at the age of four years. *British Journal of Obstetrics and Gynaecology* 87: 19–24.

Pepperell RJ, Adam WR & Dawborn JK (1970) Hemodialysis in the management of chronic renal failure during pregnancy. *Australian and New Zealand Journal of Obstetrics and Gynecology* 10: 180–186.

Pruyn SC, Phelan JP & Buchanan GC (1979) Long term propranolol therapy in pregnancy: maternal and fetal outcome. *American Journal of Obstetrics and Gynecology* 135: 485–489.

Registration Committee of EDTA (1980) Successful pregnancies in women treated by dialysis and kidney transplantation. *British Journal of Obstetrics and Gynaecology* **87**: 839–845.

Redrow M, Cherem L, Elliot J et al (1987) The use of dialysis in the management of pregnant patients with renal insufficiency. Submitted for publication.

Ringenbach M, Renger B, Beauvais et al (1978) Grossesse et accouchement J'un enfant vivant chez une patiente traitee par hemodialyse iterative. *Journal d'urologie et de nephrologie* **84**: 360–366.

Roxe DM & Parker J (1985) *Report of a Survey of Reproductive Function in Female Hemodialysis Patients.* Proceedings of the American Nephrology Nursing Association, National Meeting, New Orleans.

Rubin PC, Clark DM, Sumner DJ et al (1983) Placebo controlled trial of atenolol in treatment of pregnancy associated hypertension. *Lancet* **i**: 431–434.

Sanchez-Casajus A, Ramos I & Santos M (1978) Monitorizacion fetal en el transcurso de hemodialysis durante el embarazo. *Revista Clinic Espanola* **149**: 187–188.

Sanfilippo F, Vaughn WK, Bollinger RP & Spoto EK (1982) Comparative effects of pregnancy, transfusion and prior graft rejection on sensitization and renal transplant results. *Transplantation* **34**: 360–366.

Savdie E, Caterson RJ, Mahoney JF et al (1982) Successful pregnancies in women treated by hemodialysis. *Medical Journal of Australia* **2**: 9.

Schwartz, Post KG, Keller F & Molzahn M (1985) Value of human chronic gonadotropin measurements in blood as a pregnancy test in women on maintenance hemodialysis., *Nephron* **39**: 341–343.

Sheriff MHR, Hardman M, Lamont CAR, Shepherd R & Warren DJ (1978) Successful pregnancy in a 44-year-old hemodialysis patient. *British Journal of Obstetrics and Gynaecology* **85**: 386–389.

Surian M, Imbasciatti E, Cosci P et al (1984) Glomerular disease in pregnancy. *Nephron* **36**: 101–105.

Stempel JE, O'Grady JD, Morton MJ & Johnson KA (1982) Use of sodium nitroprusside in complications of gestational hypertension. *American Journal of Obstetrics and Gynecology* **60**: 533–538.

Thompson NM, Rigby RJ & Atkins RC (1978) Successful pregnancy in a woman on recurrent hemodialysis. *Australian and New Zealand Journal of Medicine* **8**: 243.

Unzelman RF, Alderfer GR & Chojnacki RE (1973) Pregnancy and chronic hemodialysis. *Transactions of the American Society for Artificial Internal Organs* **19**: 144–149.

Walters BNJ & Redman CWG (1984) Treatment of severe pregnancy-associated hypertension with the calcium antagonist nifedipine. *British Journal of Obstetrics and Gynaecology* **91**: 330–336.

Weisman Y, Vargas A, Duckett G, Reiter E & Root AW (1978) Synthesis of 1,25 dihydroxyvitamin D in the nephrectomized pregnant rat. *Endocrinology* **103**: 1992–1996.

15

Pregnancy in renal allograft recipients: prognosis and management

JOHN M. DAVISON

It is now almost thirty years since a healthy baby boy was delivered by caesarean section to a woman who, prior to pregnancy, had received a kidney transplant from her identical twin sister. That delivery on Monday, 10 March 1958, and the events preceding it, although not reported until much later (Murray et al, 1963), signalled the start of interdisciplinary cooperation that has now coped worldwide with over 2000 pregnancies, not all of them successful. In recent years, however, improvements in our knowledge of pregnancy physiology and advances in nephrological, transplantation and obstetric practice have drastically changed our clinical approach. Medical concern no longer just focuses on coping with established pregnancies, but also concentrates on preconception counselling, the special renal and perinatal problems in these women and the remote effects of pregnancy on both renal prognosis and the offspring. This chapter reviews the literature and highlights prevailing controversies and specific management issues.

BACKGROUND

After transplantation, renal and endocrine functions rapidly return, normal sexual activity invariably ensues and about 1 in 50 women of childbearing age with a functioning renal transplant becomes pregnant. Registry data and reviews have detailed the problems encountered, although many pregnancies, successful and unsuccessful, go unreported (Rifle and Traeger, 1975; Registration Committee EDTA, 1980; Fine, 1982; Davison and Lindheimer, 1984; Meier and Makowski, 1984; Lau and Scott, 1985; O'Donnell et al, 1985; Hadi, 1986; Penn, 1986; Davison, 1987; Evans et al, 1987). The average time between transplantation and conception was 40 months (range of 4 weeks to 13 years), with 4 of every 5 pregnancies occurring in women with cadaver grafts, the exception being the Denver series where 75% were living donor grafts (Penn, 1986). Transplants have been performed with surgeons unaware that the recipient was pregnant at the time, and obstetric success in such cases does not negate the importance of contraception counselling for all renal failure patients, including the exclusion of pregnancy prior to transplantation.

RISKS FOR THE MOTHER

Problems of early pregnancy

Spontaneous abortion occurs in about 16%, the same as for the normal pregnancy population. Between 0.2 and 0.5% of all conceptions are ectopic pregnancies. Hydatidiform mole has been reported in a transplant recipient and potential for malignant transformation is possibly enhanced by immuno-suppressive drugs (Manifold et al, 1983). Ovarian tumours in early pregnancy must be distinguished from pelvic blood vessel anomalies (Parer et al, 1984).

Therapeutic termination

This procedure is an obvious option for these women. In fact, 22% of pregnancies are terminated for various indications: psychosocial problems associated with an unplanned pregnancy, uncertainty about long-term maternal prognosis, renal dysfunction before pregnancy and deteriorating renal function and/or severe hypertension during pregnancy.

Ectopic pregnancy

Transplant patients may be at higher risk of ectopic pregnancy because of pelvic adhesions due to previous urological surgery, peritoneal dialysis or pelvic inflammatory disease. The diagnosis can be difficult because irregular bleeding and amenorrhoea accompany deteriorating renal function or even an intrauterine pregnancy (Scott et al, 1978). The main clinical problem is that symptoms secondary to genuine pelvic pathology are erroneously attributed to the transplant.

Critical factors during pregnancy

Allograft function

When preconception transplant function is adequate (plasma creatinine < 180 μmol^{-1}) then there is little or no deterioration with pregnancy. Increased glomerular filtration rate (GFR), characteristic of normal preg-nancy, is also seen in transplant recipients; the better the renal function before pregnancy, the greater the increment in GFR during pregnancy (Davison, 1985).

Transient reduction in GFR can occur during the third trimester just as in normal pregnancy. In 15% of patients, however, significant renal deterior-ation persists following delivery. As a gradual decline in function can occur in non-pregnant patients, it is difficult to identify a specific role for pregnancy. Subclinical chronic rejection may be responsible, following a bout of acute rejection or if immunosuppression becomes suboptimal.

Increases in proteinuria, often to abnormal levels (2–3 g in 24 hours), occur in the third trimester in 40% of patients, but regress postpartum and, in the absence of hypertension, are not significant (Davison, 1985) (Figure 1).

Allograft rejection

Serious rejection episodes occur in 9% of pregnant women (Rudolph et al, 1979). While this incidence of rejection is no greater than expected for non-pregnant transplant patients, it is perhaps unexpected considering the privileged immunological state of pregnancy. No factors consistently predict which patients will develop rejection during pregnancy. Occasionally rejection occurs during pregnancy in women who have had years of stable function prior to conception. More rarely it occurs in the puerperium, when it may be due to the return to a normal immune state (despite immunosuppression), or possibly a rebound effect from the altered immunoresponsiveness of pregnancy.

Chronic rejection may be a problem in all recipients. It has a progressive subclinical course but the influence of pregnancy is unknown. There may also be a non-immune contribution to chronic graft failure due to the damaging effect of hyperfiltration through remnant nephrons (Feehally et al, 1986), perhaps even exacerbated during pregnancy (the physiology and clinical implications of pregnancy hyperfiltration are discussed in Chapters 1 and 2).

In clinical practice rejection has the following hallmarks.

1. The diagnosis can be difficult.
2. The diagnosis should be considered whenever fever, oliguria, deteriorating renal function and/or renal enlargement and tenderness are present.
3. The diagnosis cannot be made with certainty without renal biopsy to exclude acute pyelonephritis, recurrent glomerulopathy, possibly pre-eclampsia and even cyclosporin-A nephrotoxicity.
4. The diagnosis must be beyond doubt before embarking upon anti-rejection therapy.

Hypertension and pre-eclampsia

Pre-eclampsia has been diagnosed clinically in 30% of pregnancies in allograft recipients. The appearance of hypertension and proteinuria in the third trimester and their relationship to deteriorating renal function, to chronic underlying pathology and to pre-eclampsia is difficult to assess. Although many of the hypertensive syndromes are quite severe, there is only one report of a woman (a primigravida) where there was rapid progress to eclampsia; interestingly, she subsequently had an uncomplicated, successful pregnancy (Williams and Jelen, 1979; Williams and Johnstone, 1982).

Unlike the situation in normal pregnant women, changes in urinary protein excretion, plasma urate levels, platelet count or liver function tests do not appear to be useful markers for either the onset or the severity of pre-eclampsia, as all of these parameters can be substantially changed in otherwise uncomplicated pregnancies.

Infection

Immunosuppression, anaemia and debility make all transplant recipients susceptible to infection. Uncommon organisms are found commonly in this population, and cultures should always be obtained when infection is suspected. Fungal and related infections occur less frequently now that transplant teams have learnt more about the limits of the various immunosuppressive regimens. *Aspergillus*, *Mycobacterium tuberculosis*, *Listeria monocytogenes* and *Pneumocystis* have all been reported. The incidence of urinary tract infection may be as high as 40%, and is said to occur in all women in whom chronic pyelonephritis was the primary cause of the renal failure. Viral infections (cytomegalovirus (CMV), herpes simplex (HSV) and HBsAg), always a potential hazard to mother and fetus, are discussed later.

Gastrointestinal disorders

Dyspepsia can cause considerable distress in any allograft recipient and in pregnancy can be more problematical. Although there is no correlation between dyspepsia and total steroid dosage, it does appear that problems are less common with low-dose immunosuppressive regimens.

Parathyroid dysfunction

Up to 20% of women with successful renal transplants develop tertiary hyperparathyroidism. If maternal hyperparathyroidism is untreated (or undiagnosed), there is the risk of maternal hypercalcaemia; because calcium concentrates differentially in the fetal compartments, with parathyroid suppression, neonatal hypocalcaemia may ensue (Schoenike et al, 1978). If parathyroidectomy is undertaken there is then the risk of hypoparathyroidism (Rabau-Friedman et al, 1982) with maternal hypocalcaemic seizures as well as congenital hypoparathyroidism or hyperparathyroidism. Calcium and phosphate levels therefore need careful monitoring during pregnancy. Supplements of calcium and vitamin D or parathyroidectomy should be considered if indicated.

Diabetes mellitus

The results of renal transplantation have been progressively improving in those patients whose end-stage renal failure was caused by juvenile onset diabetes mellitus. Inevitably pregnancies are now being reported in such patients, and it is evident that the problems experienced are at least double those in other pregnant renal allograft recipients. This may relate to the cardiovascular changes that accompany severe diabetes (Vinicor et al, 1984; Ogburn et al, 1986).

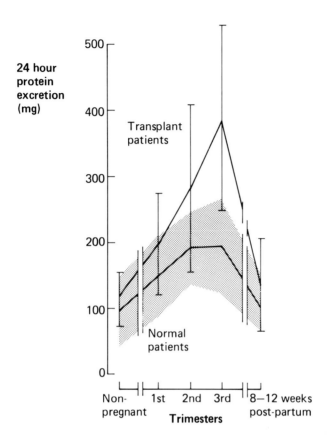

Figure 1. Alterations in 24 h urinary protein excretion in 10 healthy women (lower line) compared to 10 renal allograft recipients (upper line). Mean ± SD. (From Davison, 1985.)

Table 1. Pregnancy in renal allograft recipients: prospects.

Problems in pregnancy (%)	Successful obstetric outcome (%)	Problems in long-term (%)
46	92 (73)	11 (24)

Estimates based on 819 women in 1025 pregnancies which attained at least 28 weeks' gestation (1961–1987). Figures in brackets refer to prospects when complications developed prior to 28 weeks.

Summary

From this review of the literature certain facts emerge. About 40% of all conceptions do not continue beyond the first trimester. The overall complication rate in pregnancies continuing beyond the first trimester is 46% (Table 1). If complications (usually uncontrolled hypertension, renal deterioration or rejection) occur prior to 28 weeks' gestation then successful obstetric outcome occurs in 73%, compared to 92% when pregnancy is trouble-free prior to 28 weeks. Remote problems occur in 11% of women after delivery, but where the pregnancy is complicated prior to 28 weeks remote problems occur in 24%; although it is difficult to know whether such problems are precipitated by pregnancy or are time-dependent and would have occurred anyway.

Immunosuppressive drugs during pregnancy

The commonly used maintenance regimen is a combination of prednisone and azathioprine. Cyclosporin-A is a new immunosuppressive agent and preliminary evidence suggests that it may be more effective than the conventional drugs (Calne, 1987), but experience in pregnancy is sparse (Lewis et al, 1983; Flechner et al, 1985; Khawar et al, 1987).

Prednisone

This anti-inflammatory steroid decreases cell-mediated responses to the allograft, with the disadvantages of increased risk of infection and/or malignancy and poor healing. Additional maternal side-effects include glucose intolerance, peptic ulcer development, osteoporosis and weakening of connective tissues, which may have predisposed to uterine rupture in one patient reported in the literature (Rifle and Traeger, 1975). Prednisone crosses the placenta, and a large percentage is converted to prednisolone which, although not suppressing fetal ACTH, does have other potential adverse fetal effects (see below). Augmenting steroids postpartum to cover so-called 'rebound immunoresponsiveness' is controversial (Lau and Scott, 1985; Penn, 1986) and the consensus is that it is neither necessary nor beneficial.

Azathioprine

This purine analogue decreases delayed hypersensitivity and cellular cytotoxicity while leaving antibody-mediated responses relatively intact. In the mother the primary hazards are increased risk of infection and/or neoplasia. Azathioprine crosses the placenta, and the fetal and paediatric implications are discussed later (page 1037). In theory, the fetus should be protected from the effects of azathioprine in early pregnancy, as it then lacks the enzyme inosinate pyrophosphorylase which converts azathioprine to thioinosinic acid, the metabolite active on dividing cells (Saarikoski and Seppala, 1973).

The most sensitive method of monitoring azathioprine dosage and bioavailability is the measurement of red cell 6-thioguanine nucleotides (6-

TGN), which are metabolites of both azathioprine and 6-mercaptopurine and whose formation is catalysed by red cell thiopurine methyltransferase (TPMT). Low TPMT activity may be a risk factor for the development of thiopurine toxicity, and there certainly are large individual variations in red cell 6-TGN amongst patients receiving identical azathioprine dosage (Lennard et al, 1984, 1987). One in 300 patients lacks TPMT activity on a genetic basis; identification of such patients could be important, especially in pregnancy, if side-effects are to be avoided. A less sensitive (but nevertheless safe) approach involves adjustments in azathioprine dosage to maintain maternal leucocyte count within normal limits for pregnancy, thus ensuring that the neonate is born with a normal blood count (Davison et al, 1985a).

Cyclosporin-A

This fungal metabolite's major inhibitory effect is on the T-lymphocyte and other cells mediating allograft rejection. There is wide individual sensitivity, and it is plasma rather than whole blood drug levels that correlate best with toxicity. The widely differing accumulation seen in various human tissues is related to variations in cyclophilin, the major intracellular cyclosporin-A binding protein.

Although renal allograft survival data are better with cyclosporin-A (Calne, 1987), this drug actually reduces compensatory hyperfunction at the time of the transplant and has long-term nephrotoxic effects, so that most patients have plasma creatinine levels of 100–260 μmol l^{-1} compared to 70–180 μmol l^{-1} in those on routine immunosuppression (Thiel, 1986). Whether the usual relationship between higher plasma creatinine values and worse gestational outcome applies in patients treated with cyclosporin-A is not yet known (Davison et al, 1985b). As well as nephrotoxicity, other adverse effects include neoplasia, hepatic dysfunction, tremor, convulsions, glucose intolerance, hypertension, haemolytic uraemic syndrome and predisposition to the thromboembolic phenomena.

Little is known about either the maternal or fetal effects of this drug in pregnancy. Theoretically some of the maternal physiological adaptations could be blunted by cyclosporin-A, for example its depressive effects on extracellular volume and renal haemodynamics (Provoost, 1986; Thiel, 1986; Kaskel et al, 1987). In the few cases in the literature, however, renal function was not adequately documented, and whether the kidney in pregnancy is more vulnerable to cyclosporin-A is not known (Lewis et al, 1983; Flechner et al, 1985; Khawar et al, 1987). Interestingly, ill-defined donor factors, as well as the presence of *Escherichia coli* renal infection, can increase susceptibility to nephrotoxicity; yet absence of renal innervation, as in a transplant, possibly affords some protection (Batlle et al, 1987). More clinical and laboratory data are urgently needed to elucidate the mechanisms of nephrotoxicity in pregnancy and to rationalize cyclosporin-A usage, so that management is no longer based on clinical anecdote.

Table 2. Possible effects of immunosuppression during pregnancy.

	No. of women	Pregnancies	Oligo-hydramnios (%)	Intrauterine growth retardation (%)	In labour	
					Meconium (%)	Fetal distress (%)
Renal transplants	18	20	20	40	45	25
Controls	3410	5000	2	8	11	2

From Pirson et al (1985) with permission.

Problems at delivery

Vaginal delivery does not cause mechanical injury to the kidney transplant, which in turn does not obstruct the birth canal. Unless there are specific indications for induction then spontaneous onset of labour can be awaited.

Preterm delivery

Preterm delivery (before 37 weeks' gestation) is common (45–60%) because of intervention for obstetric reasons and the tendency to premature labour, which although commonly associated with renal impairment, is not always caused by it. It has been suggested that long-term steroid therapy weakens connective tissues and contributes to the increased incidence of premature rupture of membranes.

Average birthweights are low since most deliveries are preterm. Additionally, the incidence of intrauterine growth retardation is 20% (range 8–40% in the literature) and is not necessarily related to the severity of renal impairment, vascular disease or hypertension (Pirson et al, 1985) (Table 2). Certainly, immunogenetic disparity between conceptus and mother is advantageous, and placentas and fetuses are bigger when there is greater maternofetal histocompatibility. Thus, in the renal transplant mother, non-specific depression of the maternal immune system by immunosuppressives may contribute to fetal growth retardation. Congenital CMV infection may also be a contributory factor (Evans et al, 1975).

Caesarean section

This method of delivery is only necessary for purely obstetrical reasons. The reported section rate of about 25% is certainly much higher than expected and presumably reflects fear of the unknown, rather than certainty that vaginal delivery would be hazardous for mother and/or baby.

Pelvic problems can be recognized antenatally, so that delivery by caesarean section can be planned. Transplant patients may have pelvic osteodystrophy related to previous renal failure (and dialysis) or prolonged steroid therapy. If there is any question of disproportion or kidney

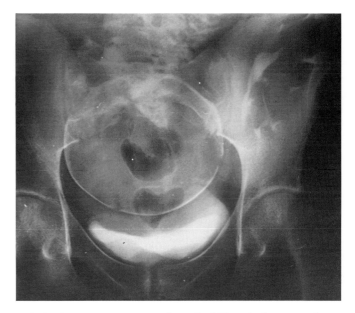

Figure 2. Single shot intravenous urogram performed at 36th week of pregnancy in a woman with a left-sided renal allograft. The kidney is in the false pelvis and would not interfere with vaginal delivery.

compression then some recommend that simultaneous intravenous urography and X-ray pelvimetry should be performed at 36 weeks' gestation (Figure 2). A lower segment approach is usually feasible but previous urological surgery may make it difficult, and care must be taken that the ureter and graft blood supply are not damaged or compromised.

RISKS TO THE FETUS AND OFFSPRING

Over 50% of liveborns have no neonatal problems. Preterm delivery is common (45–60%), small-for-dates infants are delivered in at least 20% of cases and occasionally the two problems occur together. There are some special problems in these babies such as thymic atrophy, transient leucopaenia, CMV and HBsAg infection, bone marrow hypoplasia, reduced blood levels of IgG and IgM, septicaemia, chromosome aberrations in lymphocytes, hypoglycaemia, hypocalcaemia and adrenocortical insufficiency (Rudolph et al, 1979; Rasmussen et al, 1981; Weil et al, 1985).

Congenital abnormalities

No frequent or predominant developmental abnormalities have been reported. Azathioprine is teratogenic in animals but only in large doses, equivalent to more than 6 mg kg^{-1} body weight daily, much more than the modest ones (2 mg kg^{-1} day^{-1} or less) required by women with stable renal function (Williamson and Karp, 1981; Sarramon et al, 1985). In one series, however, where birth anomalies were present in 7 out of 103 offspring, the mothers of abnormal babies had been taking a significantly higher daily dose of azathioprine than those who had normal babies: 2.64 mg kg^{-1} compared to 2.02 mg kg^{-1} (Registration Committee EDTA, 1980). This was based on a relatively small number of abnormal babies and could still be due to chance. Very large doses of steroids in experimental animals can produce congenital abnormalities, but the risk to the fetus from doses used after transplantation is small. Cyclosporin-A is embryotoxic and fetotoxic in animals when given in doses 2–5 times greater than the human dose.

Viral infections

Cytomegalovirus (CMV)

CMV infection, a major cause of morbidity in transplant recipients, can present in a variety of ways in the mother, including fever, leucopaenia, thrombocytopaenia and pneumonia, as well as liver and renal dysfunction. Of greatest importance to the pregnant transplant recipient and her fetus are the implications of congenital CMV infection (Jeffries, 1984). Therapeutic termination is not a practical approach because maternal infections are mostly symptomless, detectable only by serological monitoring; and many infants born to women with CMV infection are not seriously damaged but can be growth-retarded. If primary maternal CMV infection is responsible for the majority of damaged CMV-infected infants, then there is a case for a CMV vaccine. Live CMV vaccines are available but it is not known whether they can prevent congenital CMV infection.

Herpes hominis virus (HSV)

Primary maternal infection with HSV prior to 20 weeks' gestation is associated with an increased rate of abortion. Caesarean section should be undertaken if a cervical culture is positive for HSV at term, since the risk of neonatal infection resulting from vaginal delivery is at least 50%.

Infectious hepatitis

Renal transplant recipients, exposed to multiple blood transfusions as well as haemodialysis, may carry the hepatitis B virus. While women developing acute hepatitis in late pregnancy or within two months of delivery often transmit HBsAg and HBeAg to their offspring, the risk to children of asymptomatic carriers is much lower. When HBsAg is transmitted to the baby it invariably disappears within a few weeks after birth, only to be found later in life if active infection ever develops. This suggests that many HBsAg-positive neonates have been infected at delivery (i.e. with their mother's blood or vaginal secretions) and this maternally acquired antigen is cleared before a fresh infection is contracted (alternatively it may 'incubate' outside the blood

Table 3. Effect in mice of 6-mercaptopurine (6-MP) in pregnancy on subsequent reproduction of offspring.

6-MP dose to mother (mg/kg/d)	Weight of ovaries of offspring (mg)	No. of offspring bred	No. of offspring achieving pregnancy	No. of fetuses per pregnancy	Percentage of dead fetuses
0	8.6 ± 0.4	33	33	13.0 ± 0.4	13
0.5	8.7 ± 0.3	46	44	12.8 ± 0.3	18
1.5	7.3 ± 0.6	33	26	10.6 ± 0.5	25
3.0	2.2 ± 0.6	9	2	6.5 ± 3.5	46

Mean $\pm$ SEM.
From Reimers and Sluss (1978), with permission.

system). Further evidence of perinatal infection is that most cord-blood specimens are HBsAg negative. Without prophylaxis, a high proportion of infants of HBsAg-positive mothers become carriers within two to three months of birth, an interval that again suggests that infection first occurred during labour or delivery (Flewett, 1986).

If infection occurred during pregnancy, immunoprophylaxis initiated at birth would not be of value in preventing acquisition of the carrier state by the infant. However, hepatitis B immune globulin (HBIG) and hepatitis B virus vaccine (HBVV) given within a few hours of birth are 90% effective in reducing the HBsAg carrier state in infants, but not if administration is delayed beyond 48 hours and/or if either is given alone.

Potential long-term problems

Azathioprine can cause transient gaps and breaks in the chromosomes of lymphocytes, which disappear spontaneously in 5–32 months (Leb et al, 1971). Such anomalies, however, may not be as temporary in tissues not yet studied, and the sequelae could be the development of malignancies in the affected offspring or abnormalities in the next generation. Data to test this hypothesis will be difficult to accumulate, but there are already some disturbing observations from animal studies. For instance, fertility problems affect the female offspring of mice that have received low doses of 6-mercaptopurine, the major metabolite of azathioprine (equivalent to 3 mg kg^{-1}) (Reimers and Sluss, 1978) (Table 3). Thus exposure of the fetus to low doses of potential mutagens may not cause immediate, obvious effects such as morbidity or birth defects, but may have consequences when the otherwise normal female offspring attain reproductive age. To date, information about the general progress in infancy and early childhood of the offspring of renal transplant mothers has been reassuring, but there have been no studies of possible impairment of fertility (Rudolph et al, 1979; Korsch et al, 1980; Weil et al, 1985; Penn, 1986). With the introduction of cyclosporin-A new evaluations are urgently required, and need to be balanced against its other worrying maternal side-effects.

SPECIFIC MANAGEMENT ISSUES

Approach to counselling

Many questions arise: is contraception necessary? Which method is advisable? Is pregnancy advisable? Will pregnancy be complicated? Will pregnancy result in a healthy baby? Will pregnancy cause any long-term harm? A woman must be counselled from the time the various end-stage renal failure treatments and their potential for rehabilitation are discussed.

The option of sterilization should not be routinely offered at the time of transplantation. Even after transplantation and the joy of newfound health, stress will still be a major factor in everyday life, with its 'baseline of uncertainty'.

Long-term prospects

The ultimate measure of transplant success is the long-term survival of the patient and the graft. As it is only just over thirty years since this procedure became widely employed in the management of end-stage renal failure, there are few long-term data from sufficiently large series from which to draw conclusions. Furthermore, it must be emphasized that the long-term results for renal transplants relate to a period when several aspects of management would be unacceptable by present-day standards. Average survival figures of large numbers of patients worldwide indicate that 70–80% of recipients of kidneys from related living donors are alive five years after transplantation, and with cadaver kidneys the figure is 40–50%. Five-year survival is increased to about 80% if renal function is normal two years post-transplant, and this is probably the optimal time to contemplate pregnancy.

Many patients will choose parenthood in an effort to renew a normal life and possibly in defiance of the sometimes negative attitudes of medical and nursing establishment. Couples should be aware of all implications right down to the harsh realities of maternal survival prospects. A major concern is that even in the medium term the mother may not survive or remain well enough to rear the child she bears.

Pregnancy does not necessarily cause irreversible declines in renal function, and a recent study, albeit on a very small scale, concluded that pregnancy had no effect on graft survival or function (Whetham et al, 1983). The present review of the literature, however, indicates that 11% of women will have new, long-term medical problems after pregnancy, although it is difficult to know whether such problems are merely time-related or actually precipitated by pregnancy (Table 1). Interestingly, the incidence of later problems is doubled (24%) if pregnancy complications occur prior to 28 weeks' gestation. Registry data indicate that 10% of mothers die within 1–7 years following childbirth. More long-term studies are needed to assess this area, especially with the advent of the new immunosuppressive drugs.

Preconception guidelines

Individual centres have their own specific guidelines. Most advise a wait of about two years post-transplant. This has turned out to be good advice, because the patient will have recovered from the major surgical sequelae by then, and renal function will have stabilized with a very high probability of allograft survival at five years. Immunosuppression will also be at maintenance levels, which may account for higher birthweight babies in mothers becoming pregnant two years after transplantation compared to women becoming pregnant earlier (Cunningham et al, 1983).

A set of guidelines is given here, although the criteria are only relative.

1. Good general health for about two years post-transplant.
2. Stature compatible with good obstetric outcome.
3. No (or minimal) proteinuria.
4. No hypertension.
5. No evidence of graft rejection.
6. No pelvicalyceal distension on a recent intravenous urogram.
7. Stable renal function with plasma creatinine of 180 μmol l^{-1} or less (preferably less than 130 μmol l^{-1}).
8. Drug therapy reduced to maintenance levels: prednisone, 15 mg per day or less, and azathioprine, 2 mg kg^{-1} body weight daily or less. A safe dose of cyclosporin-A has not yet been established because of limited experience, but quoted anecdotally is 10 mg kg^{-1} daily or less, or even a change from cyclosporin-A to azathioprine before or in early pregnancy.

Antenatal strategy and decision-making

Patients must be monitored as high-risk cases, and teamwork is essential. Management should be hospital-based, and requires attention to serial assessment of renal function, blood pressure control, diagnosis and treatment of rejection, treatment of any infection and serial fetal surveillance (Table 4). It is essential to assess carefully the woman's emotional attitude and the overall support she receives from her family.

Antenatal visits should be two-weekly up to 32 weeks and weekly thereafter. The following tests should be undertaken monthly.

1. Full blood count including platelets.
2. Blood urea, creatinine, electrolyte and urate levels.
3. 24-hour creatinine clearance and protein excretion.
4. Mid-stream urine specimen for microscopy and culture.

Liver function tests, plasma protein, calcium and phosphate levels should be checked at six-weekly intervals. CMV and HSV titres should be checked in each trimester. If the patient has diabetes mellitus then a very strict management protocol is needed.

All pregnant rhesus-negative women should have serial Rh antibody screening to document the appearance of antibodies or changes in antibody titre. In selecting donors for renal transplantation Rh-antigens are usually disregarded because they are found only on red cells and not on leucocytes or other tissue cells. Nevertheless, several cases of Rh antibody response have occurred as a result of sensitization to the transplant, and it is possible for these antibodies to contribute to transplant failures since they bind to the graft. Rhesus isoimmunization and a rising antibody titre in a pregnant transplant patient could theoretically have serious consequences.

Renal function

If renal function deteriorates at any stage of pregnancy, reversible causes should be sought such as urinary tract infection, subtle dehydration or electrolyte imbalance (occasionally precipitated by inadvertent diuretic therapy), and allograft rejection must always be considered. A 15–20% decrement in function is permissible near term, which affects blood creatinine minimally (Davison, 1985). Failure to detect a treatable cause of a significant functional decrement is grounds to end the pregnancy by elective delivery. When proteinuria occurs and persists, but renal function is preserved and blood pressure normal, the pregnancy can be allowed to continue.

Blood pressure

Many of the specific risks of hypertension are mediated through superimposed pre-eclampsia, a diagnosis that cannot be made with certainty on clinical grounds alone, because proteinuria, hypertension and renal deterioration may be manifestations of underlying transplant dysfunction or even rejection. Treatment of mild hypertension is not necessary during normal pregnancy, but many would treat transplant patients more aggressively, believing this preserves renal function. It is not known whether systemic hypertension has any significant intrarenal effect in pregnancy, although in patients with a single kidney, with or without pregnancy, it could theoretically contribute further to glomerular hyperfiltration, and possibly glomerular hypertension and glomerular injury (see Chapter 2 for a further discussion of these issues).

Rejection

Rejection is difficult to diagnose clinically, and if at any time deteriorating renal function, oliguria and fever are associated with renal enlargement and tenderness, then this diagnosis has to be considered. Ultrasonography can be helpful because alterations in the echogenicity of the renal parenchyma and the presence of an indistinct corticomedullary junction are indicative of rejection (Caplan et al, 1983). Renal biopsy may be necessary, however, before any final decision is taken on the use of antirejection therapy.

Dietary counselling

The role of dietary protein in augmenting glomerular function has already been discussed in detail in Chapters 2 and 9. This issue is very important in these patients because their kidney is already hypertrophied, and it has been suggested that graft failure may be hastened by hyperfiltration. So that safe dietary recommendations can be made, more information is urgently needed about the intrarenal effects and the long-term renal sequelae of dietary protein manipulation, as well as the effect restriction might have on fetal outcome, particularly central nervous system development.

Immunosuppressive therapy

The controversies have been outlined above. Routine clinical practice is to maintain therapy at prepregnancy levels, with adjustments if there are decreases in maternal white cell and platelet counts, to ensure at least that the neonate is born with a normal blood count (Davison et al, 1985a). Azathioprine liver toxicity responds to dose reduction. Haematinics should be prescribed if the various haematological indices indicate deficiency.

Fetal surveillance and delivery

Meticulous monitoring of fetal well-being is essential, and all the current antenatal armamentarium should be utilized (Manning et al, 1987). Unless there are specific problems, spontaneous onset of labour can be awaited. Vaginal delivery is the aim, and caesarean section is only necessary for obstetrical reasons.

Augmentation of steroids is necessary to cover the stress of delivery. Maternal fluid balance, cardiovascular status and temperature must be carefully monitored. Aseptic technique is advisable at all times: any surgical procedure, however trivial, should be covered by prophylactic antibiotics. Pain relief is conducted as for healthy women.

Fetal monitoring should be undertaken. If fetal scalp blood samples are available the possibility of azathioprine-induced fetal thrombocytopaenia can be excluded; a very low fetal platelet count increases the risk of intracerebral haemorrhage, and is an indication for caesarean section.

Paediatric management

Management is the same as in neonates of other mothers, but there are some specific problems. Cord blood samples should be taken at delivery. Fetal adrenocortical insufficiency increases the risk of overwhelming neonatal infection.

Breast-feeding

Steroids are secreted in breast milk but not in sufficient quantity to affect the infant at the usual therapeutic doses. As the baby has been exposed to azathioprine and its metabolites in pregnancy and as concentrations in breast milk are minimal, it might be argued that breast-feeding is not contraindicated; but more information is needed about whether such concentrations are trivial or substantial from a biological viewpoint (Davison and Lindheimer, 1984). Cyclosporin-A is excreted in breast milk in amounts less than 2% of the maternal dose, but little is known about the potential effects of this drug in children (Flechner et al, 1985). Breast-feeding should be discouraged until more definitive data are forthcoming.

Maternal follow-up

Oral contraceptives can cause or aggravate hypertension and thrombo-embolism, and may also produce subtle changes in the immune system. This does not necessarily contraindicate their use, but careful surveillance is needed.

An intrauterine contraceptive device (IUCD) may aggravate menstrual problems, which in turn may obscure signs and symptoms of abnormalities of early pregnancy. The increased long-term risks of pelvic infection in an immunosuppressed patient with an IUCD make this method worrisome. Insertion or replacement of an IUCD is normally associated with bacteraemia in at least 1 in every 10 women, so in transplant patients antibiotic cover is essential at this time (Murray et al, 1987). Furthermore, there is a higher incidence of fungal infections with a plastic IUCD (42%) as compared to a copper-containing device (2%). The efficacy of the IUCD may be reduced by immunosuppressive and anti-inflammatory agents, possibly due to modification of the leucocyte response (Zerner et al, 1981). Nevertheless, many request this method. Careful counselling and follow-up are essential.

Gynaecological problems

There is a danger that symptoms secondary to genuine pelvic pathology may be erroneously attributed to the transplant due to its location near the pelvis. Transplant patients might be at slightly higher risk of ectopic pregnancy because of pelvic adhesions due to previous urological surgery, peritoneal dialysis, pelvic inflammatory disease or the use of an IUCD. Diagnosis can be overlooked because irregular bleeding and amenorrhoea may be associated with deteriorating renal function as well as intrauterine pregnancy.

Transplant recipients receiving immunosuppressive therapy have a malignancy rate estimated to be 100 times greater than normal, and the female genital tract is no exception (Caterson et al, 1984; Halpert et al, 1986). This association is probably related to factors such as loss of immune surveillance, chronic immunosuppression allowing tumour proliferation and/or prolonged antigenic stimulation of the reticuloendothelial system. Regular gynaecological assessment is essential and any treatment should be on conventional lines; the outcome is unlikely to be influenced by stopping or reducing immunosuppression.

SUMMARY

Renal transplantation is invariably accompanied by improvements in reproductive function. The possibility of conception in women of childbearing age emphasizes the need for compassionate and comprehensive counselling. Couples who want a child should be encouraged to discuss all the implications. Therapeutic abortion is undertaken in 22% of conceptions and the spontaneous abortion rate is about 16%, the same as for the normal population. Of the conceptions that continue beyond the first trimester, over 90% end successfully.

In most women, renal function is augmented during pregnancy, but permanent impairment occurs in 15% of pregnancies. In others there may be transient deterioration in late pregnancy (with or without proteinuria). There is a 30% chance of developing hypertension, pre-eclampsia or both. Preterm delivery occurs in 45–60%, and intrauterine growth retardation in at least 20% of pregnancies. Despite its pelvic location, the transplanted kidney rarely produces dystocia and is not injured during vaginal delivery. Caesarean section should be reserved for obstetric reasons only. Neonatal complications include respiratory distress syndrome, leucopaenia, thrombocytopaenia, adrenocortical insufficiency and infection. No predominant or frequent developmental abnormalities have been described and data on infancy and childhood are encouraging.

For the future, clinical and laboratory research are essential in order to improve prepregnancy assessment criteria, to understand the mechanisms of gestational renal dysfunction and proteinuria, to assess the side-effects and implications of immunosuppression in pregnancy and to learn more about the remote effects of pregnancy on both renal prognosis and the offspring.

REFERENCES

Batlle DC, Gutterman C, Valles A & La Pointe M (1987) Compensatory renal hypertrophy (CRH) after chronic unilateral nephrectomy (Ux): effect of cyclosporin (CyA) and renal denervation (RD). *Proceedings of the Tenth International Congress of Nephrology*, 595A. Oxford: Alden Press.

Calne RY (1987) Cyclosporin in cadaveric renal transplantation: 5-year follow-up of a multicentre trial. *Lancet* ii: 506–507.

Caplan R, Dubinsky T & Woletz PS (1983) Ultrasonography in renal transplantation and pregnancy *Medical Ultrasound* 7: 68–70.

Caterson RJ, Furber J, Murray J, McCarthy W, Mahony JF & Shiel AGR (1984) Carcinoma of the vulva in two young renal allograft recipients. *Transplantation Proceedings* 16: 559–561.

Cunningham RJ, Buszta C, Braun WE, Steinmuller D, Novick AC & Popowniak K (1983) Pregnancy in renal allograft recipients and long-term follow-up of their offspring. *Transplantation Proceedings* 15: 1067–1070.

Davison JM (1985) The effect of pregnancy on kidney function in renal allograft recipients. *Kidney International* 27: 74–79.

Davison JM (1987) Renal transplantation and pregnancy. *American Journal of Kidney Diseases* 9: 374–380.

Davison JM & Lindheimer MD (1984) Pregnancy in women with renal allografts. *Seminars in Nephrology* 4: 240–251.

Davison JM, Dellagrammatikas H & Parkin JM (1985a) Maternal azathioprine therapy and depressed haemopoiesis in babies of renal allograft patients. *British Journal of Obstetrics and Gynaecology* 92: 233–239.

Davison JM, Katz AI & Lindheimer MD (1985b) Pregnancy in women with renal disease and renal transplantation. *Proceedings EDTA-ERA* 22: 439–459.

Evans TJ, McCollum JPK & Valdimarsson H (1975) Congenital cytomegalovirus infection after maternal renal transplantation. *Lancet* i: 1359–1360.

Evans C, White D & Bone JM (1987) Is pregnancy safe after renal transplantation? *Proceedings of the Tenth International Congress of Nephrology*, 611A. Oxford: Alden Press.

Feehally J, Bennett SE, Harris KPG, Walls J (1986) Is chronic renal transplant rejection a non-immunological phenomenon? *Lancet* ii: 486–488.

Fine RN (1982) Pregnancy in renal allograft recipients. *American Journal of Nephrology* 2: 117–122.

Flechner SM, Katz AR, Rogers AJ, van Buren C & Kahan BD (1985) The presence of cyclosporine in body tissues and fluids during pregnancy. *American Journal of Kidney Diseases* 5: 60–63.

Flewett TH (1986) Can we eradicate hepatitis B? *British Medical Journal* 293: 404–405.

Hadi HA (1986) Pregnancy in renal transplant recipients: a review. *Obstetrics and Gynecology Survey* 41: 264–271.

Halpert R, Fruchter RG, Sedlis A, Butt K, Boyce JG & Sillman FH (1986) Human papillomavirus and lower genital neoplasia in renal transplant patients. *Obstetrics and Gynecology* 68: 251–258.

Jeffries DJ (1984) Cytomegalovirus infections in pregnancy. *British Journal of Obstetrics and Gynaecology* 91: 305–396.

Kaskel TJ, Devarajan P, Arbeit LA, Partin JS & Moore LC (1987) Cyclosporine nephrotoxicity: sodium excretion, autoregulation and angiotensin II. *American Journal of Physiology* 252: F733–742.

Khawar M, Pomrantz & Tejani A (1987) Two successful pregnancies in a cadaveric renal allograft recipient of cyclosporine (CsA) as the sole maintenance immunosuppressive. *Proceedings of the Tenth International Congress of Nephrology*, pp 620A. Oxford: Alden Press.

Korsch BM, Klein JD, Negrete VF, Henderson DJ & Fine RN (1980) Physical and psychological follow-up on offspring of renal allograft recipients. *Pediatrics* 65: 275–283.

Lau RJ & Scott JR (1985) Pregnancy following renal transplantation. *Clinics in Obstetrics and Gynecology* 28: 339–350.

Leb DE, Weisskopf B & Kanovitz BS (1971) Chromosome aberrations in the child of a kidney transplant recipient. *Archives of Internal Medicine* 128: 441–444.

Lennard L, Brown CB, Fox M & Maddocks JL (1984) Azathioprine metabolism in kidney transplant patients. *British Journal of Clinical Pharmacology* 18: 693–700.

Lennard L, van Loon JA, Lilleyman JS & Weinshilboum MD (1987) Thiopurine pharmacogenetics in leukemia: correlation of erythrocyte thiopurine methyltransferase activity and 6-thioguanine nucleotide concentrations. *Clinical Pharmacology and Therapeutics* 41: 18–22.

Lewis GJ, Lamour CAR, Lee HA & Slapak M (1983) Successful pregnancy in a renal transplant recipient taking cyclosporin-A. *British Medical Journal* 286: 603.

Manifold IH, Champion AE, Goepel JR, Ramsewak S & Mayor PE (1983) Pregnancy complicated by gestational trophoblastic disease in a renal transplant recipient. *British Medical Journal* 287: 1025–1026.

Manning FA, Menticoglou S, Harman CR, Morrison I & Lange IR (1987) Antepartum fetal risk assessment: the role of the fetal biophysical profile. *Clinics in Obstetrics and Gynaecology* 1: 55–72.

Meier PR & Makowski EL (1984) Pregnancy in the patient with a renal transplant. *Clinics in Obstetrics and Gynecology* 27: 902–913.

Murray JE, Reid DE, Harrison JH & Merrill JP (1963) Successful pregnancies after human renal transplantation. *New England Journal of Medicine* 269: 341–343.

Murray S, Hickey J & Houang E (1987) Significant bacteremia associated with replacement of intrauterine contraceptive device. *American Journal of Obstetrics and Gynecology* 156: 698–699.

O'Donnell D, Sevitz H, Seggie JL, Meyers AM, Botha JR & Myburgh JA (1985) Pregnancy after renal transplantation. *Australia and New Zealand Journal of Medicine* 15: 320–332.

Ogburn PL, Kitzmiller JL, Hare JW, Phillippe M, Gabbe SG, Miodovnik M et al (1986) Pregnancy following renal transplantation in Class T diabetes mellitus. *Journal of the American Medical Association* 255: 911–915.

Parer JT, Lichtenberg ES, Callen PW & Feduska N (1984) Iliac venous aneurysm in a pregnant patient with a renal transplant. *Journal of Reproductive Medicine* 29: 869–871.

Penn I (1986) Pregnancy following renal transplantation. In Andreucci VE (ed.) *The Kidney in Pregnancy*, pp 195–204. Boston: Martinus Nijhoff.

Pirson Y, Van Lierde M, Ghysen J, Squifflet JP, Alexandre GPJ & van Ypersele de Strihou C (1985) Retardation of fetal growth in patients receiving immunosuppressive therapy. *New England Journal of Medicine* **313:** 328.

Provoost AP (1986) Cyclosporine nephrotoxicity in rats with an acute reduction of renal function. *American Journal of Kidney Diseases* **8:** 314–318.

Rabau-Friedman E, Mashiach S, Cantor E & Jacob ET (1982) Association of hypoparathyroidism and successful pregnancy in kidney transplant recipients. *Obstetrics and Gynecology* **59:** 126–128.

Rasmussen P, Fasth A, Ahlmen J, Brynger H, Iwarson S & Kjellmer I (1981) Children of female renal transplant recipients. *Acta Paediatrica Scandinavica* **70:** 869–875.

Registration Committee of the European Dialysis and Transplant Association (1980) Successful pregnancies in women treated by dialysis and kidney transplantation. *British Journal of Obstetrics and Gynaecology* **87:** 839–845.

Reimers TJ & Sluss PM (1978) 6-Mercaptopurine treatment of pregnant mice: effects of second and third generation. *Science* **201:** 65–67.

Rifle G & Traeger J (1975) Pregnancy after renal transplantation: an international survey. *Transplantation Proceedings* **7:** 723–728.

Rudolph JE, Shwihizir RT & Barius SA (1979) Pregnancy in renal transplant patients: a review. *Transplantation* **27:** 26–29.

Saarikoski S & Seppala M (1973) Immunosuppression during pregnancy: transmission of azathioprine and its metabolites from mother to the fetus. *American Journal of Obstetrics and Gynecology* **115:** 1100–1106.

Sarramon JP, Lhez JM, Durand D et al (1985) Grossesse chez les transplantes renales. *Annals of Urology* **19:** 57–59.

Schoenike SL, Kaldenburgh HH & Kaplan AM (1978) Transient hypoparathyroidism in an infant of a mother with a renal transplant. *American Journal of Diseases of Childhood* **132:** 530–532.

Scott JR, Cruickshank DP & Corry RJ (1978) Ectopic pregnancy in kidney transplant patients. *Obstetrics and Gynecology* **51:** 565–568.

Thiel G (1986) Experimental cyclosporine A nephrotoxicity: a summary of the International Workshop. *Clinics in Nephrology* **25:** S205–S210.

Vinicor F, Golichowski A, Filo R, Smith EJ & Maxwell D (1984) Pregnancy following renal transplantation in a patient with insulin-dependent diabetes mellitus. *Diabetes Care* **7:** 280–284.

Weil R, Barfield N, Schröter GPT & Bauling PC (1985) Children of mothers with kidney transplants. *Transplantation Proceedings* **17:** 1569–1572.

Whetham JCG, Cardelle C & Harding M (1983) Effect of pregnancy on graft function and graft survival in renal cadaver transplant recipients. *American Journal of Obstetrics and Gynecology* **145:** 193–197.

Williams PF & Jelen J (1979) Eclampsia in a patient who had had a renal transplant. *British Medical Journal* **2:** 972.

Williams PF & Johnstone M (1982) Normal pregnancy in renal transplant recipient with history of eclampsia and intrauterine death. *British Medical Journal* **285:** 1535.

Williamson RA & Karp LE (1981) Azathioprine teratogenicity: review of the literature and case report. *Obstetrics and Gynecology* **58:** 247–250.

Zerner J, Doil KL & Drewry J (1981) Intrauterine contraceptive device failures in renal transplant patients. *Journal of Reproductive Medicine* **26:** 99–101.

Index

Note: Page numbers of article titles are in **bold** type.